Jens Hrach

**Toxicogenomic approaches to predict hepatotoxicity in vitro**

Jens Hrach

# Toxicogenomic approaches to predict hepatotoxicity in vitro

A longer-term hepatocyte sandwich culture model combined with toxicogenomic methods as an alternative early screen for hepatotoxicity

Südwestdeutscher Verlag für Hochschulschriften

**Impressum/Imprint (nur für Deutschland/ only for Germany)**
Bibliografische Information der Deutschen Nationalbibliothek: Die Deutsche Nationalbibliothek verzeichnet diese Publikation in der Deutschen Nationalbibliografie; detaillierte bibliografische Daten sind im Internet über http://dnb.d-nb.de abrufbar.
Alle in diesem Buch genannten Marken und Produktnamen unterliegen warenzeichen-, marken- oder patentrechtlichem Schutz bzw. sind Warenzeichen oder eingetragene Warenzeichen der jeweiligen Inhaber. Die Wiedergabe von Marken, Produktnamen, Gebrauchsnamen, Handelsnamen, Warenbezeichnungen u.s.w. in diesem Werk berechtigt auch ohne besondere Kennzeichnung nicht zu der Annahme, dass solche Namen im Sinne der Warenzeichen- und Markenschutzgesetzgebung als frei zu betrachten wären und daher von jedermann benutzt werden dürften.

Verlag: Südwestdeutscher Verlag für Hochschulschriften Aktiengesellschaft & Co. KG
Dudweiler Landstr. 99, 66123 Saarbrücken, Deutschland
Telefon +49 681 37 20 271-1, Telefax +49 681 37 20 271-0, Email: info@svh-verlag.de
Zugl.: Heidelberg, Ruperto-Carola University, Diss., 2009

Herstellung in Deutschland:
Schaltungsdienst Lange o.H.G., Berlin
Books on Demand GmbH, Norderstedt
Reha GmbH, Saarbrücken
Amazon Distribution GmbH, Leipzig
ISBN: 978-3-8381-0703-5

**Imprint (only for USA, GB)**
Bibliographic information published by the Deutsche Nationalbibliothek: The Deutsche Nationalbibliothek lists this publication in the Deutsche Nationalbibliografie; detailed bibliographic data are available in the Internet at http://dnb.d-nb.de.
Any brand names and product names mentioned in this book are subject to trademark, brand or patent protection and are trademarks or registered trademarks of their respective holders. The use of brand names, product names, common names, trade names, product descriptions etc. even without a particular marking in this works is in no way to be construed to mean that such names may be regarded as unrestricted in respect of trademark and brand protection legislation and could thus be used by anyone.

Publisher:
Südwestdeutscher Verlag für Hochschulschriften Aktiengesellschaft & Co. KG
Dudweiler Landstr. 99, 66123 Saarbrücken, Germany
Phone +49 681 37 20 271-1, Fax +49 681 37 20 271-0, Email: info@svh-verlag.de

Copyright © 2009 by the author and Südwestdeutscher Verlag für Hochschulschriften Aktiengesellschaft & Co. KG and licensors
All rights reserved. Saarbrücken 2009

Printed in the U.S.A.
Printed in the U.K. by (see last page)
ISBN: 978-3-8381-0703-5

# INDEX

1 **INTRODUCTION** ............................................................................................................. 5
    1.1    Endeavors of modern toxicology ........................................................................................ 5
    1.2    The liver morphology and its cell types ............................................................................. 6
    1.3    Hepatocytes and xenobiotic metabolism ........................................................................... 8
    1.4    Hepatotoxicity ................................................................................................................... 14
    1.5    *In vitro* liver models ....................................................................................................... 15
    1.6    Endpoints for the analysis of hepatocyte cultures .......................................................... 23
    1.7    Toxicogenomics ................................................................................................................ 24
    1.8    Techniques for global gene expression analysis ............................................................. 27
    1.9    Toxicoproteomics ............................................................................................................. 31
    1.10   Aim of this work .............................................................................................................. 33

2 **MATERIALS AND METHODS** ................................................................................. 34
    2.1    Materials ........................................................................................................................... 34
        2.1.1    Chemicals and reagents ................................................................................................ 34
        2.1.2    Technical equipment and auxiliary material .............................................................. 36
        2.1.3    Kits ................................................................................................................................. 38
        2.1.4    Software ......................................................................................................................... 38
        2.1.5    Culture media and supplements .................................................................................. 39
        2.1.6    Buffers and solutions ................................................................................................... 39
            2.1.6.1   Perfusion buffers for rat liver perfusion .............................................................. 39
            2.1.6.2   Buffers for SELDI-TOF-MS ................................................................................ 40
            2.1.6.3   Buffers for protein-preparation adn immunodetection ...................................... 40
            2.1.6.4   Buffers and solutions for Illumina BeadChip arrays ......................................... 41
            2.1.6.5   Buffers and solutions for Affymetrix Gene Chips® ........................................... 41
    2.2    Methods ............................................................................................................................ 43
        2.2.1    Cell culture .................................................................................................................... 43
            2.2.1.1   Isolation of primary rat hepatocytes ................................................................... 43
            2.2.1.2   Trypan Blue exclusion test ................................................................................... 44
            2.2.1.3   Preparation of culture dishes ............................................................................... 44
            2.2.1.4   Plating of cells ........................................................................................................ 45
            2.2.1.5   Culture of FaO and HepG2-cells .......................................................................... 46
            2.2.1.6   Suspension culture ................................................................................................ 46
            2.2.1.7   Precision cut liver slices ........................................................................................ 46
            2.2.1.8   Isolation of primary human hepatocytes ............................................................ 47

# INDEX

- 2.2.1.9 HepaRG cells ............................................................................................ 47
- 2.2.2 Rat *in vivo* study ............................................................................................ 47
- 2.2.3 Biochemical methods and cell viability assays ........................................... 48
  - 2.2.3.1 CellTiter-Glo® Luminescent cell viability assay ................................. 48
  - 2.2.3.2 WST-1-assay ......................................................................................... 49
  - 2.2.3.3 LDH release .......................................................................................... 49
  - 2.2.3.4 Cytochrome P450 isoform induction and activity ............................... 51
  - 2.2.3.5 Canalicular transporter activity ............................................................ 52
- 2.2.4 Molecular biological methods ........................................................................ 52
  - 2.2.4.1 Isolation of RNA and proteins ............................................................. 52
  - 2.2.4.2 Quantification and quality check of nucleic acids ............................... 53
  - 2.2.4.3 TaqMan® Low Density Arrays (TLDA) ............................................. 55
  - 2.2.4.4 Processing of RNA for Illumina and Affymetrix Chips ..................... 58
- 2.2.5 Microarray data analysis ............................................................................... 63
  - 2.2.5.1 Data extraction and quality control from Illumina BeadChip arrays .. 63
  - 2.2.5.2 Data extraction and quality control from Affymetrix arrays ............... 64
- 2.2.6 Protein separation by SDS polyacrylamide gel electrophoresis (SDS-PAGE) .............. 66
- 2.2.7 Protein detection by western blot analysis and immune detection ............. 66
- 2.2.8 SELDI-TOF analysis ..................................................................................... 68

# 3 RESULTS AND DISCUSSIONS ............................................................. 70

## 3.1 Comparison of different global gene expression platforms ..................... 70
- 3.1.1 Results of the platform comparison study .................................................. 73
  - 3.1.1.1 Experimental layout .............................................................................. 73
  - 3.1.1.2 Intraplatform comparability ................................................................. 75
  - 3.1.1.3 Interplatform comparability ................................................................. 77
  - 3.1.1.4 Biological interpretation ....................................................................... 82
- 3.1.2 Conclusions of the platform comparison study .......................................... 95

## 3.2 Establishment of a longer term cell culture of primary rat and human hepatocytes . 98
- 3.2.1 Morphological and functional characterization of primary rat hepatocytes .......... 99
  - 3.2.1.1 Morphological examinations ................................................................ 99
  - 3.2.1.2 CYP inducibility ................................................................................... 102
  - 3.2.1.3 Canalicular transport ............................................................................ 105
  - 3.2.1.4 Conclusions of the morphological and functional data ...................... 106

## 3.3 Global expression studies with different human and rat cell culture systems ......... 108
- 3.3.1 Initial changes introduced by the process of perfusion ............................. 113
  - 3.3.1.1 Primary rat hepatocytes ........................................................................ 113
  - 3.3.1.2 Primary human hepatocytes ................................................................. 115
- 3.3.2 Temporal changes in global gene expression ............................................. 118
- 3.3.3 Analysis of protein expression with SELDI-TOF ..................................... 123
- 3.3.4 Gene expression in established cell lines used as reference ..................... 126

| | | | |
|---|---|---|---|
| 3.3.5 | | Changes of gene expression early in culture - Cellular adaptation processes in primary hepatocytes...... 128 | |
| | 3.3.5.1 | Liver slices ................................................................................................................. 133 | |
| 3.3.6 | | Molecular mechanisms affected over time in culture ............................................................ 136 | |
| | 3.3.6.1 | Overview of the affected mechanisms in rat hepatocytes ................................. 136 | |
| | 3.3.6.2 | Response to wounding, oxidative stress and immune response ........................ 138 | |
| | 3.3.6.3 | ECM, cytoskeleton and tissue remodelling ....................................................... 140 | |
| | 3.3.6.4 | Metabolic competence ....................................................................................... 142 | |
| | 3.3.6.5 | Intracellular signalling and transcription factors ............................................. 144 | |
| | 3.3.6.6 | Affected mechanisms in human hepatocytes ..................................................... 146 | |
| 3.3.7 | | Confirmation of the microarray results with TaqMan PCR .................................................. 149 | |
| 3.3.8 | | Conclusions from the characterization of primary hepatocytes in culture ................................ 150 | |

**3.4 Development of an *in vitro* liver toxicity prediction model based on longer term primary hepatocyte culture .................................................................................................... 155**

| | | |
|---|---|---|
| 3.4.1 | Introduction to the *in vitro* prediction model ......................................................................... 155 |
| 3.4.2 | Short description of the test compounds ................................................................................. 155 |
| 3.4.3 | Experimental setup and dose finding ....................................................................................... 159 |
| 3.4.4 | Data Analysis and establishment of an *in vitro* prediction model for hepatotoxicity .............................. 163 |
| 3.4.5 | Analysis of the top ranked genes of the prediction model ...................................................... 169 |

**3.5 Insights into the mechanisms of action for selected compounds ................................ 171**

| | | |
|---|---|---|
| 3.5.1 | EMD X .................................................................................................................................... 172 |
| 3.5.2 | AAP ......................................................................................................................................... 175 |
| 3.5.3 | Dex ........................................................................................................................................... 178 |

**4   *CONCLUDING REMARKS AND FUTURE PERSPECTIVES* ....................... *180***

**5   *REFERENCES* ........................................................................................................... *184***

# ABBREVIATIONS

| | |
|---|---|
| % | Percentage |
| [ ] | Concentration |
| +/- FCS | With or without the addition of fetal calf serum |
| °C | Centigrade |
| µl | Micro litre |
| ALDH | Aldehyde dehydrogenase |
| AN | Accession Number |
| BNF | Beta-naftoflavon |
| bp | Basepair |
| BROD | Benzyloxyresorufin O-debenzylase |
| BSA | Bovine Serum Albumin |
| Carboxi-DCFDA | 5-(and-6)-carboxy-2',7'-dichlorofluorescein diacetate |
| CHAPS | 3-[(3-Cholamidopropyl)-dimethylammonio]-1-propanesulfonate |
| $CO_2$ | Carbonic acid |
| Da | Dalton |
| Dex | Dexametasone |
| DMSO | Dimethyl sulfoxide |
| (c)DNA | (complementary) Desoxy ribonucleic acid |
| DTT | Dithiothreitol |
| ECVAM | European Centre for the Validation of Alternative Methods |
| EDTA | Ethylenediaminetetraacetic acid |
| EROD | 7-ethoxyresorufin-O-deethylase |
| FBS | Fetal Bovine Serum |
| FC | Fresh cells (hepatocytes directly after perfusion) |
| FDA | Food and Drug Administration |
| g | Gram |
| GLP | Good Laboratory Practice |
| GSH | Glutathione |
| h | Hour |
| H&E | Hematoxylin and eosin stain |
| HepaRG | Human hepatoma cell line |
| HepG2 | Human hepatoma cell line |
| Hz | Hertz (cycles per second) |
| i.p. | intraperitoneal |
| ITS | Insulin, Transferrin, Selenit |
| IVT | In vitro transcription reaction |
| k | Kilo |
| kDa | kilodaltons |
| l | Litre |

# ABBREVIATIONS

| | |
|---|---|
| LDH | Lactate dehydrogenase |
| M | Molarity |
| mA | Mili-Ampere |
| min | Minute |
| ML | Monolayer culture |
| mm | millimetre |
| mRNA | Messenger Ribonucleic acid |
| MTD | Maximum tolerated dose |
| MW | Molecular Weight |
| nm | Nanometre |
| NRU | Neutral Red Uptake |
| OD | Optical density |
| ON | Over night |
| PAGE | Polyacrylamide gel electrophoresis |
| PB | Phenobarbital |
| PB1 | Perfusion Buffer 1 |
| PB2 | Perfusion Buffer 2 |
| PBS | Phosphate Buffered Saline |
| PCA | Principal Components Analysis |
| PCR | Polymerase Chain Reaction |
| PL | Plastic culture |
| rcf | Relative centrifugal force |
| REACH | Registration, Evaluation and Authorization of Chemicals |
| RMA | Robust multi-array average |
| (c) RNA | (complementary) Ribonucleic acid |
| rpm | rounds per minute |
| rRNA | Ribosomal Ribonucleic acid |
| RT | Room temperature |
| SDS | Sodium dodecyl sulphate |
| sec | Second |
| SELDI-TOF | Surface-enhanced laser desorption/ionization – time of flight |
| SOM | Self Organizing Map |
| Susp. | Suspension |
| SW | Sandwich culture |
| TLDA | TaqMan Low Density Array |
| WB | Washing buffer |

# 1 INTRODUCTION

## 1.1 Endeavors of modern toxicology

Toxicology is the study of adverse effects of chemical and physical agents on living organisms and the environment. The basic assumption of toxicology is that there is a relationship between the dose, the concentration at the affected site, and the resulting adverse effects. The physician Theophrast von Hohenheim (Paracelsus, 1493-1541) said: "*Alle Ding sind Gift, und nichts ohn Gift; allein die Dosis macht, daß ein Ding kein Gift ist*"[1]. As he was the first one to discover the relationship between dose and effect of substances he is often called the "father of toxicology".

The purpose of modern toxicology is to understand the character and dimension of toxic effects and to regulate the use of potentially toxic substances. Up to now, there is a general lack of knowledge regarding 99% of chemicals manufactured around the world. The distinction between so-called "existing" and "new" chemicals is based on the cut-off date of 1981. All chemicals that were on the European Community market between 1 January 1971 and 18 September 1981 are called "existing"[2]. Prior to that date, no stringent health and safety tests were needed to market chemicals, it was up to the authorities to prove that a substance posed a threat before it could be withdrawn. Since then, 3,800 so-called "new" chemicals have gone through a more stringent safety screening process. New perceptions have now introduced the possibility that the incidence of diseases, such as cancer, could be linked to this multitude of chemicals already on the market (Irigaray et al., 2007). Therefore, in June 2007, the European Parliament introduced a new system of Registration, Evaluation and Authorisation of CHemicals (REACH). Central to the system is a requirement for producers and importers of chemicals to prove that their substances are safe before put on the market (reversal of burden of proof). "Existing" chemicals will have to be screened for health and safety reasons over a period of 11 years. Therefore, defined, standardized and validated assays have to be conducted and the results regulated by national and international commissions[3].

---

[1] "All things are poisonous and nothing is without poison, only the dose permits something not to be poisonous."
[2] Around 100,000, listed in the European Inventory of Existing Commercial Chemical Substances (EINECS).
[3] Umweltbundesamt, Dessau-Rosslau, Germany; European Chemicals Agency, Helsinki, Finland

# 1 INTRODUCTION

Up to now, only few of these mandatory tests can be accomplished with animal-free alternative methods leading to the problem that a marked increase of animal testing will be of animals are required (Figure 1). This contradicts the simultaneous effort of reducing the number of animals used in experiments for ethical and cost reasons.

In 1959, Russel and Burch suggested the principle of the 3Rs in order to reduce animal experiments (Russell & Burch, 1959). It refers to the improvement of the animal welfare by reducing the number of tests realised, the refinement of existing experiments to reduce the suffering of the animals and to a replacement of animal experiments with new and alternative methods. Considering this, it is believed that *in vitro* toxicity testing methods can be a useful, time and cost-effective supplement or in some case even a replacement of toxicology studies in living animals. Certain endpoints of toxicity can be depicted quite well, although currently available *in vitro* tests are not adequate to entirely replace animals in toxicology testing. In 1991, the European Centre for the Validation of Alternative Methods (ECVAM) was founded to assist and coordinate the development and validation of alternative test methods under the guidance of the European Union.

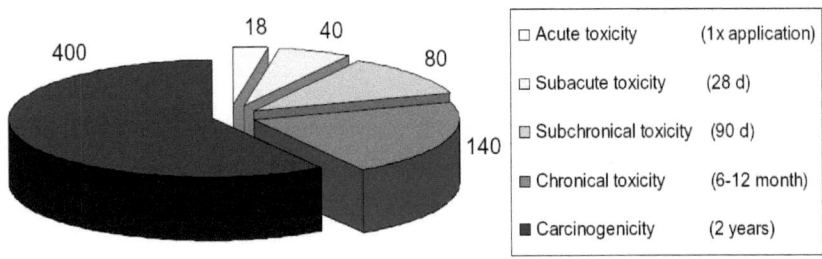

Figure 1: Increasing number of animals needed in toxicological testing procedure for one compound beginning with an acute toxicity study and ending with a 2-year carcinogenicity study.

## 1.2 The liver morphology and its cell types

The liver is the largest and most complex gland of the body. It is the main detoxifying organ in mammals, with large amounts of phase 1 and phase 2 metabolic enzymes and it is responsible for large parts of lipid and cholesterol metabolism, the production of hormones, phagocytosis of debris and bacteria as well as participating in iron metabolism. Additionally, it has an important role in many vital functions of the body, like the production of bile, the processing and storage of nutrients and Vitamin A and the synthesis of blood

# 1 INTRODUCTION

proteins including albumin, lipoproteins, transferrin, growth factors and coagulation factors (LaBrecque, 1994; Kevresan et al., 2006).

In vertebrates, the liver is divided into four lobes, with each containing thousands of equally built lobules, and is served by two distinct blood supplies. The hepatic artery supplies oxygenated blood and the hepatic portal vein feeds blood from the intestinal system (including the pancreas and the spleen) and is rich in nutrients but is low in oxygen. The blood flows out of the liver via the hepatic vein in the direction of the inferior vena cava. Thereby, xenobiotics absorbed by ingestion have to pass the hepatocytes, the predominant cell type in liver, and can be taken up, metabolised and/or detoxified (first pass effect). The metabolites are excreted partly, depending on their chemical properties, into the bile canaliculi or via the venous blood into the urine. Hepatocytes, the liver parenchymal cells, account for about 80-90% of liver mass and 65% of cell number of a normal liver, Non-parenchymal cells like Kupffer cells (15%), endothelial cells, hepatic stellate cells or pit cells make up the remaining mass (Blouin, Bolender & Weibel, 1977; Widmann, Cotran & Fahimi, 1972; Wisse, 1977a, 1977b).

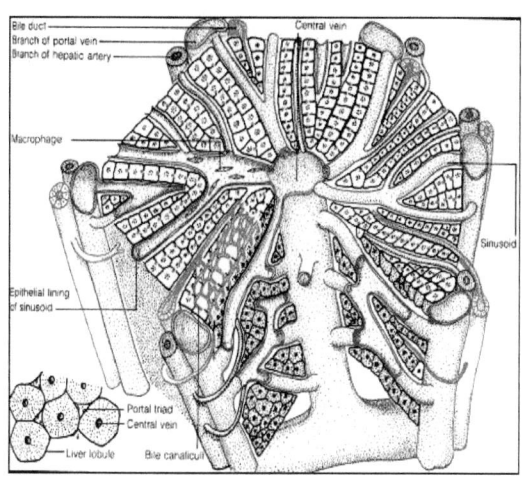

Figure 2: Schematic diagram of a normal liver lobule showing sheets of hepatocytes and the sinusoids which contain a variety of specialized cells like Ito-cells, Kupffer cells and endothelial cells. (Figure taken from www.ener-chi.com/ d_liv.htm)

In a hexagonal shaped liver lobule, the central vein is surrounded by 4-6 portal areas (Matsumoto & Kawakami, 1982) and hepatocytes are arranged in cords radiating from the central vein (Figure 2). Hepatic endothelial cells form the walls of the sinusoidal, the capillaries between the cords of hepatocytes. Unlike other endothelial cells, they lack a basement membrane and the endothelial structures possess pores called fenestrae, allowing the blood to flow directly around the hepatocytes. They express several adhesion molecules facilitating inflammatory cell migration, usually as response to activation by

# 1 INTRODUCTION

Kupffer cell signalling following liver damage (Ohira et al., 2003; Scoazec & Feldmann, 1994).

The Kupffer cells, resident macrophages in the liver, represent the second largest cell population of the liver. They are located in the hepatic sinusoids, in between or on top of endothelial cells, but they also make contact to the hepatocytes through their extensions. They exhibit several important functions, such as endocytosis of foreign material and bacteria, antigen presentation and secretion of biologically active products (e.g. nitric oxide and cytokines) and play an important role in immune and inflammatory responses involving cytokine-signalling (Winwood & Arthur, 1993).

Stellate cells are the fat-storing cells of the liver where they reside in the space of Disse between hepatocytes and endothelial cells. They store Vitamin A in lipid droplets, synthesize extracellular matrix proteins and it has been suggested that they contribute to liver fibrosis and immune response (Ogata et al., 1991; Friedman, 1997)

## 1.3 Hepatocytes and xenobiotic metabolism

As mentioned above, the liver is the main organ for endogenous and exogenous metabolism and detoxification of foreign compounds. The fenestrated endothelial allows the blood plasma to leak through the endothelial cell layer and come into close contact with the microvilli of the underlying hepatocytes in the space of Disse, providing optimal conditions for an extensive metabolic exchange (Enomoto et al., 2004). Hepatocytes are polygonally-shaped, polarized and highly differentiated cells with a turnover time *in vivo* of 300-400 days (Imai et al., 2001). There is an abundance of mitochondria and they often contain a second nucleus to manage their extensive roles in energy production, protein synthesis and metabolism/detoxification. Polyploidy is a general physiological process indicative of terminal differentiation (Sigal et al., 1999).

Each hepatocyte has a basolateral surface facing the lymph in the space of Disse and canalicular surfaces facing the bile duct. The basolateral membrane is rich in microvillus and expresses many transporters for uptake of organic anions, cations (OATPs and Oct1-3 respectively) and bile salts (NTCP, OST $\alpha$ and $\beta$). The canalicular membrane of neighbouring hepatocytes is sealed by tight junctions generating fine channels that run around the cells (Figure 3).

# 1 INTRODUCTION

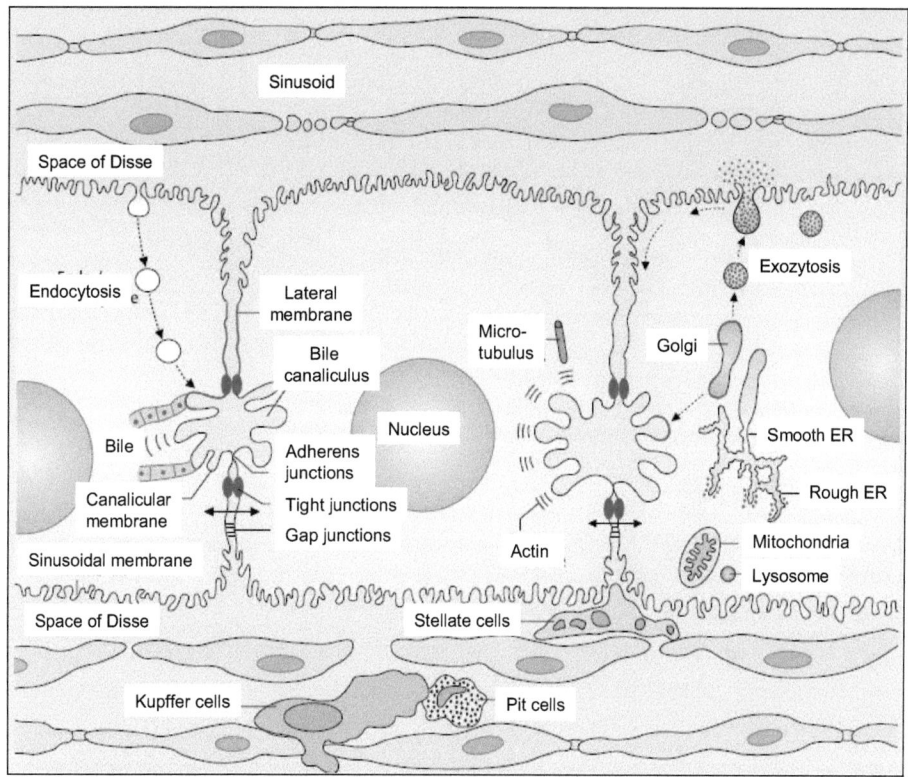

Figure 3: Ultrastructure of hepatocytes as polarized, secretory active cells with basolateral and apical surrounding (Figure adapted from Siegenthaler & Blum, 2006).

The hepatocyte membranes accommodate transporters which have overlapping substrate specify (MDR 1-3, OATP) and are responsible for the export of bile salts or products of metabolic pathways (Figure 4). Hepatic export into the bile is an important function for the detoxification of foreign compounds entering the body and is therefore often referred to as phase 3 of xenobiotic metabolism (Makowski & Pikuła, 1997; Yamazaki, Suzuki & Sugiyama, 1996). MRPs 1, 3 & 4 and OST α, β are basolaterally located, ATP-dependent, transporters. The shading of these transporters in Figure 4, and the white arrows in the pathways leading to and through them, symbolize their low activity in the normal hepatocyte. With hepatocellular disease or cholestasis, they are greatly up regulated, increasing the export of organic anions, thus limiting accumulation of toxic organic anions (e.g. bilirubin, bile salts) within the hepatocyte.

# 1 INTRODUCTION

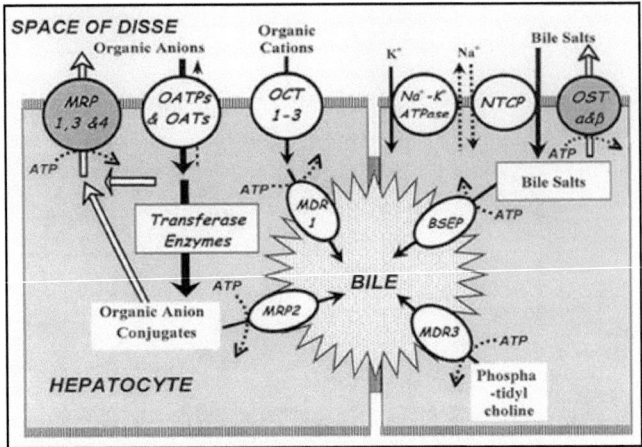

Figure 4: Schematic diagram of transport processes in hepatocytes. Shown are influx transporters, such as OATPs, OATs, NTCP and OCTs at the sinusoidal membrane, and efflux transporters, such as MDR1, MDR3, MRP2 and BSEP at the canalicular membrane. Additional efflux transporters such as MRP3, MRP4, and MRP6 at the basolateral membrane are not shown (Figure taken from www.uwgi.org/ gut/liver_05.asp).

There are different requirements, which the hepatocytes, as xenobiotic metabolizing cells, have to accomplish. The cells have to transform non-polar, lipophilic xenobiotics to more hydrophilic metabolites to facilitate their excretion into the bile or the urine (Figure 5). The resulting metabolites should be less biologically active (detoxificated) and the metabolizing enzymes must have a broad, overlapping specificity so new and unknown compounds can be metabolized (Marquardt et al., 1999). For this reason, hepatocytes express a variety of metabolic enzymes, which are responsible for different types of reactions.

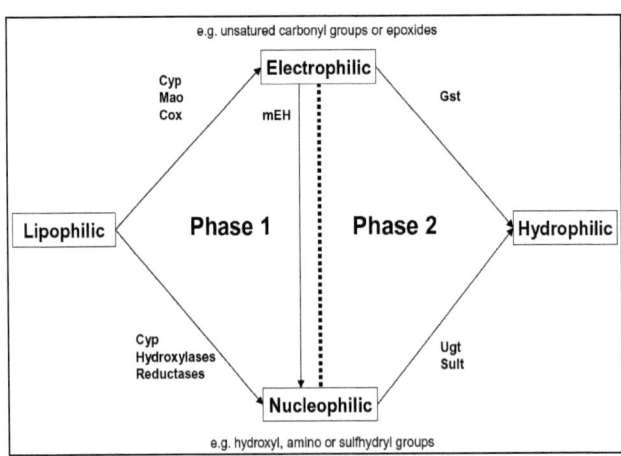

Figure 5: Phase model of xenobiotic metabolism. Lipophilic compounds are sequentially metabolized over electrophilic or nucleophilic intermediates to hydrophilic products that can afterwards be excreted renally or biliary. (Figure adapted from Marquardt & Schäfer, 2004).

# 1 INTRODUCTION

Two main processes usually occur sequentially called phase 1 and phase 2. The former leads to an activation of the compound by introducing functional groups into the compound by oxidation, reduction or hydrolysis reactions. This is followed by phase 2 reactions, the conjugation of the active metabolite with a highly polar ligand like glucuronic acid or glutathione, leading to more hydrophilic products. As mentioned above, the directed transport of metabolites out of the cells by specialized transporters is often referred to as phase 3 of xenobiotic metabolism.

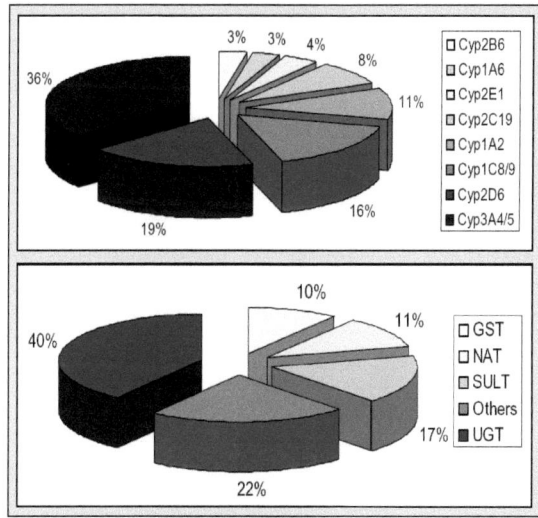

Figure 6: Proportion of drugs metabolized by cytochrome P450 isoenzymes (upper figure) and phase 2 enzymes (lower figure). Figures adapted from (Evans & Relling, 1999) and (Wrighton & Stevens, 1992).

Typical phase 1 enzymes are listed in Table 1. The CYP enzymes, the predominant group of phase 1 enzymes in mammals, consist of at least 17 gene families with 50-60 individual isoforms (Guengerich, 2003; Waxman, 1999). The major human CYP enzymes involved in metabolism of drugs or exogenous toxins are Cyp3A4, Cyp1A1, Cyp1A2, Cyp2D6 and Cyp2C (Figure 6). The amount of each of these enzymes present in the liver reflects their importance in drug metabolism (Goodman et al., 1996).

Depending on the chemical properties of the introduced functional groups, phase 1 products can be classified as electrophilic or nucleophilic metabolites. Strong electrophilic metabolites are able to covalently bind to biological molecules like DNA, RNA or proteins and therefore have inherent cytotoxic or mutagenic potential (Besaratinia & Pfeifer, 2005). In contrast to this, nucleophiles can show biological activity by binding to cellular receptors

# 1 INTRODUCTION

and activating downstream reactions. Thus, the metabolic activity of cells can lead not only to a detoxification but also, in certain cases, to a toxification of compounds.

The activation reaction is in most cases followed by a detoxifying phase 2 conjugation reaction. Thereby, the water solubility is increased allowing the cells to excrete the conjugates into the bile canaliculi and/or the blood plasma. Enzymes catalyzing phase 2 reactions are e.g. sulfotransferases (SULT), acetyltransferases (AT), glucoronyltransferases and Glutathione-S-Transferases (GST) (Figure 6).

| Phase-1-Enzymes |
|---|
| Cytochrom-P450-dependent monooxygenases (CYP) |
| Oxidoreduktases |
| Flavin-dependent monooxygenases (FMO) |
| Monoaminoxidases (MAO) |
| Cyclooxygenases (COX) |
| Dihydrodioldehydrogenases |
| Alcohol- and aldehyddehydrogenases (ADH, ALDH) |
| Esterases |
| Amidases |
| Glucuronidases |
| Epoxidhydrolases (EH) |
| DT-Diaphorase (NQOR) |
| Hydrolases |

| Phase-2-Enzymes |
|---|
| Transferases |
| Glutathiontransferases (GST) |
| UDP-glucuronosyltransferases (UGT) |
| Sulfotransferases (SULT) |
| Acetyltransferases (NAT) |
| Methyltransferases |
| Aminoacyltransferases |

| Phase-3-Enzymes |
|---|
| OATCs |
| MDRs |
| MRPs |

Table 1: Examples of enzyme classes involved in the three phases of xenobiotic metabolism.

Several factors can influence the efficiency of xenobiotic metabolism. The activation and inhibition of enzyme activity and the induction and repression of gene expression are the main elements of regulation. Inducers usually affect multiple enzymes from different steps of xenobiotic metabolism. Thereby, an entire metabolism cascade can be activated leading to the detoxification of the compound (Elias & Mills, 2007; Xu, Li & Kong, 2005). Responsible for this coordinated gene expressions are several forms of nuclear receptors which act in concert with other regulatory proteins (Figure 7). In their inactive form, they are present in the cytoplasm and, after binding of a substrate, are translocated into the nucleus in their active form as homo- or heterodimers. By binding to the DNA at different hormone response elements (HRE´s) and recruiting other proteins, so called co-regulators, their effect can be modulated in various ways.

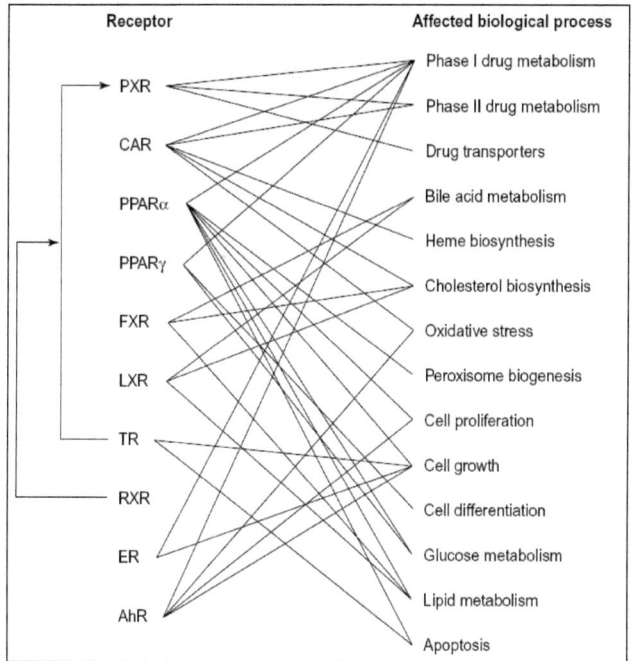

Figure 7: interaction of cellular transcription factors and their influence on several biological processes (Taken from Ulrich 2003).

Some receptors, so-called orphan receptors, do not have any known endogenous ligands but can bind metabolic intermediates with low affinity (Benoit et al., 2006). They are therefore thought to function as metabolic (*Peroxisome Proliverator activated receptors* (PPAR)) or xenobiotic (*pregnane X receptor* (PXR), *constitutively active receptor* (CAR)) sensors. Ligands for these kinds of receptors include lipophilic substances like hormones or xenobiotic compounds. They often build heterodimers with the *Retinoic X receptor* (RXR) or the *AHR-nuclear translocator* (Arnt) to activate the transcription of a wide range of metabolizing enzymes which in turn are often needed for further metabolisation of the initial substrate. This whole mechanism builds up an autoregulatory metabolic feedback-loop.

The expression of most metabolic enzymes, especially the CYP enzymes, is regulated in this way with the exception being CYP2E1, which is regulated in an even more complex

1 INTRODUCTION

manner. It is regulated on not only transcriptional but also pre-translational, translational, and posttranslational level with the stabilization of mRNA and protein as the most important steps (Ingelman-Sundberg et al., 1994).

## 1.4 Hepatotoxicity

Because of the central role the liver plays in the metabolism of xenobiotic compounds, hepatotoxicity is a major issue in pharmaceutical drug development (Ballet, 1997). Drug-induced liver injury is the major reason for attrition in clinical studies (Wysowski & Swartz, 2005) and hepatotoxic side effects are the main reason for drug withdrawals from the market (31%). A broad variety of liver pathophysiologies have been reported, including steatosis (fatty liver), cholestasis (obstruction of bile secretion), fibrosis (increased production and deposition of extracellular matrix components), hepatitis (inflammation), necrosis (cell death) or the formation of liver tumours. These pathological findings may arise from diseases affecting the liver, but also from xenobiotics, alcohol abuse or undesired drug-drug interactions. The pathological symptoms of certain liver diseases allow conclusions about the affected intracellular organelles. Although different histological changes can appear, a compound-class often displays a typical clinical or pathological appearance.

Xenobiotics administered orally first pass through the liver before entering the general blood circulation (first pass effect). Because the liver has multiple functions for the homeostasis of the whole body, drug induced liver toxicity can have severe consequences. Thirty to fifty percent of acute liver failures and fifteen percent of liver transplantations are related to chemical-induced hepatotoxicity (Andrade et al., 2004; Kaplowitz, 2001; Lewis, 2002).There is often a lack of reasonable understanding of the general molecular mechanisms of most drug-induced hepatoxicities (Boelsterli, 2003; Jaeschke et al., 2002; Lee, 2003). The inhibition of mitochondrial function, disruption of intracellular calcium homeostasis, activation of apoptosis, oxidative stress, inhibition of specific enzymes or transporters and the formation of reactive metabolites that cause direct toxicity or immunogenic responses are some mechanisms that have to be considered.

The drug development process comprises a variety of steps to assess whether a test compound has adequate efficacy, appropriate physicochemical properties, metabolic stability, safety and bioreactivity in humans. Hepatotoxicity in humans has a poor correlation with regulatory animal toxicity tests (Olson et al., 1998; Olson et al., 2000). However, if assays identified a compound as a human liver-toxicant, there is more than 80% correlation to the corresponding findings in animals (Xu, Diaz & O'Brien, 2004). While *in vivo* models, limited by animal welfare/ethical concerns, are used to investigate systemic influences, cell culture models provide systems that can investigate specific mechanisms in a precisely controlled environment (Ulrich et al., 1995).

Although there are ways to analyse the many toxicological parameters individually *in vitro*, most have low predictive value for the detection of human hepatotoxicity. The poor predictivity and sensitivity of standard *in vitro* cytotoxicity assays is due to several reasons, including strong inter-species variation, the lack of a true physiological environment of *in vitro* experiments or the insufficient culturing conditions, resulting in a loss of e.g. metabolic capabilities (Olson et al., 1998). The *in vitro* assays usually measure lethal events in late stages of toxicity, but toxicity may not always be lethal per se. Cytotoxicity may take several days to appear (Olson et al., 1998; Slaughter, Thakkar & O'Brien 2002; Schoonen et al., 2005), demanding repeated drug administration. In contrast to directly active compounds (primary toxins), some compounds elicit their toxic potential only as a metabolite (secondary toxins) and usually cause damage in the organ where they are produced.

This of course raises the need for metabolically active long-term *in vitro* models that facilitate extended exposure times. Several models have been used for the detection of acute toxicity, but sub-chronic and chronic toxicities have not been addressed so far. Furthermore, standard tests generally investigate only one parameter whereas hepatotoxicity can develop via many different mechanisms and is considered a multi-factorial process. In order to improve sensitivity it will be necessary to analyse several morphological, biochemical and functional endpoints in parallel. Finally, tests should be performed not only with high concentrations, causing acute toxicity, but also with *in vivo* pharmacological concentrations.

## 1.5  *In vitro* liver models

*In vitro* tests have the advantage of allowing multiple testing of different compounds, doses and/or time points simultaneously under well-defined conditions. The simplicity of some *in vitro* systems, besides saving time, money and animals used for experimentation, provides the ability to specifically manipulate and analyze a small number of well-defined parameters. The most commonly used test systems include, the isolated perfused liver, liver slices, primary hepatocytes in suspension or culture, cell lines, transgenic cells and sub-cellular fractions such as S9 mix, microsomes, supersomes or cytosol (Table 2). The reduction in the complexity of the system and the increase in throughput offer the ability to

# 1 INTRODUCTION

study specific parameters more closely but create inherent constraints for each model (Figure 8). However, this limits their widespread use and acceptance by the regulatory authorities as an alternative for *in vivo* testing (Brandon et al., 2003). Although studies have shown that *in vitro* cytotoxicity data can be used to identify appropriate doses for *in vivo* studies (Scholz et al., 1999).

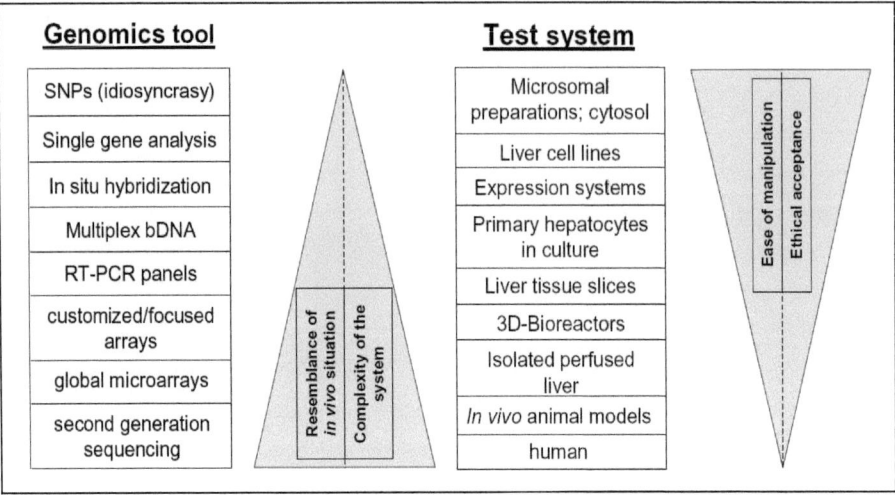

Figure 8: Models and genomic tools used for drug development, ordered by the correlation of the complexity of experiments conducted, the expressiveness, and the complexity of *an in vitro* model (Adapted and modified from Brandon et al., 2003).

One major obstacle for some *in vitro* models is their limited metabolic competence, mainly due to the down regulation of CYP enzymes over time (Ching et al., 1996; De Smet et al., 1998). This is especially important since phase 1 and phase 2 metabolic conversions of chemicals can greatly influence their toxicity (Holme, 1985). To overcome these problems, new and innovative strategies are being developed in order to find reliable markers that are involved not only in early toxic responses but also in chronic toxicities, also occurring at sub-lethal doses of a test compound. Furthermore, there is a strong need for a robust long-term *in vitro* screening system that allows the characterisation of drug/chemical induced toxicities and helps to reduce the use of animals in toxicity testing.

*Isolated perfused liver*

Ideally, an *in vitro* test system should adequately represent the *in vivo* situation as closely as possible. Most liver specific features are preserved in whole isolated and perfused

# 1 INTRODUCTION

livers, first developed in 1972 by Gordon and colleagues (Gordon et al., 1972). Especially, the three-dimensional architecture of the liver, the cell-cell, cell-matrix interactions and functional bile canaliculi are maintained. Additionally, all liver cell types are present and the communication between them can play an important role in mediating toxicity. Despite all these advantages, the isolated perfused liver model is difficult to handle and retains its functional integrity for only a few hours. Moreover, reproducibility is low, the use of animals is not significantly reduced and human organs are rarely available.

*Precision-cut liver slices*

First used in 1923 by Otto Warburg and improved over the following decades (Warburg, 1923; Krumdieck, dos Santos & Ho, 1980), precision-cut liver slices have the advantage of partially conserved liver cyto-architecture, cell-cell, cell-matrix contacts and the presence of different cell types (Lerche-Langr & Toutain, 2000). The preparation of slices from different parts of the liver facilitates lobe and zone specific analysis of metabolism and toxicity. In addition, since many slices can be prepared from the same human or animal donor, reproducibility and throughput can be increased significantly. Another major advantage is the possibility to conduct histopathological examinations, as well as biochemical and molecular biological studies from the same tissue. Due to the thickness of liver slices, 200-250 µm resembling 10-20 cell layers, the adequate supply of nutrients and oxygen from the incubation medium is only maintained for the outer cell layers. Therefore, liver slices are only useful for short-term toxicity studies due to their limited viability and the rapid decline of liver specific functions. The metabolic activity of tissue slices are reported to be preserved for 1-2 days in culture (Ekins et al., 1995).

*Cell lines and sub-cellular fractions*

Cell lines, isolated hepatocytes or whole liver cell suspensions are used as the starting material for a variety of *in vitro* models of different complexity and throughput. The simplest liver *in vitro* models are sub-cellular fractions, such as organ homogenates, microsomes, mitochondria or nuclei. Most sub-cellular fractions can be prepared and separated relatively easily by homogenisation of the tissue and sequential centrifugation. They are commercially available for a large number of species, including human. Nevertheless, they are only suitable for short-term studies with specific questions, such as enzyme inhibition, covalent binding or clearance studies. For example, liver supernatants ("S9") are used as an activation system for xenobiotics in *in vitro* genotoxicity assays (e.g., Ames-assay

# 1 INTRODUCTION

(Ames, Lee & Durston, 1973)). Mitochondria are added for the analysis of drug effects on respiration, ATP-synthesis and fatty acid oxidation. To acquire increased metabolic activity, animals are often induced by treatment with Arochlor 1254 or a Phenobarbital/beta-naphthoflavone (PB/BNF) mixture prior to S9 preparation (Callander et al., 1995), leading to elevated and unphysiological expression levels of metabolic enzymes. Most systems are supplemented with cofactors to preserve enzymatic activity. Other disadvantages include the absence of complete enzyme systems like for phase 2 enzymes in microsomes.

The usage of different cell lines is one step forward in complexity. They are used for a variety of toxicological applications, but since most hepatic cell lines originate from tumours, they have lost the high degree of differentiation seen in hepatocytes and their gene expression pattern is distinctively different from normal liver cells. In addition, many cell lines display genetic instability. For example, the frequently used human hepatoma cell line HepG2 lacks expression of several CYP isoforms and phase 2 enzymes, making them insensitive to secondary toxic compounds (Knasmüller et al., 2004). To complicate matters, different sources of HepG2 cells can have very different enzyme profiles (Hewitt & Hewitt, 2004). Several transfected variants of HepG2 have been constructed which express increased levels of drug metabolising enzymes, including CYP1A1, CYP1A2, CYP2E1 and glutathione-S-transferases (Knasmüller et al., 2004), but *in vivo* relevance may not always be assumed because expression of the cloned enzymes is not at physiological levels and only single enzyme functions can be analyzed. Recently, the human hepatoma cell line HepaRG has been described. It is a naturally immortalized cell line from human liver with liver progenitor properties (Parent et al., 2004). After application of a differentiation protocol (Chapter 2.2.1.9, Page 47), HepaRG cells display hepatocyte like morphology and expression of drug metabolising enzymes at near *in vivo* levels (Gripon et al., 2002; Parent & Beretta, 2008). However, these novel cell lines still have to be confirmed and validated as a reasonable alternative cell-based assay for use in toxicological studies.

*Cultures of isolated primary liver cells*

To overcome the dilemma of non physiological gene expression and genomic instability, freshly isolated hepatocytes are often used for toxicological research. Although these are mostly mono-factorial systems which do not take into account the interactions between cell types or even whole organs in the body, cultures of primary rat and human hepatocytes are used in a variety of pharmacological and toxicological experiments, for example the

# 1 INTRODUCTION

evaluation of hepatic drug uptake and metabolism, drug-drug interactions and hepatotoxicity (Brandon et al., 2003; Gebhardt et al., 2003; Cross & Bayliss, 2000).

Fresh liver cells can be obtained by different procedures, all of which involve perfusion of the liver with $Ca^{2+}$-free buffers combined with enzymes/proteases which disintegrate the extracellular matrix, leading to the separation of the cells from each other (Seglen, 1976; Howard et al., 1967). The isolation of liver cells is routinely performed for many species used in toxicity testing, but also with tissue from partial liver resections and non-transplantable whole livers from human donors (LeCluyse et al., 2005; Richert et al., 2004).

In suspension, the survival of cells is short lived, normally not longer than 6 hours. Although the system is relatively high throughput, easy to use and preserves most of the metabolising enzymes at *in vivo* levels for a short time, it is only useable for acute toxicology or metabolism studies because the loss of contact to surrounding cells and the ECM environment has severe influence on the defined cell polarization and shape (Gebhardt et al., 2003). By capturing the cells into beads of alginate, the survival time can be prolonged to 24 hours. However, the lack of functional bile canaliculi, cell polarity and cell-cell contacts limits the use of alginate-embedded cells for drug transporter studies (Rialland et al., 2000).

The survival time in culture can be increased if hepatocytes are cultured on adhesive surfaces, for example, tissue culture dishes coated with ECM components. The most commonly used models are the monolayer culture (ML) where hepatocytes are usually attached to dried films of collagen I or Matrigel, a laminin-rich preparation from the Engelbreth-Holm-Swarm mouse sarcoma (Berthiaume et al., 1996).

During the perfusion procedure the cells are already primed for proliferation and can easily be forced to proliferate by the addition of mitogenic compounds, for example epidermal growth factor (EGF), allowing longer culturing (Etienne et al., 1988). However, this causes a down regulation of metabolic enzymes and thereby induces dedifferentiation associated with a loss of many liver specific functions and defined cell polarity (Luttringer et al., 2002; Skett & Bayliss, 1996; Paine & Andreakos, 2004; LeCluyse et al., 2000). Additionally, it is known that the typical phenotypic change of hepatocytes in monolayer culture, the "spreading" of the cells, has a negative effect on liver specific gene expression (Miranti, 2002). Intracellular signalling is closely connected to the interaction between ECM, cell-adhesion molecules and the cytoskeleton and therefore has a major impact on gene expression and the metabolic capacity of the cells. Altogether, this processes lead to a

# 1 INTRODUCTION

loss of up to 80-90% of phase 1 and about 50% of phase 2 metabolic activity during the first 24h in culture (Rodríguez-Antona et al., 2002; Wilkening, Stahl & Bader, 2003).

Culturing hepatocytes in a sandwich configuration (SW), embedded between two layers of gelled ECM proteins (e.g., collagen I or Matrigel), has prolonged the time in culture displaying hepatocyte-specific functions dramatically (LeCluyse et al., 2000; Dunn, Tompkins & Yarmush, 1991; Richert et al., 2002; Dunn et al., 1989). Cells adapted and maintained their physiologically occurring polygonal shape and bile canalicular-like structures could be observed for up to 14 days in culture (Tuschl & Müller, 2006). The same study showed less alterations of known stress-markers like Gadd45$\alpha$ in serum free sandwich culture compared to others and the expression of some marker genes involved in hepatocyte function were more stable. Additionally, SW cultured hepatocytes were successfully used for metabolism and induction studies (Kern et al., 1997; LeCluyse et al., 1999) indicating that the collagen overlay does not interfere with the test compounds. The development of long-term primary hepatocyte cultures is an essential step towards the study of chronic effects *in vitro*.

Another factor greatly influencing the morphological development and cell survival of hepatocytes in culture is the medium formulation and the addition/omission of serum, specified hormone mixtures or other supplements (Sidhu, Liu & Omiecinski, 2004; Pascussi et al., 2000; Turncliff, Meier & Brouwer, 2004). Among the most frequently used basal media, Dulbecco's modified Eagle medium (DMEM), modified Chee's medium (MCM) and Williams' medium E (WME), the DMEM/F12 mix seems most appropriate to maintain liver-specific functions and to help rebuild bile canaliculi (Turncliff, Tian & Brouwer, 2006). In culture, the addition of the glucocorticoid dexamethasone (DEX), at nanomolar concentrations, is essential for the long-term preservation of hepatocyte specific functions like polygonal hepatocyte morphology, structural integrity of cytoplasmic membranes, bile canaliculi-like structures and by maintaining the expression of liver specific transcription factors. Insulin enhances the glucose uptake of cells and contributes to maintaining liver specific gene expression. Selenium, a structural component of the enzyme glutathione peroxidase, which plays an essential role in the neutralization of metabolically generated peroxides, has also been shown to be beneficial when added to the medium (Yamada et al., 1980; Laishes & Williams, 1976; Müller & Pallauf, 2003). Since it is well known that serum enhances the surface attachment ability of hepatocytes (Williams, Bermudez & Scaramuzzino, 1977), cells are generally seeded in medium containing fetal calf serum, regardless of the subsequent culture conditions.

# 1 INTRODUCTION

*Co-cultures, spheroid cultures and 3 d bioreactor cultures*

Hepatocytes make up about 60-70% of the cells in the intact liver. However, liver toxicity may not always originate from these cells. Therefore, co-cultures of hepatocytes with other non-parenchymal liver cells, such as endothelial, Kupffer, or stellate cells and also stable cell lines or fibroblasts can be applied to reflect a more physiological situation. For example, the excretion of $TNF\alpha$ or nitric oxide by Kupffer cells can lead to inflammatory reactions or apoptosis (El-Bahay et al., 1999; Kmieć, 2001).

Spheroids (spherical multicellular aggregates) will form if a crude liver cell suspension is prevented from adherence to the surface by continuous shaking. Cell-cell contacts are re-established, hepatocytes are located on the inside, non-parenchymal cells on the outside and the deposition of ECM is seen throughout the spheroids. Alginate or other materials can be added to make up the internal structure of the spheres. Several studies showed the positive effect of this culture method on the expression of hepatotypic genes and the maintenance of metabolic capacity (Guigoz et al., 1987; Landry et al., 1985). The maintenance of prolonged functional activity has been related to the restoration and stability of cell polarity and close cell-to-cell contacts (Lu et al., 2005). However, the formation of these spheroids leads to hypoxic and necrotic cells dying at their centre. Additional problems arise from the accumulation of bile in the centre of spheroids.

Another skilful attempt to mimic a liver-like environment *in vitro* is the bioartificial liver system (3 d-bioreactors). Their major advantage is the re-establishment of the 3 d liver cyto-architecture with cell-cell contacts and a three-dimensional ECM environment, combined with continuous medium perfusion, providing a constant supply of oxygen and nutrients. Today a variety of culture systems are being used for bioreactor setups (Bader et al., 1998; Powers et al., 2002). Different studies have shown an improvement in some hepatocyte-specific functions in co-culture with other cell types, in spheroids and in 3D-bioreactors (Sivaraman et al., 2005). A very new and promising attempt to transfer and rebuild liver specific properties was developed by Linke et al (Linke et al., 2007). They co-cultured primary hepatocytes and microvascular endothelial cells by seeding them into a decellularized porcine jejunal segment with preserved vascular structures. The supply with nutrients was accomplished by perfusion of the blood vessels with culture medium. Biochemical testing showed metabolic and morphological stability for up to three weeks. However, the preparation of these cultures is quite elaborate, therefore their use as a high throughput tool for toxicological screening tests is unlikely.

# 1 INTRODUCTION

| Model | Advantages | Disadvantages |
|---|---|---|
| Isolated Perfused Liver | - liver specific functions close to *in vivo*<br>- three dimensional cytoarchitecture<br>- functional bile canaliculi<br>- lobular structure preserved<br>- collection of bile possible<br>- short-term kinetic studies | - not a high throughput system<br>- hepatic function only preserved for a few hours<br>- complicated to use<br>- study of human liver difficult/impossible<br>- best suited for liver of small animals<br>- no significant reduction in the number of animals used |
| Liver Tissue Slices | - *in vivo* cytoarchitecture preserved<br>- reasonably high throughput<br>- functional drug metabolising enzymes, transporters and bile canaliculi<br>- zone specific metabolism and toxicity may be studied<br>- lobular structure preserved, selective effects detectable<br>- human tissue slices more easily available than whole organs | - hepatic function preserved for no more than 24 h<br>- bile cannot be collected and analysed<br>- necrotic cells / scar tissue at edges of the slice<br>- presence of necrotic cells might affect the performance of the culture |
| 3 d-Bioreactors (Bioartificial Liver Systems) | - long-term use possible<br>- re-establishment of 3 d cytoarchitecture<br>- continuous perfusion with medium<br>- specific gene expression closer to *in vivo* than in hepatocyte cultures | - very low throughput<br>- difficult to standardize |
| Spheroids | - re-establishment of 3 d cytoarchitecture<br>- presence of non-parenchymal cells on outer layer of and extra-cellular matrix throughout the spheroids | - necrotic and hypoxic cells in centre of spheroids<br>- accumulation of bile in centre of spheroids possible<br>- not usable for long-term investigations (disaggregation and dedifferentiation) |
| Primary Hepatocyte Cultures | - reasonably high throughput<br>- viability and differentiation preserved for up to 2 weeks<br>- potential for use of long-term cultures in chronic toxicity<br>- analysis of human samples possible<br>- functional drug metabolising enzymes, transporters and bile canaliculi,<br>- co-culture with other liver cells possible | - culture may need special supplements in media<br>- survival, differentiation status and function depends on culture conditions<br>- no culture system is able to preserve all the different liver specific functions *in vitro*<br>- difficult to regain cells for FACS analysis |
| Hepatocytes in Suspension | - reasonably high throughput<br>- most drug metabolising enzymes well-preserved at in vivo levels<br>- zone specific metabolism and toxicity may be studied<br>- cryopreservation possible<br>- analysis of human samples possible | - limited use for drug transporter studies<br>- lack of functional bile canaliculi<br>- short-term viability (2-4 h.)<br>- lack of cell-cell and cell-matrix contacts<br>- variations in samples from different human donors |
| Cell Lines | - unlimited availability<br>- some liver specific functions have been shown to be maintained<br>- easy to use<br>- reasonably high throughput | - lacks in vivo phenotype<br>- only a small set of hepatic functions expressed at levels different from liver<br>- genotypic instability |
| S9-Mix | - contains microsomal and cytosolic fractions<br>- phase 1 and phase 2 activity | - cofactors required for activity<br>- lower enzyme activity compared to microsomes or cytosol |

# 1 INTRODUCTION

| Model | Advantages | Disadvantages |
|---|---|---|
| Microsomes, Supersomes, Baculosomes, | - high throughput system<br>- maintain expression of phase 1 enzymes<br>- can be recovered from frozen tissue<br>- production of metabolites for structural analysis possible<br>- use for drug inhibition, covalent binding and clearance studies<br>- available from several species (including human)<br>- one or more human enzymes (CYPs, UGTs) can be specifically expressed | - lacks phase 2 and other cytosolic enzymes<br>- short-term studies<br>- cofactors required for activity<br>- inadequate representation of the diversity of hepatic functions<br>- UGT-reaction partly impaired |
| Mitochondria | - high throughput<br>- analysis of the effect of drugs on respiration, ATP synthesis and fatty acid oxidation | - only very short-term studies |
| Cytosol | - soluble phase 2 enzymes (GST, ST, NAT) can be studied separately depending on added cofactors | - cofactors required for activity<br>- no CYPs, UGTs |
| Cloned Expression Systems | - high throughput<br>- one or more human enzymes can be specifically expressed<br>- unlimited cell number | - studies may lack *in vivo* relevance<br>- no physiologic levels of expressed enzymes<br>- only single (some) enzymes can be analyzed |
| The Virtual Hepatocyte | - mathematical modelling of cellular events<br>- prediction of unknown interactions may be possible | - limited computational power<br>- still in experimental stage |

Table 2: Overview of *in vitro* methods used for toxicology (adapted and expanded from Sahu, 2008)

## 1.6 Endpoints for the analysis of hepatocyte cultures

The list of tests used to gain insight into the effect of a test-substance on cells and to assess functional and biochemical parameters of cultured cells is extensive. These range from standardised tests, e.g. cell viability measurements or morphology-based approaches, to hepatocyte specific activity tests such as bile production, CYP activity or drug transport. In addition, the analysis of gene or protein expression with established molecular methods like real-time PCR, microarray technologies, mass spectrometry or immune detection is commonly applied.

Some chemically induced changes in cellular functions may be irreversible, ultimately leading to cell death, whereas others may be transient. Irreversible endpoints include the induction of apoptosis, measured by increased caspase activity, or the loss of plasma membrane integrity. Plasma membrane damage can be analysed by the detection of cytoplasmic enzyme release (e.g., lactate dehydrogenase, LDH) or the uptake of specific dyes such as neutral red and trypan blue into the cytoplasm. In addition, alterations in general hepatocyte functions like albumin synthesis and urea or bile secretion provide information on the impairment of cellular processes. The energy status of the cell is often used to determine cytotoxicity by studying the ATP content of cells or the mitochondrial or enzymatic capacity to reduce tetrazolium salts (XTT, MTT, WST) (Berridge, Herst & Tan,

1 INTRODUCTION

2005). Compound induced oxidative stress can lead to glutathione (GSH) depletion. GSH is considered one of the primary antioxidant molecules for sustaining the intracellular redox status by scavenging peroxides and the reduction of oxidized molecules. Additionally, it is used in phase 2 reactions for neutralizing strong oxidants, by the formation of glutathinyl adducts which is catalyzed by various glutathione S-transferases (GSTs) and plays a vital role in rescuing cells from apoptosis. The cytosolic GSH content can be measured with specific glutathione detection kits. Drug transport is studied by fluorescent dyes or with the analysis of the bile acid transport by HPLC (High Performance Liquid Chromatography) (Kostrubsky et al., 2003; Liu et al., 1999).

## 1.7    Toxicogenomics

Traditional toxicological studies, e.g. the 2-year carcinogenicity rodent study, are time consuming and expensive together with a high requirement for laboratory animals. They focus on evaluating classical endpoints like gain of body- or organ-weight, death rate, tumour incidence, serum markers or histological changes, making safety assessment one of the bottlenecks in the pharmaceutical drug developmental process. New methods and processes like genomics, proteomics, lipidomics or metabonomics are being used to improve the drug development process (Ballet, 1997; Brandon et al., 2003) and the "-omics" field is rapidly growing. Toxicogenomics is defined as a scientific sub-discipline that combines toxicology (the study of the nature and effects of poisons) with genomics (the investigation of the way that our genetic make-up, the genome, translates into biological functions). It is the study of the structure and output of the genome as it responds to adverse xenobiotic exposure and the identification of their putative mechanisms of action. The analysis of changes in gene expression caused by exposure to a test-compound together with strong bioinformatics and toxicological knowledge form the basis of toxicogenomics (Khor, Ibrahim & Kong, 2006; Nuwaysir et al., 1999; Chin & Kong, 2002). Central to genomic studies in toxicology is the assumption that compounds with a common endpoint can be classified based on related changes in gene expression. This allows extrapolation of toxic effects from known model compounds to unknown compounds by comparison of their expression profiles (Hamadeh et al., 2002a; 2002b; Zidek et al., 2007; Ellinger-Ziegelbauer et al., 2004). Several open source or commercial attempts (e.g., GENELOGIC (USA), ICONIX Biosciences Inc. (USA)) have been made to develop databases based on expression profiles of reference compounds in order to classify chemicals. It should not be forgotten that many internal databases in the pharmaceutical industry are only used for in house purposes and are not made accessible to the public (Mattes et al., 2004). There are several statistical methods to discriminate compounds on the basis of their gene expression profiles, some of which are discussed later (Page 29). In principle, they try to find single genes or gene sets that can discriminate between different treatment groups. These highly informative gene clusters can then be used to predict the class membership of a new unknown sample (Hamadeh et al., 2002a; Simon et al., 2003). The reported results are very encouraging but also show the need for large gene expression databases and effective analysis models to allow their future implementation into the drug development process.

Mechanistic studies are performed to increase the understanding of the function and regulation of genes that lead to compound specific toxicity. In most cases, the changes in gene and protein expression precede the physiological effects. This means that there is a great potential to extrapolate from changes in gene expression to long term toxicological endpoints such as liver necrosis, inflammation, steatosis or tumour neogenesis (Pennie, 2000; Burchiel et al., 2001; Fielden & Zacharewski, 2001). The detection of both the underlying mechanism of toxicity and the molecular basis of the response to exposure in an early stage of drug development will have a great impact on safety evaluation. Recent studies showed the possibility to define different toxic mechanisms, including tumour formation, inflammatory effects, oxidative stress, impairment of cellular signalling and induction of apoptosis (Bulera et al., 2001; Lettieri, 2006). Warring and his coworkers have shown a correlation between a physiological response to a toxicant and changes in the genomic profile, allowing the interpretation of gene expression data with respect to specific organotypic endpoints. This concept is referred to as "phenotypic anchoring" (Waring et al., 2001; Orphanides, 2003).

There have been numerous attempts to find new biomarkers for the early identification of hepatocarcinogenesis with the use of toxicogenomics and proteomics methods (Ellinger-Ziegelbauer et al., 2004; Fella et al., 2005). There is hope that these new methods will make it possible to detect intrinsic changes in the molecular pattern ("genetic fingerprint") that are indicative of the pathological endpoint before he becomes histopathologically detectable (Aardema & MacGregor, 2002). Besides the improvement of the drug development process, this could also facilitate a considerable reduction in the time needed to obtain results and the number of animals used in toxicity testing (Kroeger, 2006). Although most data is generated from *in vivo* liver samples, there are efforts to build databases for the screening of hepatotoxicity based on primary hepatocyte cell culture

# 1 INTRODUCTION

experiments by genomic and proteomic approaches. Therefore, it is necessary to carefully characterise the cell culture model used.

In order to understand the mechanisms behind any compound induced change of gene expression, it is essential to know the basal gene expression in the test system. In the case of primary hepatocytes, it is not only the individual differences but also the effects of time and the conditions of culturing which have to be taken into account. Therefore, a comprehensive analysis of gene expression changes in rat and human hepatocytes and different cell culture systems (liver slices, suspension culture, primary hepatocytes cultured on plastic surface, on collagen I ML and in SW culture as well as different cell lines) has been carried out as part of this thesis.

Not every cell culture system is appropriate for every toxicological endpoint, as liver specific functions gradually decrease over time. *In vivo*, they are supported by liver architecture, cell-cell and cell-matrix interactions and the complex hormonal signalling of the body. It is impossible to mimic these conditions in culture and great endeavours are being made to maintain liver specific functions and attributes for as long as possible (LeCluyse et al., 2005; Richert et al., 2004; Turncliff et al., 2006; Vinken et al., 2006). Evaluating the basal gene expression pattern will help to understand the processes of dedifferentiation and will allow the interpretation of gene expression changes caused by xenobiotics and to extrapolate to mechanisms *in vivo*.

However, one has to be aware of the limitations of these techniques. Some compounds directly effect cellular macromolecules causing damage without changing gene expression. Often expression changes may reflect secondary effects following after the primary direct toxicity of the compound. The dimension of changes in gene expression is also dependent on dose, duration of exposure to the toxicant and on time from dosing to sampling (Gatzidou, Zira & Theocharis, 2007). Not all changes in gene expression have a direct impact on the corresponding protein content of a cell. Due to the variety of epigenetic control mechanisms there can be significant differences in gene and protein expression. Additionally, changes in protein activity, caused for example by phosphorylation or ubiquitinylation, can not be addressed and other, proteomic techniques have to be considered (Pennie et al., 2000; Merrick & Madenspacher, 2005). With this in mind, toxicogenomics can be a powerful tool. The extrapolation from data generated from animals to potential human activity could be enhanced by finding species-overlapping biomarkers (Aardema & MacGregor, 2002). Even the generation of human data is achievable and relatively straight forward.

## 1.8 Techniques for global gene expression analysis

The new and developing field of microarray technology evolved from E.M. Southerns realization that labelled nucleic acid molecules can be hybridized to their counterparts and therefore be used to detect their existence and amount in the original sample (Southern, 1975). The sequencing of whole genomes from human, as well as of many "laboratory" animal species, quickened the development of new technologies for the measurement of several thousand genes in a single experiment (Brown & Botstein, 1999; Schena, 1996). Meanwhile, these microarray technologies are used for a wide spectrum of issues, like drug discovery, basic research and target discovery, biomarker determination, pharmacology, toxicology, target selectivity, development of prognostic tests and disease-subclass determination (Butte, 2002). A wide range of different platforms for global gene expression are currently available. Although they all are either cDNA or oligonucleotide based, they differ in distinct properties such as the type of probes (short/long oligonucleotides, cDNA), the number of genes, probe selection and design, competitive versus non-competitive hybridization, labeling methods or the methods of production (*in situ* polymerization, spotting, microbeads). In the following paragraphs, the bead chip technology of Illumina Inc. and the Affymetrix Gene Chip, used during this work, are introduced.

*Illumina BeadChip arrays*

Illumina Inc. developed in 2003 a bead based technology for global gene expression analysis (Gunderson et al., 2004). The chips are based on a silicon wafer with 3 µm sized beads on their surface and covalently bound 50mer oligonucleotide probes. One single probe-type representing one gene is bound to each bead type with more than 100,000 copies per bead. All the bead types are pooled and put onto the surface of a silicon wafer (Figure 9). This wafer was previously prepared by plasma etching to provide wells at a regular distance of 5 µm. Each array contains about 900,000 beads so statistically on a whole genome array, each bead-type is represented ~30 times on average. This redundancy allows up to 30,000 genes to be detected simultaneously per array. Because of the random arrangement of the beads, local area effects (scratches, impurity and intensity variation) are of minor consequence, but this feature also raises the need for an initial decoding step. Therefore, the probes consist not only of the gene specific part (50 nts) but also of a 23 nt-long address sequence. Decoding is performed by Illumina Inc and is at the same time an important step for quality control (Gunderson et al., 2004).

# 1 INTRODUCTION

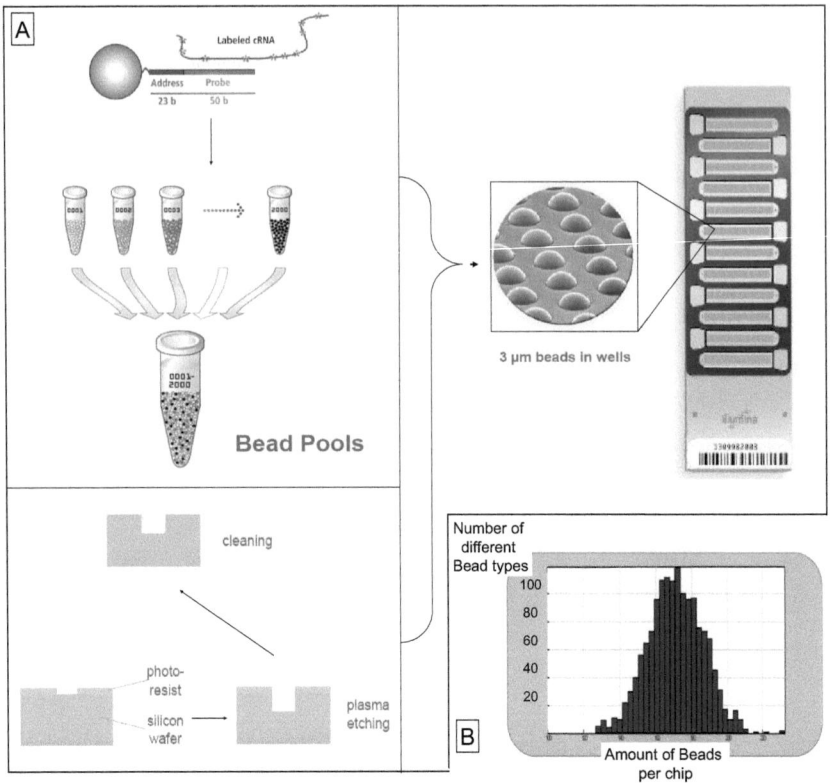

Figure 9: The production process of an Illumina BeadChip array. A) Depicts the structure of a single bead, the generation of a bead pool and the combination with a previously etched silicon wafer to a complete BeadChip. B) Histogram of the average abundance of bead types per chip.

*Affymetrix gene expression arrays*

Affymetrix arrays are based on in situ synthesis of oligonucleotides directly on to the array surface. The probes are 25 nt long and are directly synthesized onto a silicon wafer via a combination of photolithography and combinational chemistry (McGall & Fidanza, 2001). For each gene, Affymetrix uses 11 to 20 probe sets, a probe set consisting of a 25 nt perfect match and a 25 nt mismatch oligonucleotide, to guarantee statistical relevance and certainty. After scanning, the intensity differences between perfect match and mismatch probes are calculated to give both quantitative (signal intensity) and qualitative (statistical significance) measurements (Figure 10).

# 1 INTRODUCTION

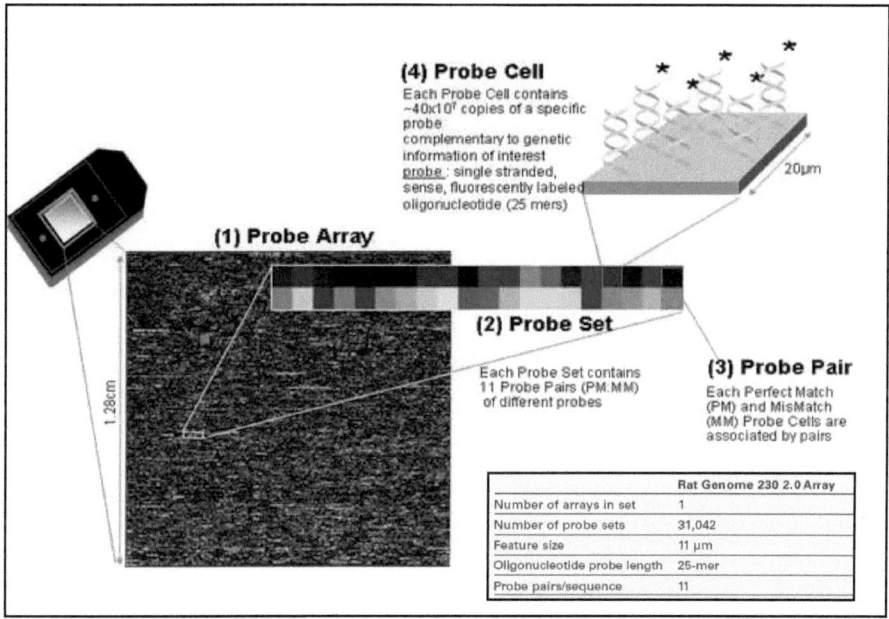

Figure 10: Scheme of the process and the architecture of an Affymetrix gene expression array (Taken from the Affymetrix homepage, www.affymetrix.com).

The RNA samples have to be isolated from the sample and reverse transcribed in order to produce biotinylated cRNA before hybridizing them to arrays of both suppliers, Illumina and Affymetrix. This procedure allows detection and quantification which otherwise wouldn't be possible. After scanning, raw data must be preprocessed before statistical analysis and the relative expression level of each gene can be determined by comparing the intensities of the genes to each other or to a control. With respect to the technical aspects and the experiment layout, each set of microarray data has to be normalized in an appropriate way. Further details of both techniques used will be discussed in detail in chapter 3.1.

*Methods of data analysis*

DNA microarray technology has made it possible to generate millions of data-points in a relatively short time. The analytical steps needed to convert the noisy data into reliable and interpretable biological information are challenging and error prone. Due to their great number, only an overview of the most common and important methods and algorithms

# 1 INTRODUCTION

used during these studies are presented. In principle, there are two main statistical approaches to identify genes or patterns of interest from microarray data. Supervised methods are used to identify patterns of gene expression, e.g. for the identification of marker genes or the classification of compounds. Unsupervised methods identify signatures in the data set without input of data specific knowledge and can be used to summarize and to reduce the complexity of the multidimensional data. Important unsupervised tools include Principal Components Analysis (PCA), Hierarchical Clustering, Correlation and Self Organizing Maps (SOM) (Butte, 2002).

PCAs are an attempt to reduce the multi-dimensional data of microarrays. Therefore, vectors (so called "Eigenvektoren") are calculated, each representing the greatest amount of variance of the data cloud within one certain experiment (Figure 11). The largest, and therefore statistically most relevant, Eigenvektoren are plotted resulting in one single point per sample in two- or three-dimensional space and is therefore a good tool for data reduction and display (Yeung & Ruzzo, 2001).

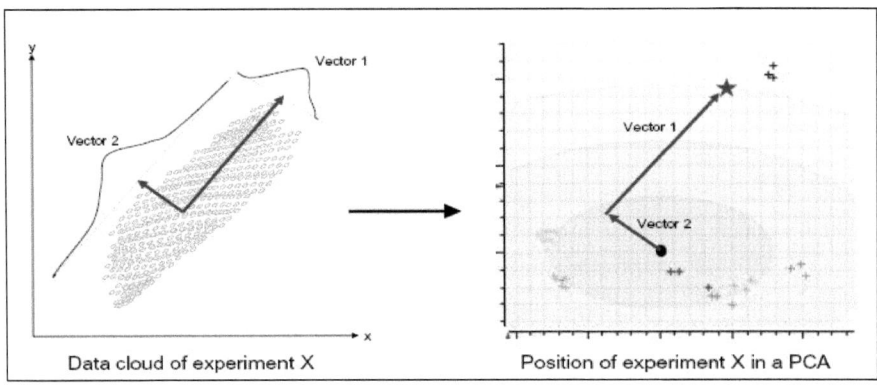

Figure 11: Graphical representation of a PCA transformation in two dimensions (x and y). The variance of the data in the original space (x, y) is best captured by the basis vectors v1 and v2, which in turn are used as basis for the localization of the experiment in the appertaining PCA.

Several different algorithms can be applied depending on the structure of the dataset and the aim of the analysis. Hierarchical clustering calculates the distance of the sample or gene profiles from each other and visualizes this in form of a dendrogram-tree. Experiments closer to each other are more similar to each other than those further away. During a correlation analysis, the correlation of samples or genes to each other are calculated and then visualized in a heat map with a defined colour code. A two

# 1 INTRODUCTION

dimensional output is also produced by SOM Clustering, also termed as Kohonen-Maps after its inventor (Kohonen, 1997). This statistical method is a type of artificial neural network that is trained using unsupervised learning. During the presented work SOM was used to group genes according to their expression profile (Nikkilä et al., 2002).

Supervised methods include t-test and the Analysis of Variance (ANOVA). T-test was applied to detect differences between empirical mean values of two datasets giving statistical confidence to the detected values. ANOVA was used to identify genes in a multivariate model whose expression is significantly altered between different biological samples. First described by R.A. Fisher in the 1920s, an ANOVA partitions the observed variance into components due to different explanatory variables and allows the effects of two or more treatment variables to be studied simultaneously. Other supervised methods include classification methods, such as Support Vector Machine or K-nearest-neighbour analysis. These algorithms "learn" to classify the data into preset categories from a training set and are able to match new data to the existing classifier (Raudys, 2000). Additionally, the minimum amount of genes needed for this discrimination can be calculated by ranking.

## 1.9     Toxicoproteomics

Marc Wilkins first used the term "proteome" in 1994. He defined it as the totality of all proteins produced at a certain moment by a cell and encoded by a genome. Like the transcriptome it depends on broadly diverse factors and is highly dynamic. The analysis of proteins, of the total proteome especially, is very challenging because of its extreme heterogeneity. Proteins range from relatively small peptides to large multi-enzyme complexes and are built up out of amino acids, which can, due to their side chains, develop multiple interactions and carry different charges. Several mechanisms of post-translational modification are known which enhance and increase this complexity of the proteome. It is believed that about 30,000 genes are encoded by the human genome. These genes result, via alternative splicing, in about 100,000 different transcripts. Further modifications are achieved by mechanisms such as nuclear transport, posttranscriptional modifications, gene silencing, changes in mRNA stability and in post-translational modifications like glycosylations, phosphorylations, methylations, enzymatic cleaving, changes in protein stability or intracellular transport mechanisms.

The abundance of proteins in the cell can be very heterogeneous. Some proteins are present only in a low copy number (e.g. some cellular receptors) whereas others are highly abundant (e.g. structural proteins) (Smith, 2000). The dynamic range of protein expression

# 1 INTRODUCTION

encompasses more then seven orders of magnitude (Anderson & Anderson, 2002). It is obvious then that the analysis of the proteome has high demands on the techniques applied for their exploration. To date none of the techniques can acquire the analysis of the whole proteome. Each method has certain advantages and drawbacks and depicts only a small part of the whole picture.

Similar to genomic studies, proteomic methods can be used to examine early changes due to treatment with xenobiotics on a molecular level. Occurring prior to changes on histopathological level or classical toxicological endpoints, these changes can help in candidate selection, mechanistic studies, finding new biomarkers or the classification of compounds (Bandara & Kennedy, 2002). The classification of compounds is possible even without further mechanistic knowledge on the basis of "molecular signatures" (Wetmore & Merrick, 2004). One technique to collect such signatures of protein expression is the Surface Enhanced Laser Desorption and Ionisation (SELDI) Chip Technology (Bio-Rad, Hercules, CA, USA). This method was invented in 1993 by Hutchens and Yip and is a mixture of chromatographic surfaces and mass spectrometry (Hutchens & Yip, 1993). Samples of proteins are bound to a chromatographic surface (e.g. anionic, cationic, hydrophobic, hydrophilic or metal-binding) due to their physical properties and are afterwards analyzed via time of flight mass spectrometry. The resulting spectrum of masses resembles a so called "proteomic fingerprint" (Veenstra & Conrads, 2003).

A drawback of this method is the lack of fragmentation of the proteins. Therefore, an identification of the proteins detected with SELDI is complicated and needs additional efforts. Complex mixtures of proteins, like cell lysates, have to be intensely cleaned up as far as possible and enzymaticaly digested. Afterwards, they can be used for downstream analysis with "normal" MS or MS/MS techniques.

# 1 INTRODUCTION

## 1.10    Aim of this work

The aim of this work was the development and characterization of the sandwich culture of primary rat and human hepatocytes as a tool for in *in vitro* toxicology studies. Moreover, the gene expression changes in response of compound treatment of the cells in culture were addressed and used to build a predictive classification model.

Primarily, a thorough optimization of the culture conditions was performed with the main goal to enhance the differentiation status of cells and to prolong their time in culture. Besides the insurance of cells displaying liver-typical functionality over a long period of time, a clear definition of changes over time on different levels, the cell morphology and viability, gene and protein expression, metabolic activity and inducibility, were part of this project.

The main part of this work was concerned with the extensive characterization of the global gene expression changes over time in culture. Therefore, several culture systems were analyzed and compared with regard to their similarities and differences in gene expression over time.

The ability to establish a predictive hepatotoxicity model was examined by conducting toxicological studies with the new sandwich *in vitro* culture system. Cells were dosed with reference compounds (Chapter 3.4.2, Figure 57), changes in gene expression were analyzed and used to calculate a novel predictive model based on the global expression profile. Additionally, a predictive subset of discriminative genes should be found. The gene expression profile of two blinded compounds should be conducted as a preliminary verification of this model.

As the new platform from Illumina was used for these experiments, it was important to compare the results gained from these experiments to a well established platform (Affymetrix) and to TaqMan PCR, as the quality standard, in terms of reliability, sensitivity and concordance.

## 2 MATERIALS AND METHODS

### 2.1 Materials

#### 2.1.1 Chemicals and reagents

| Chemical/ Reagent | Provider |
|---|---|
| Secondary antibodies (Rabbit, Sheep) | GE Healthcare Europe GmbH, Freiburg, Germany |
| ECL Detection-Reagents and Hyperfilm | GE Healthcare Europe GmbH, Freiburg, Germany |
| Neutral Red | Sigma-Aldrich, Taufkirchen, Germany |
| Carboxi-DCFDA | Invitrogen, Karlsruhe, Germany |
| Acetic Acid ($CH_3CO_{2h}$) | Invitrogen, Karlsruhe, Germany |
| Ammonium bicarbonate ($NH_4HCO_3$) | Merck KGaA, Darmstadt, Germany |
| Ammonium persulfate (($NH_4)_2S_2O_8$) | Merck KGaA, Darmstadt, Germany |
| Anti-Streptavidin Antibody (goat), biotinylated | Vector Laboratories, Burlingame, USA |
| Benzyloxy-Resorufin | Sigma-Aldrich, Taufkirchen, Germany |
| Biotin-16-UTP, 10 mm | PerkinElmer Life and Analytical Sciences, Waltham, USA |
| Bovine serum albumin (BSA), acetylated, 20 mg/ml | Ambion - An Applied Biosystems Business, Austin, USA |
| Calcium chloride hexahydrate ($CaCl_2 \cdot 6 H_2O$) | Sigma-Aldrich, Taufkirchen, Germany |
| CHAPS ($C_{32}h_{58}N_2O_7S$) | Merck KGaA, Darmstadt, Germany |
| Chloroform LiChrosolv® ($CHCl_3$) | Merck KGaA, Darmstadt, Germany |
| Coomassie Brilliant Blue G250 | Serva, Heidelberg, Germany |
| E1BC Buffer | Buffer Illumina, San Diego, USA |
| ECL-Detection Kit | Amersham, Buckinghamshire, UK |
| EDTA-Solution (0.5M) | Ambion - An Applied Biosystems Business, Austin, USA |
| Ethanol LiChrosolv® ($CH_3CH_2OH$) | Merck KGaA, Darmstadt, Germany |
| Ethoxy-Resorufin | Sigma-Aldrich, Taufkirchen, Germany |
| Cy3™ labelled streptavidin (1 mg/ml) | Amersham Biosciences, Buckinghamshire, UK (GE Healthcare) |
| Formamide, deionised ($HCONH_2$) | Ambion - An Applied Biosystems Business, Austin, USA |
| HEPES ($C_8H_{18}N_2O_4S$) | Merck KGaA, Darmstadt, Germany |
| Hering sperm DNA (10 mg/ml) | Promega Corporation, Madison, USA |
| HybE1 Buffer | Buffer Illumina, San Diego, USA |
| NuPage 4-12% Bis-Tris Gel | Invitrogen - Molecular Probes, Eugene, USA |
| Isopropanol, LiChrosolv® (($CH_3)_2CHOH$) | Merck KGaA, Darmstadt, Germany |
| Calcium chloride ($CaCl_2$) | Sigma-Aldrich, Taufkirchen, Germany |
| Potassium sulfate ($KH_2SO_4$) | Sigma-Aldrich, Taufkirchen, Germany |

## 2 MATERIALS AND METHODS

| Chemical/ Reagent | Provider |
|---|---|
| Potassium chloride (KCl) | Merck KGaA, Darmstadt, Germany |
| Potassium phosphate monobasic ($KH_2PO_4$) | Merck KGaA, Darmstadt, Germany |
| Liberase Blendzyme 2 | Roche Applied Biosciences, Basel, Suisse |
| Magnesium sulfate ($MgSO_4$) | Sigma-Aldrich, Taufkirchen, Germany |
| MES (2-[N-Morpholino]ethanesulfonic acid, $C_6H_{13}NO_4S$) | Sigma-Aldrich, Taufkirchen, Germany |
| Magnesium sulfate monohydrate ($MgSO_4 \cdot 7\ H_2O$) | Sigma-Aldrich, Taufkirchen, Germany |
| Sodium phosphate dibasic ($Na_{2h}PO_4$) | Sigma-Aldrich, Taufkirchen, Germany |
| Sodium chloride (NaCl) | Sigma-Aldrich, Taufkirchen, Germany |
| Sodium acetate ($CH_3COONa$) | Merck KGaA, Darmstadt, Germany |
| Sodium hydrogen carbonate ($NaHCO_3$) | Merck KGaA, Darmstadt, Germany |
| Sodium hydroxide (NaOH) | Merck KGaA, Darmstadt, Germany |
| Trypan Blue 0.5% (w/v) in PBS | Biochrome AG, Berlin, Germany |
| Nuclease free water | Ambion - An Applied Biosystems Business, Austin, USA |
| Pentoxy-Resorufin | Sigma-Aldrich, Taufkirchen, Germany |
| RNA 6000 Ladder | Ambion - An Applied Biosystems Business, Austin, USA |
| Hydrochloric acid (HCl) | Merck KGaA, Darmstadt, Germany |
| ß-Mercaptoethanol | Sigma-Aldrich, Taufkirchen, Germany |
| SSPE (3 M NaCl, 0.2 M $NaH_2PO_4$, 0.02 M EDTA) | BioWhittaker Molecular Applications, Rockland, USA |
| Streptavidin Phycoerythrin (SAPE) | Invitrogen - Molecular Probes, Eugene, USA |
| Trichloroacetic acid (TCA, $Cl_3CCOOH$) | Merck KGaA, Darmstadt, Germany |
| Triton X-100 | Serva, Heidelberg, Germany |
| TRI Reagent™ | Sigma-Aldrich, Taufkirchen, Germany |
| Tween20 (10%) | Merck KGaA, Darmstadt, Germany |

## 2 MATERIALS AND METHODS
## 2.1.2 Technical equipment and auxiliary material

| Equipment | Provider |
|---|---|
| PBSII ProteinChip Reader | Ciphergen |
| ABI Prism 7000 | Applied Biosystems, Foster City, USA |
| Agilent 2100 Bioanalyzer | Agilent Technologies, Waldbronn, Germany |
| Autoclave | H&P Labortechnik, Oberschleißheim, Germany |
| Axon GenePix® 4000B Microarray Scanner | Molecular Devices (Axon Technologies), Union City, USA |
| Bead Station 500 | Illumina, San Diego, USA |
| BeadChip® Hyb Cartridge | Illumina, San Diego, USA |
| BeadChip® Hyb Wheel | Illumina, San Diego, USA |
| BeadChip® Staining Dish | Illumina, San Diego, USA |
| BeadChip® Wash Trays | Illumina, San Diego, USA |
| Bottle-top filter, 0.2µm | Nalge Nunc International, Rochester, USA |
| Syringes | MT Braun, Melsungen, Germany |
| Cell scraper (25 cm, sterile) | Greiner-Bio One, Frickenhausen, Germany |
| Centrifuge 5415R | Eppendorf, Hamburg, Germany |
| Fluidic Station 450 | Affymetrix, Santa Clara, USA |
| Digital camera CC 12 | Olympus, Hamburg, Germany |
| iBlot™ Dry Blotting System | Invitrogen, Karlsruhe, Germany |
| Fluorescent-Spectralphotometer (RF-1502) | Shimadzu Europa, Duisburg, Germany |
| Fuchs-Rosenthal-Chamber (Neubauer improved) | Paul Marienfeld GmbH & Co., Lauda-Königshofen, Germany |
| Gene Chip® Fluidic Station 450 | Affymetrix, Santa Clara, USA |
| Gene Chip® Human Genome U133 Plus 2.0 Array | Affymetrix, Santa Clara, USA |
| Gene Chip® Rat Expression Array (RAE) 230 2.0 | Affymetrix, Santa Clara, USA |
| Gene Chip® Scanner 3000 | Affymetrix, Santa Clara, USA |
| Glassware | Schott Glas, Mainz, Germany |
| Heat block Thermo Stat Plus | Eppendorf, Hamburg |
| HP GeneArrayTM Scanner | Affymetrix, Santa Clara, USA |
| HumanRef-8 v2 Expression BeadChip | Illumina, San Diego, USA |
| NuPAGE® MES Running Buffer | Invitrogen, Karlsruhe, Germany |
| *NuPAGE® Novex* Bis-Tris-Gele | Invitrogen, Karlsruhe, Germany |
| NuPAGE® Reducing Agent | Invitrogen, Karlsruhe, Germany |
| Hybridization Oven 650 | Affymetrix, Santa Clara, USA |
| Incubator | Kendro Laboratory, Hanau, Germany |
| Krumdieck-Tissue-Slicer | Alabama R&D Corp., Munford, USA |
| Microscope | Zeiss, Jena, Germany |
| Microtiterplates (96 well, 24 well and 6 well) | Nalge Nunc, Rochester, USA |
| Molecular Imager | BIORAD, München, Germany |

## 2 MATERIALS AND METHODS

| Equipment | Provider |
|---|---|
| NanoDrop ND-1000 | NanoDrop Technologies, Wilmington, USA |
| Nitrocellulose membrane | Schleicher & Schuell, Dassel, Germany |
| Microscope Olympus IX70 | Olympus, Hamburg, Germany |
| Peristaltic Pump 313S | Watson-Marlow, Birmingham, UK |
| Petri-dishes TC (100 mm, 60 mm) | Greiner-Bio One, Frickenhausen, Germany |
| pH-Meter | Knick, Berlin, Germany |
| Pipettboy | Hirschmann Laborgeräte, Eberstadt, |
| Plastic ware | Nalge Nunc, Rochester, USA |
| Plastic tubes | 15/50 ml Greiner-Bio One, Frickenhausen, Germany |
| RatRef-12 Expression BeadChip | Illumina, San Diego, USA |
| Reaction-cups (0.2 / 1.5 / 2 ml), Nuclease free | Eppendorf, Hamburg, Germany |
| Scale | Sartorius, Göttingen, Germany |
| Sentrix BeadChip custom array | Illumina, San Diego, USA |
| Speed-Vac Concentrator 5301 | Eppendorf, Hamburg |
| Spectrophotometer TM3000 | Bio-Rad, Hercules, USA |
| Steel beads | Qiagen, Hilden, Germany |
| Sterile Workbench | Kendro Laboratory, Hanau, Germany |
| Sterile filters (0.2 µM) | Nalge Nunc, Rochester, USA |
| Surgical instruments | Braun, Melsungen, Germany |
| Thermocycler | Eppendorf, Hamburg, Germany |
| TissueLyser | Qiagen, Hilden, Germany |
| Multifuge® 3 S-R | Thermo Fisher Scientific (Heraeus), Waltham, USA |
| U-RFL-T Power Supply Unit | Olympus, Hamburg, Germany |
| Vortex | Scientific Industries, Bohemia, USA |
| Varioclav Steam Sterilyzer | ThermoFisher Scientific, Schwerte, Germany |
| Water bath | Lauda GmbH & Co. KG, Lauda, Germany |
| Water bath SW 21 | Julabo Labortechnik, Seelbach, Germany |
| Centrifuge | Kendro Laboratory, Hanau, Germany |

# 2 MATERIALS AND METHODS

## 2.1.3 Kits

| Chemical/ Reagent | Provider |
|---|---|
| Apo-ONE® Homogeneous Caspase-3/7 assay | Promega Corporation, Madison, USA |
| BeadChip Buffer Kit | Illumina, San Diego, USA |
| CellTiter-Glo® Luminescent Cell Viability Assay | Promega Corporation, Madison, USA |
| CytoTox-ONE™ Homogeneous Membrane Integrity Assay | Promega Corporation, Madison, USA |
| Gene Chip® Hybridization Control Kit | Affymetrix, Santa Clara, USA |
| Gene Chip® IVT Labeling Kit | Affymetrix, Santa Clara, USA |
| Gene Chip® One-Cycle cDNA Synthesis Kit | Affymetrix, Santa Clara, USA |
| Gene Chip® Poly-A RNA Control Kit | Affymetrix, Santa Clara, USA |
| Gene Chip® Sample Cleanup Module | Affymetrix, Santa Clara, USA |
| Glutathione (GSH) Detection Kit | Chemicon International, Tamecula, CA |
| MessageAmpTM II aRNA Amplification Kit | Ambion- An Applied Biosystems Business, Austin, USA |
| P450Glo® (3A4 and 2C9) Assay Kit | Promega Corporation, Madison, USA |
| Primer and Probes for TaqMan®-RT-PCR | Applied Biosystems, Foster City, USA |
| QIAquick PCR Purification Kit | Qiagen, Hilden, Germany |
| RNA 6000 Nano LabChip® Kit | Agilent Technologies, Waldbronn, Germany |
| RNeasy Mini Kit | Qiagen, Hilden, Germany |
| WST-1-Assay | Roche, Mannheim, Germany |

## 2.1.4 Software

| Software | Provider |
|---|---|
| GECOS | Affymetrix, Santa Clara, USA |
| AnalySIS cell imaging | Soft Imaging System, Münster, Germany |
| 2100 Expert Software | Agilent Technologies, Waldbronn, Germany |
| ABI Prism 7000 SDS | Applied Biosystems, Foster City, USA |
| BeadScan | Illumina, San Diego, USA |
| BeadStudio | Illumina, San Diego, USA |
| Expressionist®Pro | Genedata, Basel, Swisse |
| Gene Chip® Operating Software (GCOS) | Affymetrix, Santa Clara, USA |
| GenePixTM Pro | Molecular Devices, UnionCity, USA |
| KC4 | Bio-Tek Instruments, Vermont, USA |
| MetaCoreTM | GeneGO, St. Joseph, USA |
| OriginLab | OriginLab, Northampton, USA |

## 2 MATERIALS AND METHODS

### 2.1.5 Culture media and supplements

| Media/ Supplement | Provider |
|---|---|
| After-shipment media for HepaRG-cells | Biopredic international, Rennes, France |
| Albumin Solution 35% | Sigma-Aldrich, Taufkirchen, Germany |
| Bovine serum albumin (BSA) | Merck KGaA, Darmstadt, Germany |
| Collagen I (Rat Tail) | Roche, Mannheim, Germany |
| D-MEM/F-12 (1:1) (1X), liquid - with GlutaMAX™ I | Invitrogen, Karlsruhe, Germany |
| D-MEM/F-12 (1:1) (1X), liquid - with L-Glutamine, without Phenol Red | Invitrogen, Karlsruhe, Germany |
| D-MEM/F-12, powder, 1:1 | Invitrogen, Karlsruhe, Germany |
| DMSO (($CH_3$)$_2$SO) | Sigma-Aldrich, Taufkirchen, Germany |
| Fetal Bovine Serum (Research Grade) | HyClone, South Logan, USA |
| HEPARG culture medium | Biopredic international, Rennes, France |
| Insulin | Novo Nordisk Pharma, Mainz, Germany |
| ITS | Invitrogen, Karlsruhe, Germany |
| L-Glutamine | Ferak, Berlin, Germany |
| PBS | Invitrogen, Karlsruhe, Germany |
| Penicillin [10000 U/ ml] | Sigma-Aldrich, Taufkirchen, Germany |
| Streptomycin [10 mg/ml] | Sigma-Aldrich, Taufkirchen, Germany |

### 2.1.6 Buffers and solutions

#### 2.1.6.1 Perfusion buffers for rat liver perfusion

| Stock solution | |
|---|---|
| 6.30 g | NaCl |
| 0.32 g | KCl |
| 0.27 g | $MgSO_4 \cdot 7\ H_2O$ |
| 0.15 g | $KH_2PO_4$ |
| 1.81 g | $NaHCO_3$ |
| 3.58 g | HEPES |
| 1.50 g | D-Glucose |
| Add $H_2O$ to 1 l | |

| For Perfusion Buffer 1, add | |
|---|---|
| 0.038 g | EGTA |
| Calibrate to pH 7.2 | |

| For Perfusion Buffer 2, add | |
|---|---|
| 0.58 g | $CaCl_2 \cdot 2\ H_2O$ |
| Calibrate to pH 7.2 and add Liberase Blendzyme to 300 ml | |

| Washing buffer | |
|---|---|
| 0.58 g | $CaCl_2 \cdot 2\ H_2O$ |
| 20.00 g | BSA |
| Add $H_2O$ to 1 l and calibrate to pH 7.2 | |

| Trypan-blue solution | |
|---|---|
| 500 µl | Trypanblue-Solution (0.5 %) |
| 500 µl | Wash buffer |

## 2 MATERIALS AND METHODS

| modified Williams' Medium E | |
|---|---|
| 1 mg | Ampicilline |
| 125 mg | Gentamicine |
| 29.2 mg | L-Glutamine |
| 345 mg | Insulin |
| 10 mg | Tylosin |
| Add 100 ml Williams' Medium E and calibrate to pH 7.4 | |

| Krebs-Henseleit-Buffer | |
|---|---|
| 60 mm | NaCl |
| 2.4 mm | KCl |
| 0.6 mm | $KH_2PO_4$ |
| 0.6 mm | $MgSO_4 \times 7\ H_2O$ |
| 12.5 mm | $NaHCO_3$ |
| 0.625 mm | $CaCl_2 \times 6\ H_2O$ |
| 12.6 mm | HEPES |
| 50 mg/l | Gentamycine |
| Add $H_2O$ to 1 l and calibrate to pH 7.4 | |

### 2.1.6.2 Buffers for SELDI-TOF-MS

| Pre-activation buffer WCX | |
|---|---|
| 10 mM | HCl (1 M) |
| Add $H_2O$ to 1 l | |

| Binding buffer WCX | |
|---|---|
| 0.1 M | Natriumacetat pH 4.5 |
| 0.05% (v/v) | Triton X-100 |

### 2.1.6.3 Buffers for protein-preparation adn immunodetection

| Lysis buffer for resuspending of Proteins | |
|---|---|
| 6.3 g | Urea |
| 2.3 g | Thio-urea |
| 0.48 g | CHAPS |
| 600 µl | DTT (1 M) |
| 300 µl | Spermin (1 M) |
| Add $H_2O$ to 12 ml | |

| PBS-Tween-Buffer | |
|---|---|
| 10% (v/v) | PBS (10x) |
| 0,1-5% (v/v) | Tween 20 |
| 85-89,9% | Aqua purificata |

| Coating-Solution | |
|---|---|
| 5% (m/v) | dry milk - powder |
|  | PBS-Tween-Buffer |

## 2 MATERIALS AND METHODS

### 2.1.6.4 Buffers and solutions for Illumina BeadChip arrays

| First strand synthesis mastermix (8 samples) | |
|---|---|
| 2.2 µl | T7(dT)Primer, 10 pmol/µL |
| 4.4 µl | 10X 1st-strand buffer |
| 8.8 µl | dNTP mix |
| 2.2 µl | RNase Inhibitor |
| 2.2 µl | Reverse Transcriptase |
| 24.2 µl | Nuclease free water |

| Second strand synthesis mastermix (8 samples) | |
|---|---|
| 22 µl | 10X 2nd-strand buffer |
| 8.8 µl | dNTP mix |
| 4.4 µl | DNA polymerase |
| 2.2 µl | RNaseH, 2U/µL |
| 140 µl | nuclease free water |

| Heat Wash buffer | |
|---|---|
| 50 ml | Heat wash buffer |
| 450 ml | Nuclease free water |

| IVT-Reaction | |
|---|---|
| 8.8 µl | 10X reaction buffer |
| 8.8 µl | ATP, 75 mM |
| 8.8 µl | CTP, 75 mM |
| 8.8 µl | GTP, 75 mM |
| 4.4 µl | UTP, 75 mM |
| 33 µl | Biotin-16-UTP, 10 mM |
| 8.8 µl | T7 Enzyme Mix |
| 6.6 µl | nuclease free water |

| Wash buffer E1BC | |
|---|---|
| 1.5 ml | E1BC Buffer |
| 500 ml | Nuclease free water |
| Heat to 55°C over night | |

| Cy3 staining solution | |
|---|---|
| 2 ml | Blocker™ Casein in PBS (1% m/v) |
| 2 µl | FluoroLinkTM CyTM3 labelled streptavidin (1 mg/ml) |

### 2.1.6.5 Buffers and solutions for Affymetrix Gene Chips®

| first strand mastermix | |
|---|---|
| 4 µl | 5x First Strand Reaction Mix Buffer |
| 2 µl | DTT [0.1M] |
| 1 µl | dNTP Mix [10 mM] |

| IVT Mastermix | |
|---|---|
| 4 µl | 10x IVT Labeling Buffer |
| 12 µl | IVT Labeling NTP Mix |
| 4 µl | IVT Labeling Enzyme Mix |

| Second strand Mastermix | |
|---|---|
| 30 µl | 5x Second Strand Reaction Mix Buffer |
| 3 µl | dNTP Mix [10 mM] |
| 1 µl | E. coli DNA Ligase (10 U/µl) |
| 4 µl | E. coli DNA Polymerase I (10 U/µl) |
| 1 µl | RNase H (2 U/µl) |
| 91 µl | nuclease free water |

## 2 MATERIALS AND METHODS

| Hybridization mix | |
|---|---|
| 20 µl | fragmentede cRNA (15 µg) |
| 5 µl | Control-Oligonucleotide B2 (5 nm) |
| 3 µl | Herring-sperm DNA [10 mg/ml] |
| 15 µl | 100x Control-cRNA-Cocktail |
| 3 µl | acetylated BSA [50 mg/ml] |
| 150 µl | MES-Hybridising buffer |
| 104 µl | DEPC-$H_2O$ |
| Add $H_2O$ to 12 ml | |

| MES-buffer for chip staining | |
|---|---|
| 41.7 ml | 12x MES |
| 92.5 ml | 5 M NaCl |
| 2.5 ml | Tween20 (10 %) |
| Add $H_2O$ to 1 l | |

| SAPE- buffer | |
|---|---|
| 600 µl | 2x MES-buffer |
| 120 µl | acetylated BSA (20 mg/ml) |
| 12 µl | SAPE (1 mg/ml) |
| 468 µl | Nuclease free Water |
| Centrifuge 5 min at 9,000 x g | |

| Non-stringent washing buffer | |
|---|---|
| 300 ml | 20x SSPE |
| 1 ml | Tween20 (10 %) |
| Add $H_2O$ to 1 l | |

| Stringent washing buffer | |
|---|---|
| 83.3 ml | 20x SSPE |
| 5.2 ml | 5 M NaCl |
| 1.0 ml | Tween20 (10 %) |
| Add $H_2O$ to 1 l | |

| Antibody detection solution | |
|---|---|
| 300 µl | 2x MES-buffer |
| 60 µl | acetylated BSA (20 mg/ml) |
| 6.0 µl | Goat IgG (10 mg/ml in 150 mM NaCl) |
| 3.6 µl | Anti-Streptavidin Antibody, biotinylated (0.5 mg/ml) |
| 230.4 µl | nuclease free water |

## 2.2 Methods

### 2.2.1 Cell culture

#### 2.2.1.1 Isolation of primary rat hepatocytes

Male Wistar-rats with a weight between 200 to 300 g were used for the isolation of hepatocytes. The animals were kept according to animal welfare regulations[4] and the perfusion was done with authorization from the local authorities[5]. The rats had free access to food and water and were kept at a constant temperature of 20°C and a light dark circle of 12 h each.

The perfusion was carried out using a modification of the two-step perfusion method described by Seglen (Seglen, 1976). Before that, the rats were weighed, and anesthetised by a mixture of Ketanest S and Rampun 2% at a concentration of 100 mg/kg bodyweight and 15 mg/kg bodyweight, respectively. The anesthesized rats were mounted facing backwards and the abdominal wall was opened. A syringe was inserted into the portal vein and fixed with a ligature. The syringe was connected to a pumping system and the perfusion buffers by a flexible tube.

During the first step of perfusion the liver was flushed with perfusion buffer 1 (PB1) with a flow rate of 50 ml/min for 2 min and afterwards with a flow rate of 40 ml/min for another 3 min. To guaranty the complete removal of blood and to allow the perfusion buffers to flow trough the liver, the inferior vena cava, which is located behind the liver, was opened. PB1 is $Ca^{2+}$ free and contains EGTA, which complexes the remaining $Ca^{2+}$-ions which are important for cellular adhesion. During this procedure, the colour of the liver changes from red to pink.

Secondly, perfusion buffer 2 (PB2) was used at a flow rate of 45 ml/min for 5-7 min. PB2 contains Liberase Blendzyme 2, a mixture of Thermolysin (a neutral protease) and a collagenase. The dissociation of the tissue and thereby the separation of the cells was indicated by the appearance of a fine network on the surface of the liver. The liver was transferred into an ice cold washing buffer (WB), the liver capsule was opened and the separated cells were released. The cell suspension was filtered through a coarse gaze to remove bigger cell clumps. To remove non-parenchymal cells, the cell suspension was three times centrifuged (500rpm, 4°C for 2 min) to pellet the hepatocytes, the supernatant

---

[4] Deutsches Tierschutzgesetz
[5] Approval-Nr. v54-19c20/15 [DA4/Anz271E]

## 2 MATERIALS AND METHODS

containing the other cell types of the liver was aspirated and the pellet was resuspended with cold WB.

### 2.2.1.2 Trypan Blue exclusion test

Cell viability and cell number of freshly isolated hepatocytes was assessed by the trypan blue exclusion test. It is based on the principle that live cells possess intact cell membranes that exclude trypan blue, whereas dead cells do not.

50 µl Cell suspension was incubated with 1 ml trypan blue solution (500 µl Trypan blue, 0.5% + 500 µl WB1) for 1 min at RT. Afterwards, viable and dead cells were counted in a Fuchs-Rosenthal-Chamber by counting 3 fields with 16 squares each. The determined numbers of living and dead cells were used to calculate the viability, as well as the total number of cells.

$$Cells/ml = Cells_{Viable} \bullet D \bullet 5000 \qquad \%_{(Viability)} = \frac{Cells_{Viable}}{Cells_{Dead}} \bullet 100$$

D= Dilution Factor

The outcome per perfusion usually was in between $5 \times 10^8$ and $1 \times 10^9$ hepatocytes and the viability had to be greater than 85% for the cells to be used for further studies.

### 2.2.1.3 Preparation of culture dishes

Cells were plated onto either uncoated or collagen I coated culture plates for the plastic- and monolayer cultures and on a collagen-gel for sandwich cultures. This required different pre-processing of the culture dishes, except for the plastic cultures, were the culture-dishes were used as delivered.

The dishes for the monolayer cultures (ML) were coated by adding an acidic collagen I solution [10µg/ml] and letting it dry either over night (ON) or for two days (Table 3).

| Cell culture plate | Area/well | Volume | Concentration | Time to dry |
|---|---|---|---|---|
| 96 well plate | 0.32 cm² | 110 µl | 20 µg/ml | 2 d |
| 24 well plate | 2 cm² | 125 µl | 100 µg/ml | ON |
| 6 well plate | 9.6 cm² | 600 µl | 100 µg/ml | ON |
| 60 mm dish | 28 cm² | 1.8 ml | 100 µg/ml | ON |

Table 3: Scheme of pipetting for coating of culture dishes for monolayer culture

## 2 MATERIALS AND METHODS

For the sandwich cultures (SW) a layer of gelled collagen had to be prepared prior to the seeding of the cells. An ice-cold acidic solution of collagen I [83 µg/ml] was mixed with 1/10$^{th}$ volume 10x DMEM-F12 media resulting in a final collagen-concentration of 75 µg/ml. This was then neutralized to a pH of 7.2 to 7.4, with a 1M sodium hydroxide solution and directly transferred to the culture dishes/plates (Table 4). By incubation in an incubator at 37°C for at least 30 min, the collagen was allowed to gelatinize.

| Cell culture plate | Volume |
|---|---|
| 24 well plate | 75 µl |
| 6 well plate | 200 µl |
| 60 mm dish | 500 µl |

Table 4: Volume of collagen I solution used for each layer of sandwich culture.

### 2.2.1.4 Plating of cells

After isolation, hepatocytes were plated as fast as possible. Cells were mixed with plating media (DMEM/F12 medium (Gibco)) supplemented with 10% (v/v) FBS, sodium pyruvate, antibiotics and insulin and dispensed uniformly onto the dishes (Table 5).

| Cell culture plate | Cells/ ml | Volume | Total number of cells |
|---|---|---|---|
| 96 well plates | 500 *10$^3$ | 100 µl | 50 *10$^3$ |
| 24 well plates | 500 *10$^3$ | 0.5 ml | 250 *10$^3$ |
| 6 well plates | 1 *10$^6$ | 1.5 ml | 1.5 *10$^6$ |
| 60 mm dishes | 1.5 *10$^6$ | 3 ml | 4.5 *10$^6$ |

Table 5: The media volumes and the amount of cells used for seeding.

Cells were allowed to attach to the culture surfaces at 37°C and 5% $CO_2$ in a humidified atmosphere for 4 h. Cultures were subsequently washed with cooled PBS to remove dead and damaged cells. Specific media, according to the experiment type, was added (medium with FBS (above) or serum-free medium supplemented with 0.1% BSA, dexamethasone and ITS) and cells were cultured in an incubator as described above.
After attachment (3-6 h) SW cultures were overlaid with a second layer of collagen I in the same manner as the first layer and incubated at 37°C for additional 30 min to allow the second layer to gelatinize. Medium was added afterwards and either changed daily for the

## 2 MATERIALS AND METHODS

time course experiments or every second day for the experiments with compound treatment.

### 2.2.1.5 Culture of FaO and HepG2-cells

The human hepatoma cell line HepG2 and the rat hepatoma cell line FaO were grown in DMEM/F12 medium (Gibco) supplemented with 10% (v/v) FBS, sodium pyruvate, antibiotics and insulin at 37°C and 5% $CO_2$ in a humidified atmosphere to 90% confluency, washed with PBS and lysed with Trizol for subsequent RNA isolation.

### 2.2.1.6 Suspension culture

The preparation and cultivation of rat and human suspension cultures was performed by Biopredic International. After perfusion, rat and human hepatocytes were purified, suspended in DMEM supplemented with fetal calf serum (5%), insulin (4 mg/l), hydrocortisone ($10^{-6}$ mM), and gentamycin (50 mg/l) and incubated at 37 °C, 5% $CO_2$ on a mixer at 300 rpm. At each time point used for later analysis, cells were collected, shock frozen in liquid nitrogen and stored for subsequent RNA isolation with Trizol.

### 2.2.1.7 Precision cut liver slices

The preparation and cultivation of rat liver slices was performed in the laboratory of Prof. Müller[6]. 33-40 Day old male Wistar-rats from the institutes own breeding facility were kept according to the actual rules of animal welfare[7] at a light dark rhythm of 12 h, 22°C and free access to water and food (Altromin 1316, Altromin GmbH, Lage, Germany). Animals were sacrificed by decapitation after being anaesthetized with ether and liver slices were cut according to the method of Müller (Müller et al., 1998).

Briefly after dissection, the liver was flushed with and then transferred into ice-cold Krebs-Henseleit-Buffer. Cylinders of 8 mm diameter were cut out and a Krumdieck-Tissue-Slicer was used to cut liver slices with a thickness of about 200-250µm. Four slices per 25 ml Erlenmeyer flask were incubated in 5 ml modified Williams´E Medium for 2 h, 6 h, 1 d and 2 d at 37°C, gassed with carbogen (95% $O_2$ and 5% $CO_2$) and bidirectionally shaken (100 hz). Change of media was made after 2 h and 24 h. At the mentioned time points, liver slices were transferred into 1.5 ml reaction tubes, shock-frozen in liquid nitrogen and stored at -80°C until RNA isolation.

---

[6] Institute of Pharmacology and Toxicology of the Friedrich-Schiller-University of Jena
[7] Deutsches Tierschutzgesetz

## 2 MATERIALS AND METHODS

### 2.2.1.8 Isolation of primary human hepatocytes

Primary human hepatocytes were prepared from lobectomy segments resected from adult patients for medically required purposes by KaLy Cell[8]. Cells were checked for viability and seeded in culture wells in either ML culture or on a collagen gel as preparation for SW configuration. After incubation over night to ensure attachment of the cells, they were sent to Merck KGaA and used for further analyses. Cells designated for SW cultures were overlaid with a second layer of collagen gel as described in 2.2.1.4 and cells were incubated for another night at 37°C to allow the cells to recover from the transport procedure.

### 2.2.1.9 HepaRG cells

Cells were seeded and pre-incubated by Biopredic International[9] and delivered as confluent ML cultures. After receipt, the media was changed to "after-shipment" media and cells were incubated at 37°C and 5% $CO_2$ in a humidified atmosphere for three days to allow regeneration. Following this incubation, media was changed to either basal media or to basal media supplemented with 2% DMSO and incubated for another two days. During this time, cells differentiated to their "hepatocyte-like" phenotype and were then used for time course experiments.

### 2.2.2 Rat *in vivo* study

Liver samples from rats treated with tetracycline (Tet) or vehicle control were taken from a short term toxicity study performed by phase-1 Molecular Toxicology Inc.[10] The study was run according to the official guideline of animal welfare[11] and "Good laboratory Practices" (GLP)[12] compliance.

Male Sprague Dawley (Crl:CD®) rats with a body weight between 300 g and 400 g were kept under regular light-dark cycle of 12:12 hours with food (PMI Feeds Inc., Purina Milla,

---

[8] KaLy Cell, 2500 Besançon, France
[9] Biopredic International, 35000 RENNES, FRANCE
[10] PHASE 1 MOLECULAR TOXICOLOGY INC., Santa Fe, USA
[11] United States Department of Agriculture (USDA) Animal Welfare Act (9 CRF Parts 1, 2, 3)
[12] Good Laboratory Practice refers to a system of management controls for laboratories and research organisations to ensure the consistency and reliability of results as outlined in the OECD Principles of GLP and national regulations. The FDA has rules for GLP in 21CFR58

## 2 MATERIALS AND METHODS

Richmond, USA) and water ad libitum. The rats were separated in groups of three animals per time point. Each group was treated once with vehicle control (sodium chloride solution), low or high doses of tetracycline by i.p. injection. The high dose was 150 mg/kg and as low dose, one third of it was chosen (50 mg/kg). Dose finding was done by phase-1 Molecular Toxicology Inc. and was based on both published and unpublished data.

Treatment groups of three rats were sacrificed at 6 h, 1 d or 3 d by exposure to $CO_2$. After bleeding of the rats, the livers were withdrawn and divided into two pieces and cut into small pieces, shock-frozen in liquid nitrogen and stored at -80°C for later RNA extraction.

### 2.2.3 Biochemical methods and cell viability assays

There are a variety of assays to test for the number of dead cells (cytotoxicity assays), the number of living cells (viability assays), the total number of cells or the mechanism of cell death (e.g., apoptosis). Here, a number of different tests were used to address several of these different parameters. These tests were used to assess hepatocyte viability after perfusion (Trypan blue Test) or to characterize the different cell-cultures and their change over incubation time and to determine the kinetics of cell death caused by compound treatment. Results of the latter experiments were used to calculate the final concentrations used in the gene expression experiments.

#### 2.2.3.1 CellTiter-Glo® Luminescent cell viability assay

For the detection of cell viability, the CellTiter-Glo® Luminescent Cell Viability Assay was used. This test is based on a luciferase reaction (Figure 12) to measure the amount of ATP in cells. This correlates directly with the number of cells and their viability because cells lose the ability to synthesize ATP directly after e.g. loss of membrane integrity or a cytotoxic event. The protocol was adapted to 24 well plates and to the different culture conditions resulting in a standardized protocol which is described below. Cell lysis, inhibition of endogenous ATPases and detection of ATP was performed by adding the CellTiter-Glo® Reagent to the culture wells. Per well, 100 µl reagent were mixed with the same volume of DMEM-F12 Medium. Lysing of the cells took place by 10 min incubation at RT and moderate shaking. Three times 50 µl cell lysate was transferred into a white 96 well plate to eliminate stray light, and the bioluminescence was measured.

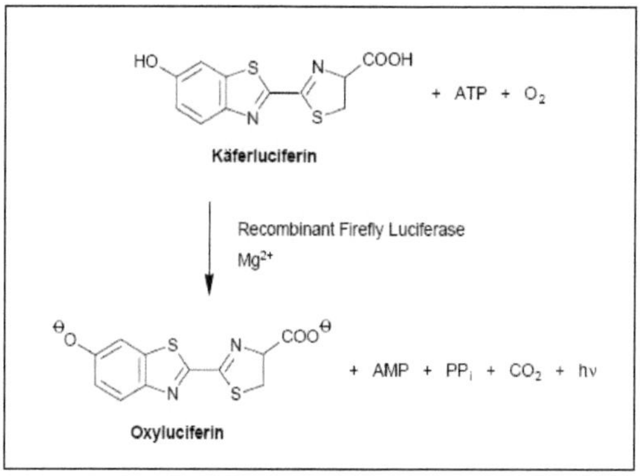

## 2 MATERIALS AND METHODS

Figure 12: Chemical reaction of the CellTiter-Glo® Luminescent Cell Viability Assay. The reagent contains recombinant luciferase that uses the likewise contained luciferin as a substrate and reacts under the consumption of cellular ATP with the release of luminescence (Adapted from Assay Manual).

#### 2.2.3.2 WST-1-assay

This test is based on the reduction of a tetrazolium salt that can be used for cell proliferation or cell viability assays. The rate of WST-1 cleavage by mitochondrial dehydrogenases correlates with the number of viable cells in the culture (Figure 13).

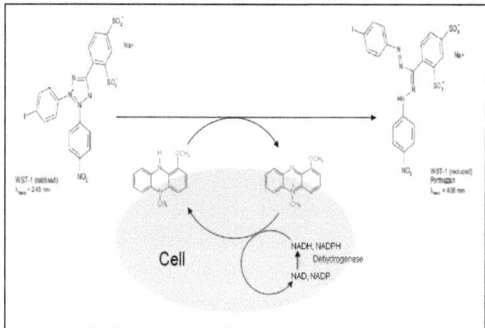

Figure 13: Assay mechanism of WST-1 conversion by dehydrogenases in viable cells. The water-soluble tetrazolium salt WST-1 is reduced to the coloured dye formazan by mitochondrial dehydrogenase enzymes with the intermediate electron acceptor PMS (Adapted from Assay Manual).

After aspiration of the culture wells, 350 µl of a mixture of DMEM F-12 media and WST-1 reagent (1/10th volume) was added to the cells and, following 4 hours incubation at 37°C, absorbance at 450 nm was measured.

#### 2.2.3.3 LDH release

If cells get damaged or die, they loose their membrane integrity, releasing, among others, cytoplasmic proteins like lactate dehydrogenase (LDH) into the surrounding media. Based on the CytoTox-ONE™ Homogeneous Membrane Integrity Assay, a standardized protocol

## 2 MATERIALS AND METHODS

was developed to measure the release of LDH from damaged hepatocytes as an indicator of cytotoxicity.

LDH catalyzes the conversion of lactate to pyruvate with the simultaneous production of NADH. The CytoTox-ONE™ Reagent contains substrates as well as cofactors for this reaction and for the conversion of resazurin to resorufin using NADH as an energy source. The emerging fluorescence is relative to the amount of LDH released into the media and was optically measured at 544 nm excitation and 595 nm emission wavelengths (Figure 14).

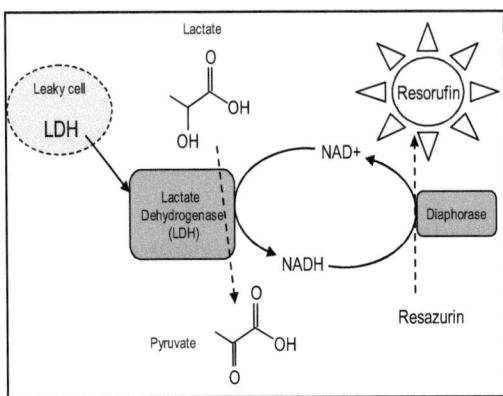

Figure 14: Principal behind the CytoTox-ONE™- Homogeneous Membrane Integrity Assay. Released LDH of damaged cells catalyzes the conversion of Lactate to Pyruvate under production of NADH in the culture media. This NADH is used to drive the diaphorase-catalyzed production of the resorufin product from resazurin.

Three times 50 µl culture media per well were transferred to a black 96 well plate, mixed with the same volume of CytoTox-ONE™ Reagent and incubated for 10 min at RT. The reaction was stopped by adding 25 µl Stop Solution and the fluorescence intensity was measured. Meanwhile, the remaining reaction media was aspirated and cells were lysed with 200 µl 0.1%TritonX100 in PBS (v/v) for 10 min at RT. Again, three times 50 µl were transferred to a black 96 well plate, the reaction was carried out and the fluorescence was measured as described above.

The LDH content of treated cells relative to the controls (time matched or fresh cells), which is an indication for the membrane integrity and cell viability, was calculated as follows:

$$\%LDH_{retained} = \left(\frac{LDH_{released}}{LDH_{released} + LDH_{cellular}}\right)_{Control} \div \left(\frac{LDH_{released}}{LDH_{released} + LDH_{cellular}}\right)_{Sample} \bullet 100$$

## 2 MATERIALS AND METHODS

### 2.2.3.4  Cytochrome P450 isoform induction and activity

#### 2.2.3.4.1  Induction of Cyp isoforms

Hepatocytes in ML and SW culture were induced with known inducers for the expression of CYP 1A, 2B, 2C and 3A isoforms. Cells were cultured as previously described and dosed at 0 h, 3 d and 9 d with the appropriate inducer for 48 h. CYP 1A1 was induced with β-naphthoflavone (BNF; 10µM), CYP 2B and 2C with phenobarbital (PB; 500µM) and CYP 3A with dexamethasone (Dex; 50µM). The concentrations of the inducers used in this experiment were selected based on preliminary experiments to obtain the largest enzyme induction without causing toxicity (data not shown).

#### 2.2.3.4.2  Detection of Cytochromes P4503A7 and 2C9 isoform activity

The activity and induction of cytochrome P450s 3A7 and 2C9 were measured with the P450-Glo™ Assays (Promega). These tests are based on the CYP450-isoenzyme specific conversion of derivatives of beetle luciferin to a luciferin product that can be detected in a second reaction with a Luciferin Detection Reagent via the generation of luminescence. The amount of light produced is proportional to the activity of the CYP450-isoform (Figure 15).

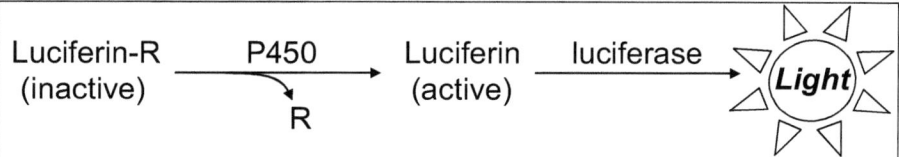

Figure 15: Conversion of P450-Glo™ substrate by cytochrome P450. Cytochrome P450 isoenzymes act specifically on a substrate to produce a luciferin product that generates light with the Luciferin Detection Reagent (modified from assay-manual).

The luciferin substrate (5 mM) was diluted in an appropriate Media (1:50) and culture media was replaced by 100 µl of this mixture. Cells were incubated for 4 h at 37°C and 5% $CO_2$ for the progress of the biochemical reaction. Afterwards 2x 40 µl were transferred into a white 96 well plate and the same volume of the P450-Glo™ Luciferin Detection Reagent was added. The reagent simultaneously stops the CYP450 reaction and initiates a luminescent signal, which was measured after 20min incubation at RT with a luminescence plate reader.

### 2.2.3.4.3 Detection of Cytochromes P450 1A1 and 2B6 isoform activity

Cytochrome P450 1A1 and Cytochrome P450 2B6 isoform activities and induction were characterized with either 7-ethoxyresorufin-O-deethylase (EROD) or benzyloxyresorufin-O-debenzylase (BROD). The reaction product was measurable with an excitation wavelength of 544 nm and an emission wavelength of 595 nm (Burke et al., 1985).

The cell culture media of cells cultured in a 24 well plate was aspirated and replaced by 150 µl salicylamide solution (0.3M). Cells were incubated for 10 min at 37°C and 5% $CO_2$ and subsequently 150 µl substrate solution was added (concentration of EROD was 5 µM, BROD was 10 µM). After 20 min incubation at 37°C, 3x 75 µl were transferred into a black 96well plate and fluorescence was measured in a fluorescence plate reader.

### 2.2.3.5 Canalicular transporter activity

The functional activity of the canalicular transporter multidrug resistance associated protein (Mrp2) was studied with carboxy-DCFDA. This diacetate exhibits only weak fluorescence but is, after penetrating through the plasma membrane, rapidly metabolized to the fluorescent product carboxydichlorofluorescein. This fluorescent bile acid is known to be a substrate for this hepatocellular transporter (Heredi-Szabo et al., 2008) and therefore the dye efflux from hepatocytes cultured in either ML or SW culture could be determined over time.

Per well of a 24 well plate, the culture media was replaced by 500 µl carboxy-DCFDA (diluted in PBS to a concentration of 5 µM). The cells were incubated for 20min at 37°C and 5% $CO_2$, subsequently washed three times with warm PBS and observed with a fluorescence microscope at an excitation wavelength of 480 nm and a 530 nm filter for detection of the emitted light.

## 2.2.4 Molecular biological methods

### 2.2.4.1 Isolation of RNA and proteins

The isolation of RNA and proteins was conducted with TRI Reagent. TRI Reagent contains phenol and guanidine thiocyanate to maintain nucleotide and protein integrity during cell/tissue homogenization while at the same time disrupting and breaking down cells and cell components. All steps of the procedure were conducted according to the manufacturers' manual (Sigma).

## 2 MATERIALS AND METHODS

Cells in culture were lysed by replacing the culture media with the appropriate volume of TRI reagent and the lysate was transferred into a 15 ml reaction tube. Tissue slices were homogenized by the addition of a nuclease free steel bead and the appropriate volume of TRI reagent with the Tissue Lyzer for 1 min with a frequency of 25 Hz. All samples were incubated for 10 min at RT, afterwards 200 µl chloroform per 1 ml TRI reagent were added, mixed by shaking and incubated for another 10 min. For the separation of the phases, this mixture was centrifuged for 15 min at 12,000 x g and 4°C. The upper aqueous phase containing the RNA was transferred into new reaction tube containing 500 µl ice cold isopropanol per ml TRI reagent, mixed by vortexing and incubated for 10 min at RT. Another centrifugation step precipitated the RNA. The pellet was washed with 1.5 ml ethanol (75%), the supernatant discarded, the pellet dried for 5-10 min and finally resolved in nuclease free water.

The proteins, which are contained in the organic lower phase, were isolated by discarding the white interphase containing the genomic DNA, precipitated by adding 1.5 ml isopropanol per 1 ml of TRI reagent used for initial homogenization and incubation for 10 min at room temperature. The proteins were sedimented by centrifugation at 12000 x g for 10 min at 4°C. The protein pellet was washed 3 times for 20 min at RT in 0.3 M guanidine hydrochloride in 95% ethanol (2 ml per ml TRI reagent) and once in 100% ethanol with centrifugation steps of 7500 x g for 5 min at 4°C to re-acquire the pellet. After this final wash step, the protein pellet was air dried for 5-10 min at RT and resuspended in 200-300 µl lysis buffer by using the tissue lyzer. After complete solubilization, the protein solution was stored at -20°C.

### 2.2.4.2 Quantification and quality check of nucleic acids

The quantification of isolated nucleic acids and the check for absence of protein was done by measuring the absorbance at 260 nm and 280 nm with a UV-spectrophotometer (NanoDrop ND-1000). The ratio between the two resulting values must be 1.8 or higher to guarantee a protein-free solution. With the help of the Lambert-Beer-Law and the molar extinction-coefficient, the concentration of the RNA in solution was calculated as follows:

# 2 MATERIALS AND METHODS

$$c = \frac{\log_{10} \frac{I_0}{I}}{\varepsilon \bullet d}$$

c= Concentration, $I_0$ = Intensity of the initial light beam, I = Intensity of the transmitted light, $\log_{10} I_0/I$ = Absorption, $\varepsilon$ = Extinction coefficient, d = Thickness of the cell

The quality of the nucleic acids was checked with the RNA 6000 Nano LabChip Kit II on the Agilent 2100 bioanalyzer according to the manufacturers' recommendations. This assay is based on capillary electrophoresis so the RNA was separated according to their length and detected by fluorescent labeling. The resulting electropherograms ( Figure 16) were checked for signs of RNA degradation.

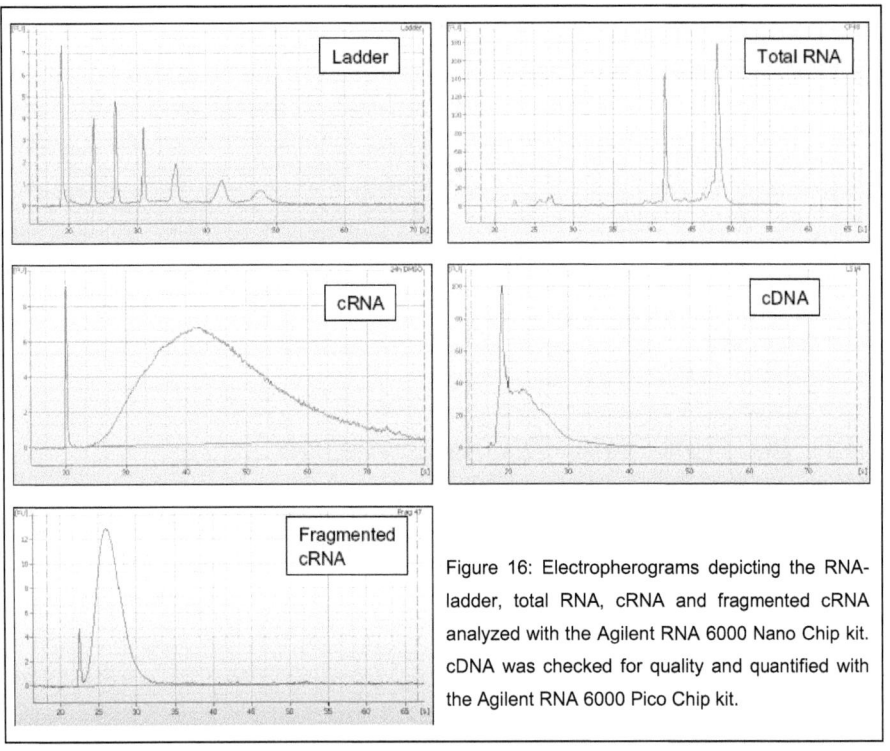

Figure 16: Electropherograms depicting the RNA-ladder, total RNA, cRNA and fragmented cRNA analyzed with the Agilent RNA 6000 Nano Chip kit. cDNA was checked for quality and quantified with the Agilent RNA 6000 Pico Chip kit.

2 MATERIALS AND METHODS

### 2.2.4.3 TaqMan® Low Density Arrays (TLDA)

#### 2.2.4.3.1 Quantification of mRNA with TaqMan® Low Density Arrays (TLDA)

TaqMan real time PCR is based on the principle of a linear amplification and the 5' exonuclease activity of DNA polymerase during the PCR (Lawyer et al., 1993). TaqMan® probes contain a reporter dye (6-FAM™) linked to the 5' end of the probe and a non-fluorescent quencher (NFQ) at the 3' end of the probe. When the probe is intact, the proximity of the reporter dye to the quencher results in suppression of the reporter fluorescence, primarily due to Förster energy transfer (Förster, 1948).

During PCR, the TaqMan® probe anneals specifically to the middle of the amplified sequence. These probes are cleaved by the 5' exonuclease activity of the DNA polymerase during amplification whereby the reporter dye is separated from the quencher, resulting in an increase in fluorescence (Figure 17). The amount of fluorescence produced is measured at each amplification cycle, providing a real-time estimation of the amount of mRNA. This increase in fluorescent signal occurs only if the probe was bound to the target sequence which is amplified during PCR. The assays are designed to span exon junctions to eliminate the possibility of detecting genomic DNA, which may still be present in the cDNA sample.

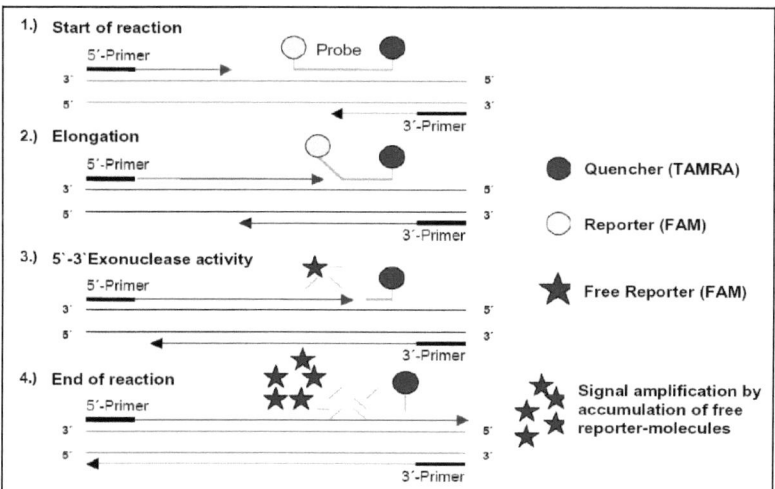

Figure 17: Principle of TaqMan-PCR. Additionally to the two amplification primers, a third gene specific primer, carrying a reporter and a quencher, hybridizes to the amplified gene. During amplification, this primer is degraded by the exonuclease activity of the Taq-polymerase, the reporter separates from the quencher and a fluorescent signal can be measured (modified from assay-manual).

## 2 MATERIALS AND METHODS

TLDA´s are a high throughput application of TaqMan PCR. A 384 well micro fluidic card enables 384 simultaneous real-time PCR reactions to be run in parallel across 12 to 384 targets. They are pre-loaded with optimized primers and probes and can be customized. A list of genes measured for the verification of microarray experiments can be found in the Appendix (Appendix 5 and Appendix 6).

### 2.2.4.3.2   cDNA synthesis for TaqMan® Low Density Arrays (TLDA)

For cDNA synthesis, the Transcriptor First Strand cDNA Synthesis Kit for RT-PCR (AMV) was used with random hexamers. 1 µg Total RNA in a volume of 11 µl was mixed with 9 µl reverse transcription mastermix and transcribed as follows:

| Incubation | 10 min | 25°C |
|---|---|---|
| Reverse transcription | 60 min | 50°C |
| RT-Inactivation | 5 min | 85°C |

Table 6: cDNA synthesis reaction for TaqMan® by RT-PCR

The success of the reverse transcription was reviewed and cDNA was quantified with the Agilent 2100 Bioanalyzer using the RNA 6000 Pico LabChip Kit according to the manufacturers manual (
Figure 16).
The area under the curve (AUC) from the ladder and samples was used to calculate the concentrations of cDNA. One µl Ladder represents an AUC of 100 and a cDNA concentration of 1 ng/µl.

$$[cDNA] = 10\,pg/\mu l \bullet \frac{AUC_{Ladder}}{100} \bullet AUC_{Sample}$$

## 2 MATERIALS AND METHODS

### 2.2.4.3.3 Conduction of TaqMan® Low Density Arrays (TLDA)

10 ng cDNA of each sample were made up to 50 µl with nuclease free water, mixed with the same volume qPCR™ Mastermix Plus (Eurogentec) and transferred into the sample reservoirs of the TLDA card. By centrifugation (2 min at 331 g), the samples were distributed into the sample wells and finally, the card was sealed to avoid mixing of the samples and reagents.

The cards were measured using the ABI Prism 790 hT Sequence Detection System controlled by the AB Prism 7900 h SDS Software 2.1 according to the manufacturers' recommendations (Applied Biosystems). Following time scale was used with 45 cycles:

| Initial phase | 2 min | 50°C |
| --- | --- | --- |
| Activation of Taq-Polymerase | 10 min | 94.5°C |
| Denature cDNA | 30 sec | 97°C |
| Annealing and Elongation | 1 min | 59.7°C |

Table 7: Cycle-scheme of TLDA-cards, step 2-4 were repeated 45 times.

### 2.2.4.3.4 Evaluation of TaqMan® Low Density Arrays (TLDA)

Changes in gene expression were calculated relative to a constitutively expressed housekeeping gene such as 18s ribosomal RNA, and additionally compared to a control sample of fresh liver or a time matched vehicle control. Under optimal conditions, the amplification is exponential corresponding to a doubling of the amplified sequence during each cycle. Because this is not always the case, the efficiency corrected $_\Delta$CT method of Pfaffl was used (Pfaffl, 2001). The CT value is defined as the number of cycles in the exponential phase of amplification

$$Ratio = \frac{(E_{T\arg et})^{\Delta CT_{Target}(Control - T\arg et)}}{(E_{Control})^{\Delta CT_{Control}(Control - T\arg et)}}$$

$\quad$ E $\quad$ = Efficiency of reverse transcription
$\Delta$CT = Change in the number of cycles between sample and control

## 2 MATERIALS AND METHODS

To calculate the efficiency of reverse transcription, a titration series of a standard cDNA over four orders of magnitude (0.1 ng - 100 ng) was prepared and amplified. The resulting CT values for each gene were plotted against the amount of cDNA inserted and a standard curve for each gene was calculated. The slope of this curve (m) was used to caculate the transcription efficiency as follows:

$$E = 10^{(-\frac{1}{m})}$$

### 2.2.4.4 Processing of RNA for Illumina and Affymetrix Chips

To enable signal detection and quantification after hybridization to the microchips, the sample RNA has to be labelled. In this case, this was done for both techniques used (Affymetrix and Illumina) by incorporation of biotin-labelled nucleotides during an *in vitro* transcription reaction after an initial cDNA generation from total RNA. The labeling kits were purchased and enzymatic reactions were carried out as recommended by the suppliers.

#### 2.2.4.4.1 cRNA Synthesis from total RNA for Illumina BeadChips

For the cRNA synthesis, the MessageAmp II aRNA Amplification Kit (Ambion Inc.), the RNeasy® MiniKit and the QIAquick® PCR Purification Kit (both Qiagen) were used. Per sample, 500ng total RNA were dried in a 0.2 ml PCR tube in a vacuum centrifuge concentrator at RT prior to the first strand synthesis.

## 2 MATERIALS AND METHODS

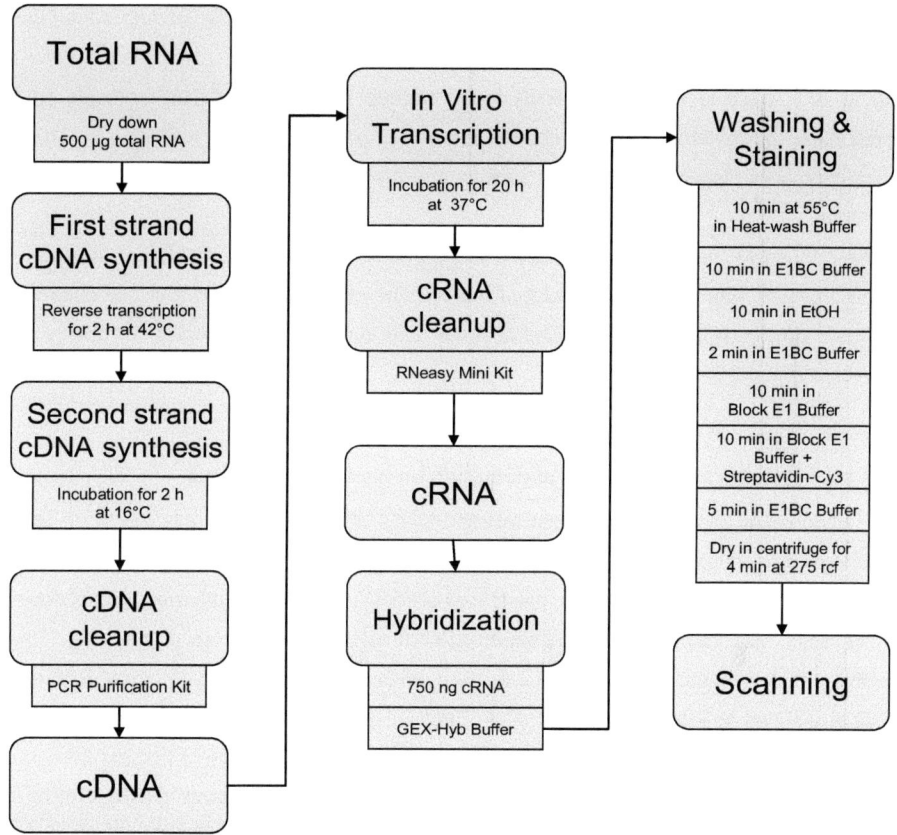

Figure 18: Workflow for the conduction of Illumina BeadChip arrays

During the first strand synthesis step, a single stranded cDNA from the mRNA-containing total RNA sample was synthesized with oligo-dT-primers and a reverse transcriptase. 5µl 1st strand synthesis master mix were dispensed into each sample tube, mixed to dissolve the dried RNA and incubated at 42°C for two hours.

In the 2nd strand synthesis step, the single stranded cDNA from the previous step was converted to double-stranded cDNA; the second strand master mix was prepared directly prior to use. 20 µl of this solution were dispensed into each sample tube and samples were incubated at 16°C for a further two hours.

For the clean up of the sample, the QIAquick PCR Purification Kit was used according to the manufacturers' instructions up to the point of elution which was done with 50 µl

## 2 MATERIALS AND METHODS

nuclease free water. The double stranded cDNA was dried down in a vacuum centrifuge concentrator at RT prior to *in vitro* transcription (IVT).

During IVT, multiple copies of cRNA were created from every cDNA molecule and additionally, biotinylated UTP-nucleotides were incorporated into the cRNA. 10 µl IVT mastermix were dispensed into each sample and the reaction was incubated at 37°C for 20 hours.

Following the IVT, samples were cleaned using the RNeasy Mini Kit (QIAGEN) according to the provided manual up to the point of elution. The cRNA was eluted from the columns by washing twice with 50 µl nuclease free water and quantified and checked for quality as described under 2.2.4.2.

### 2.2.4.4.2 Hybridizing, staining and detection on Illumina BeadChips

For hybridization, 750ng of the biotin labelled cRNA of each sample was made up to a volume of 5 µl with Nuclease free water and mixed with 10 µl GEX-HYB buffer (provided by Illumina). Each mixture was then preheated at 65°C for 5 minutes, allowed to cool down to RT again and dispensed into a separate sample port on the chip (Figure 19). The RatRef-12_v1 chip allows 12 samples to be hybridized simultaneously, Human_RefSeq-8_v2 arrays can be loaded with 8 samples. Each BeadChip simultaneously assays 22,523 probes per sample, targeting genes and known alternative splice variants derived from the National Center for Biotechnology Information Reference Sequence (NCBI RefSeq) database (Build 36.2, Release 22 for human and Release 16 for rat)

Each BeadChip was placed into a BeadChip hybridization chamber, prepared with 200µl GEX HCB in each of the two humidifying buffer reservoirs. Hybridization chambers were sealed and incubated for 20 hours at 58°C with a rocker speed of 5.

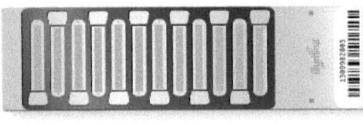

Figure 19: The RatRef-12 Expression BeadChip with IntelliHyb Seal contains 12 rat specific whole genome gene expression arrays, allowing 12 samples to be hybridized to a single chip. Each array probes 21,910 genes and contains 22,523 probes.

To guarantee a consistent quality and fluorescence intensity, several washing steps were performed after hybridization. A high stringency washing step with high temperature wash buffer to remove unbound and mismatched cRNA, low stringency washing steps with Wash E1BC solution and ethanol, a blocking step with Block E1 buffer, the detection with

# 2 MATERIALS AND METHODS

Prepare Block E1 buffer containing streptavidin-Cy3 [1 mg/ml] and final wash steps with Wash E1BC solution were performed according to the manufacturers protocol. Finally, the BeadChips were dried by centrifugation at 275g at RT for 4 minutes. Scanning was done directly afterwards with the Illumina BeadStation500x at 532 nm and a resolution of 3μm. Three BeadChips could be scanned at once, data extraction was performed simultaneously during the scanning process by the BeadScan control software and the intensity data was exported.

### 2.2.4.4.3  cRNA synthesis from total-RNA for Affymetrix microarrays

During the whole process of generating cRNA the Gene Chip® One-Cycle cDNA Synthesis Kit, the Gene Chip® Sample Cleanup Module and the Gene Chip® IVT Labeling Kit supplied by Affymetrix were used. All enzymes and buffers used were included in these kits and all steps were accomplished according to the manufacturers' recommendations.

For the reverse transcription, 5μg of total RNA were used in 8 μl nuclease free water. 2 μl Poly-A RNA spike in controls and 2 μl T7 Oligo(dT) Primer [50 mM] were added to make a final volume of 12 μl and incubated for 10 min at 70°C.

7 μl First strand mastermix was added and the mixture was heated up to 42°C for 2 min. Finally, 1 μl enzyme (Superscript II™ [200μM]) was added and the reaction was incubated for 1 h at 42°C.

The single stranded cDNA resulting from the first strand synthesis reaction was used completely for the second strand synthesis. Therefore, 130 μl second strand synthesis mastermix was added and the reaction was incubated for 2 h at 16°C. The reaction was started by adding 2 μl T4-DNA-polymerase (5U/ μl), incubation for another 5 min at 16°C and stopped by the addition of 10 μl EDTA-solution (0.5 M). The clean up was done with the Gene Chip® Sample Cleanup Module and the cDNA was eluted from the columns with 14 μl nuclease free water.

Based on the double stranded cDNA, the biotinylated cRNA was synthesized with the Gene Chip® IVT Labeling Kit. 12 μl cDNA were made up to 20 μl with nuclease free water, mixed with 20 μl IVT-mastermix and incubated for 16 h at 37°C. The cleanup was again performed with the Gene Chip® Sample Cleanup Module and the elution was done in two steps with 11 μl and 10 μl nuclease free water. Quantification and quality control of the synthesized cRNA was performed as described in 2.2.4.2.

Prior to hybridization, the cRNA was fragmented to 200–300mers by metal-induced hydrolysis in fragmentation buffer (supplied with Sample Cleanup Module). 15μg cRNA

## 2 MATERIALS AND METHODS

was made up to 32 µl with nuclease free water, mixed with 8 µl 5x Fragmentation Buffer and heated up to 94°C for 35 min. The fragmentation was checked on the Agilent Bioanalyzer 2100.

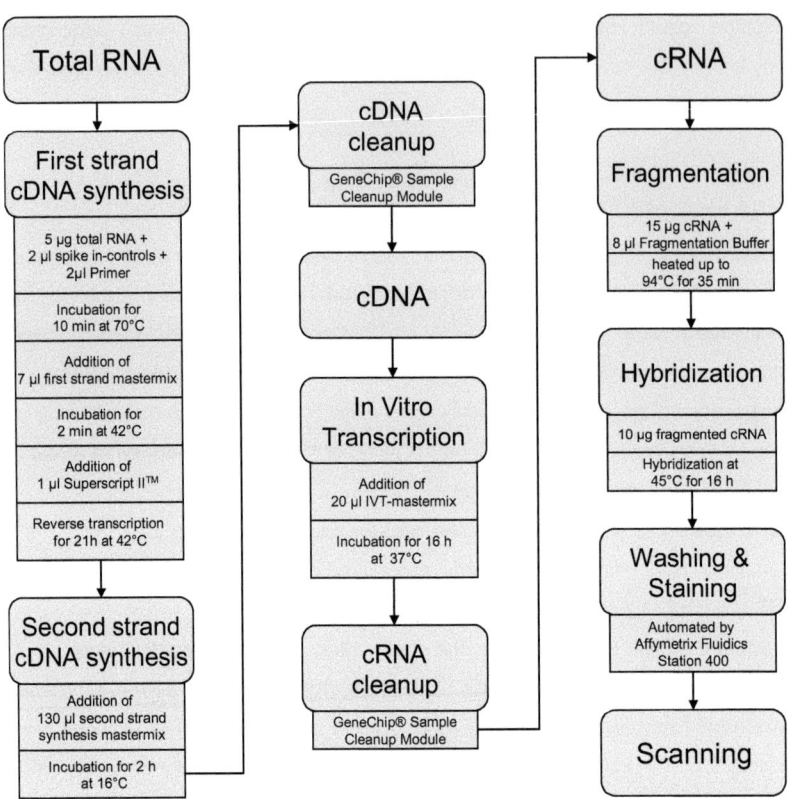

Figure 20: Scheme of the whole workflow for the conduction of Affymetrix Gene Chips®.

#### 2.2.4.4.4 Hybridizing, staining and detection on Affymetrix microarrays

15µg fragmented cRNA (40 µl) were mixed with 260 µl hybridization mastermix, incubated for 5 min first at 99°C followed by 5min at 45°C and afterwards centrifuged at maximum speed for 5 min. The Affymetrix Chips used (either Gene Chip® Rat Expression Array(RAE) 230 2.0 or Gene Chip® Human Genome U133Plus 2.0Array) were pre-hybridized with 200 µl 1x MES-Hybridization Buffer for 10 min at 45°C and at a rotation speed of 60rpm. The 1 x MES-Hybridization Buffer was replaced by 200 µl of the cRNA-hybridization-mastermix (10 μg) and the Chips were hybridized for 16 h at the same rotation speed.

The washing and staining steps were performed automatically by the Affymetrix Fluidics Station 400. Therefore, the precast washing program EukGE WS5, including the initial low and high stringency wash steps with wash buffers A and B, staining with SAPE-staining solution, antibody solution and a final wash step again with wash buffer A (Figure 20), was used.

The scanning took place in a Gene Chip® Scanner 3000 at 570 nm wavelength and a resolution of 3 μm controlled by the GCOS-Software which was used for data extraction and quality control afterwards, too.

### 2.2.5 Microarray data analysis

The data extraction for Illumina BeadChips and for Affymetrix Genome arrays was performed with specific vendor software.

#### 2.2.5.1 Data extraction and quality control from Illumina BeadChip arrays

Data extraction for Illumina BeadChips was performed by the supplied BeadScan software during the process of scanning and data was exported. The intensity values for every bead were aligned with the decoding data, which was delivered together with each chip (Gunderson et al., 2004, Chapter 1.8). The data from all beads with the same probe bound to their surface were condensed to one value. Simultaneously, for each bead type, a p-Value was calculated indicating the probability to be able to discriminate between negative controls and the samples. Each array on the BeadChips contained also various controls which could be analyzed and used to confirm the quality of the data. Three different hybridization controls with low, medium and high concentration, contained in the hybridization buffer, were used to identify the over all quality of the hybridization, independent from the sample cRNA. Perfect match and mismatch controls were used to detect unspecific hybridizations and, together with a GC-rich probe, to ensure the stringency of the hybridization. Also contained in the hybridization buffer were two biotin-labelled oligonucleotides to control the fluorescence intensity and negative controls with random sequences to identify the background intensity level. Arrays which did not fulfil defined quality parameters were removed and sample hybridization was repeated. In some cases the BeadStudio software was used to normalize the data. Further statistical

## 2 MATERIALS AND METHODS

analyses were conducted in the software Expressionist®Analyzer of Genedata and will be discussed in later chapters.

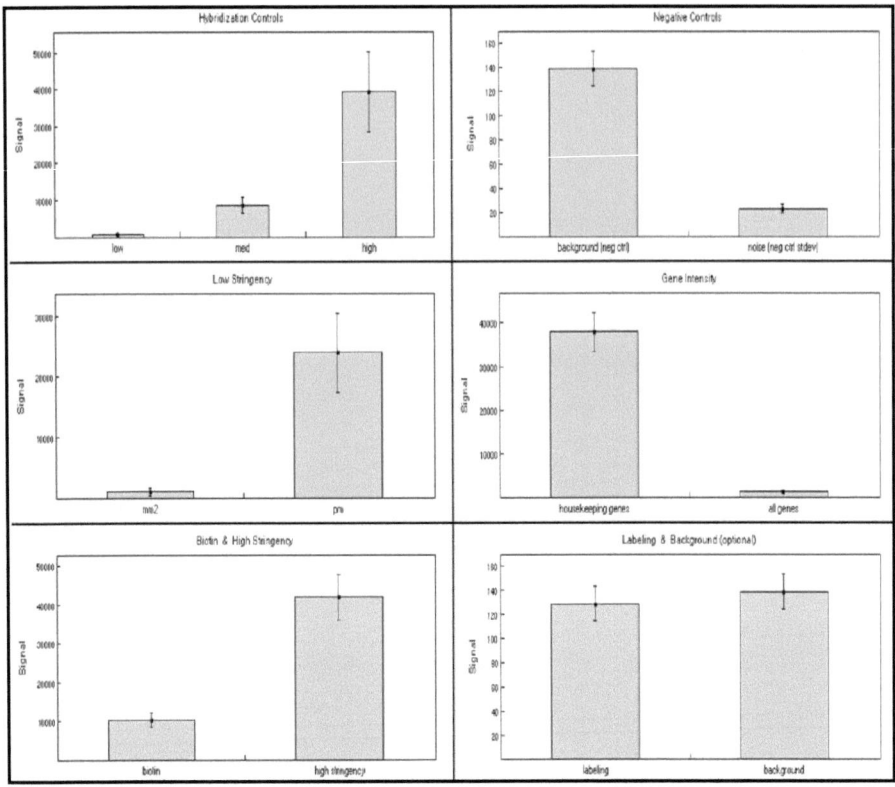

Figure 21: Overview of the hybridization controls for Illumina BeadChips. Mean values for all arrays analyzed are shown together with the standard deviation for low, medium and high abundant controls, a perfect and a mismatch control, a biotin control, the background intensity and the overall intensity for housekeepers and all genes. Together, these controls ensure the high quality of the data used for later analyses.

### 2.2.5.2 Data extraction and quality control from Affymetrix arrays

For each probe cell on the array, a single value was generated by the GCOS software. Because of the layout with eleven perfect match and eleven mismatch probe-cells per gene, a condensing step was included in the data extraction process, so only a single value per probe set was computed. The overall intensity and the intensity of the spike-in controls were visualized and checked for quality. The created .cel-files were uploaded into and processed with the Expressionist®Refiner software from Genedata. Therein, an

## 2 MATERIALS AND METHODS

automated workflow, including several quality controls and a RMA-normalization, was performed (Irizarry et al., 2003). This normalization method uses only the perfect match data to perform background correction, normalization and expression value estimation. This results in lower variation coefficients and enhances the comparability between experiments (Irizarry et al., 2003).

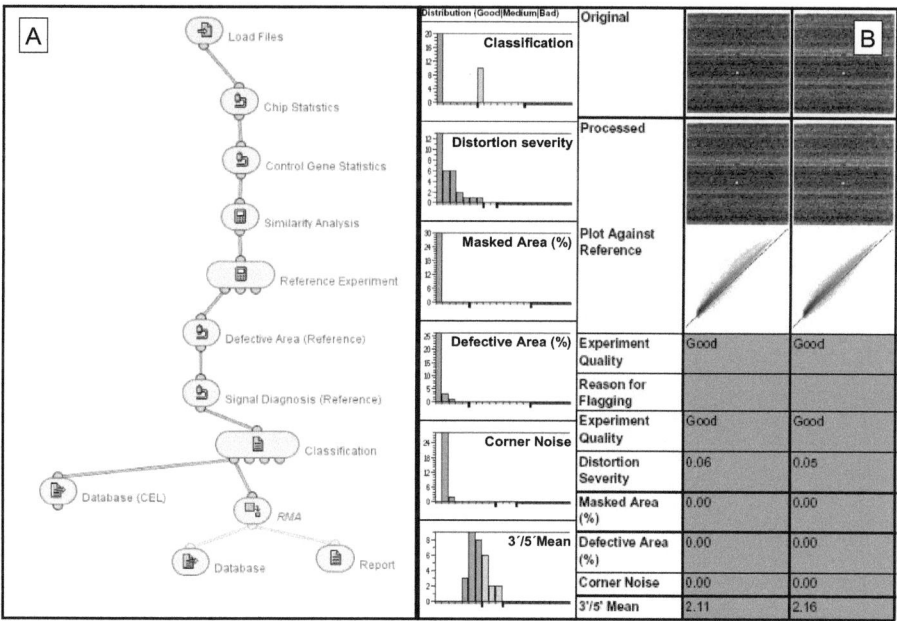

Figure 22: A) Overview of the Refiner workflow including chip statistics, quality controls, classification and RMA-normalization. B) Detail of the result report of a refiner analysis. The classification indicates the overall quality with a colour code; additional details for each Chip are shown on the right side.

At the end of each workflow and as a result of the controls, each Array was classified by the software in the quality parameters as either good, medium or bad (Figure 22). Chips classified as good were used in the analysis, chips classified as bad were repeated. The medium classification was checked manually and the decision if the data was used was made on a case-by-case basis.

## 2 MATERIALS AND METHODS

### 2.2.6 Protein separation by SDS polyacrylamide gel electrophoresis (SDS-PAGE)

Isolated proteins and cell lysates were separated by SDS-PAGE. 5-50 µg Protein with a volume of 20-25 µl were mixed with 5 µl LDS sample buffer and 2 µl of reducing agent and heated for 10 min at 70°C. Each sample was transferred into a pocket of a NuPAGE® Novex 4-12% Bis-Tris-gel in an incubation tray assembled in accordance with the manufacturers' recommendations (Invitrogen). The separation was performed at 200 V and 125 mA per gel for 60 min. 10 µl Molecular marker were always run in one slot of the gel to allow an estimation of protein size.

### 2.2.7 Protein detection by western blot analysis and immune detection

Blotting of proteins from polyacrylamide gels to nitrocellulose membranes (0.2 µm) was performed with the iBlot™ Dry Blotting System (Invitrogen) according to the manufacturers´ recommendations. This system enables rapid protein transfers by the use of a shortened distance between electrodes, high field strength and high currents. The ion reservoirs are incorporated into the gel matrix instead of the buffer tanks or soaked papers. Transfer membranes and the copper electrodes (anode and cathode) are included into the iBlot™ Gel Transfer Stacks (Figure 23).

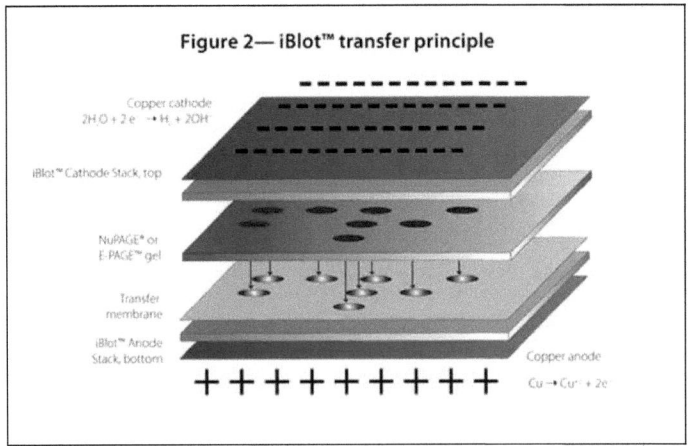

Figure 23: Principle of the iBlot™ Dry Blotting System (taken from the system manual).

## 2 MATERIALS AND METHODS

Membranes were blocked by incubation with coating solution (5% milk solution in PBS-Tween buffer) for 1 h. The primary antibodies were diluted and incubated together with the membranes as follows:

| Antibody | Organism | Provider | Time of incubation | Dilution |
|---|---|---|---|---|
| **Primary antibodies** | | | | |
| Cytochrome P450 3A1 | Mouse | abcam | 1h | 1:3,000 |
| Cytochrome P450 2B1/2 | Mouse | abcam | 1h | 1:3,000 |
| Cytochrome P450 1A1 | Rabbit | abcam | 1.5h | 1:3,000 |
| **Secondary antibodies** | | | | |
| Peroxidase conjugated (HRP) anti-rabbit IgG | Sheep | GE Healthcare (#329616) | | 1:5,000 |
| Peroxidase conjugated (HRP) anti-mouse IgG | Rabbit | GE Healthcare (#328634) | | 1:5,000 |

Table 8: Antibodies used for immunodetection.

The membrane was washed with PBS-Tween buffer 3x 10 min, incubated with the adequate secondary antibody, also diluted in PBS-Tween buffer, for another hour and finally washed again as previously mentioned.

The detection was performed with freshly prepared ECL solution according to the manufacturers´ recommendations (ECL-Kit, Amersham Biosciences). A chemoluminescent signal is produced by an enzymatic reaction between the secondary antibody-coupled horseradish peroxidase and the ECL-reagent which can be used to detect and quantify the specific protein.

The ECL solution was spread out on the membrane and incubated for 1min. The membrane was put into a film cassette together with a detection Film (Hyperfilm ECL, Amersham Biosciences), the time of exposure ranged from 2 min to 5 h. The processing of the films was performed automatically with a hyper processor (Amersham Biosciences).

## 2 MATERIALS AND METHODS

### 2.2.8 SELDI-TOF analysis

SELDI-TOF (Surface-enhanced laser desorption/ionization - time of flight) retains the target proteins on a solid-phase chromatographic surface array, were they are vaporized by ionization using a laser and fly through a "time-of-flight" tube where they separate based on mass and charge ( Figure 24). To allow ionization, sinapinic acid was applied to each array. As the solvent evaporates, the proteins co-crystallize with the sinapinic acid. By absorbing the laser energy these crystals raise ionized proteins which can then be detected. In these experiments cation exchange ProteinChip CM10 arrays were used to bind and analyse positively charged proteins.

The chip surface was pre-activated for 10 min with 50 µl pre-activation binding buffer, afterwards 50 to 500 µg isolated protein sample were applied onto the chip surface in 150 µl citrate binding buffer and centrifuged in a special chip processor for 1 h at 270 rpm and RT. The chip surface was washed three times with 300 µl binding buffer for 7 min at 270 rpm to remove unbound proteins. Washing was finalized by incubation with 300 µl $H_2O$ for 1 min and drying for 15 – 20 min. Two times 0.5 µl sinapinic acid, freshly diluted in a 1:1 mix of acetonitrile and TFA [1%] were applied onto the chip surface and allowed to dry.

After drying, chips were placed into the *PBSII ProteinChip Reader* (Ciphergen) and measured in the linear mode. The ionisation of the sample was achieved with a $N_2$-laser beam at (337 nm) with one warming shot with energy of 2,100 nJ and 10 data shots with 2,000 nJ. The mass range accomplished was 2 to 30 kDa, with a focus mass of 10 kDa. These settings were kept constant across all chips in an experiment.

The ProteinChip Reader is directly linked to the *ProteinChip Software* for data analysis. The generated protein profiles were analysed by a multiple comparison of all spectra's. The *Biomarker Wizard*, a software tool, allows clustering of the detected mass to charge (m/z) signals for all spectra. Similar m/z signals were matched to a cluster and afterwards relatively quantified. Significant intensity changes of single mass-ion-peaks were detected using non-parametric Mann–Whitney statistical analysis (p-Value ≤ 0.01). Signals with a deregulation of more than two fold were accepted as differentially expressed. The visualisation of the differences between different groups was accomplished by plotting the signal intensities against the m/z-values of the clusters.

# 2 MATERIALS AND METHODS

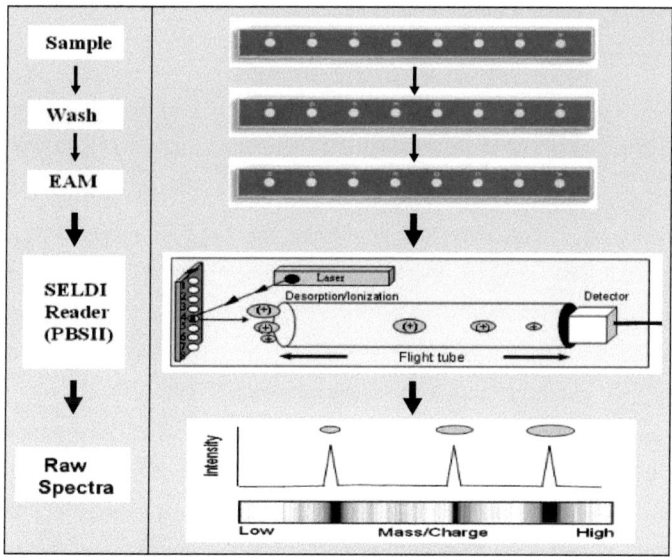

Figure 24: Scheme of the SELDI-workflow.

# 3 RESULTS AND DISCUSSIONS

## 3.1 Comparison of different global gene expression platforms

Microarray technology is one of the fastest evolving and most promising fields in molecular biology. Over the last decade, this technology has basically changed the way of addressing biological interrogations and opens new perspectives in monitoring cellular mechanisms and processes on a global level. There are applications in almost every field of biology and medicine and the number is still growing. The analysis of genomic data has become more and more important in modern toxicology and drug development, enabling researchers to identify changes in global gene expression as well as specifically affected pathways. Also the computing power was no longer a limitation, allowing the implementation of larger and more realistic models The FDA and the EPA (US Environmental Protection Agency) have defined pharmaco- and toxicogenomics as key opportunities to personalized medicine and risk assessment (Dix et al., 2006; Lesko & Woodcock, 2004).

The use of microarrays to obtain insight into cellular processes and to monitor molecular interactions is a well-established method and has enabled scientists to understand cellular mechanisms in extreme detail and complexity. The amount of data in public databases, together with the molecular knowledge has tremendously increased over the last years. In the past, there were no official guidelines for conducting these types of experiments and so, the vast majority were performed without internal controls or accepted standards. The comparison of data within each platform and of results gained with other platforms gave quite conflicting results, showing either agreement (Li, Pankratz & Johnson, 2002; Parrish et al., 2004) or disagreement (Kuo et al., 2006; Mah et al., 2004) between the outcomes. This fact has driven the development of more rigid quality standards and guidelines not only in the manufacturing process but also on the handling and processing of the resulting data. The Implementation of MIAME (Minimal Information About a Microarray Experiment) was the first step towards a common standard. The FDA initiated a comprehensive project to look at microarray quality control and cross-platform comparisons (MAQC). The aim of this study was to learn how to handle existing microarray data in respect to reliability, comparability, repeatability and how the various sources of variance, like intra- and interplatform and interlaboratory differences, affect the resulting data (Shi et al., 2006).

# 3 RESULTS AND DISCUSSION

Several providers have developed diverse variants of this technique and although the basic principle, measuring the amount of transcripts, is elementary, there are various differences in commercially available microarray platforms. Variability can be caused by multiple factors like the type of probes (*in situ* polymerization, spotting, microbeads), the probe selection and design, the number of probes (short/long oligonucleotides, cDNA), different labeling methods or competitive versus non-competitive hybridization. Affymetrix and Illumina both provide platforms allowing one sample to be hybridized per array. Array-to-array variability is minimized by highly standardized manufacturing and hybridization procedures. The degree of variation between replicates is an important issue for the experimental design and the interpretation of the results.

Results of gene expression experiments are often used for the development of large databases. Right now, great efforts are taking place to test the ability of integrating data generated with different types of platforms (Roter, 2005). An important aspect is the understanding of the influence that the technology has on the data itself, data handling and processing and of course the overlap of genes common to these technologies. Therefore, the reliability and accuracy of gene expression measurements are a quality attribute and an elementary requirement.

With this study, we wanted to investigate the comparability of a new global rat gene expression platform provided by Illumina Inc. with the well-established and accepted technique provided by Affymetrix. We therefore analyzed data generated from samples simultaneously on Illumina RatRef-12 Expression BeadChips (Illumina) and the Affymetrix Gene Chip® Rat Genome 230 2.0 Arrays.

The study comprised two sets of samples to elucidate the technical and biological differences/similarities. A titration series with RNA extracted from control liver and kidney was generated for the more technically based comparison to test the linearity and the detection sensitivity of both platforms. Additionally, we investigated liver samples from rats treated with the model compound tetracycline as well as primary rat hepatocytes treated with tetracycline hydrochloride (both will be called Tet in the following to simplify reading). This setup enabled not only the direct comparison of results of both platforms but also to compare the changes in gene expression *in vivo* with the reaction of the hepatocytes cultured *in vitro*.

Our study design gave us the option to analyze the comparability of both platforms by means of technical concordance but also on the level of the biological interpretation of the data. The evaluation of intra-laboratory variation is important for future experimental design as are the number of replicates (biological and technical) needed. Additionally, by

# 3 RESULTS AND DISCUSSION

comparing *in vivo* and *in vitro* data, we gained deeper insights into the compound-specific mechanism of action and the possibility to mimic these effects *in vitro*.

The key questions of this study were:

1) Do we find a high concordance in the results of both platforms and if not, to what extent do they vary?
2) Is the biological interpretation of the data nevertheless the same?
3) Are both types of gene expression platforms equally qualified to measure samples with such a variety of origins?

Tet is an antibiotic that is produced by streptomycetes in nature. It inhibits bacterial growth by reversibly binding to the 16S subunit of the bacterial ribosome, inhibiting the binding of amino-acyl-tRNA to the ribosomal A site and thereby translation. In higher doses, this effect has been proven to take place in mammalian cells (McKee et al., 2006). In addition, Tet and its derivates exert anti-inflammatory and immunomodulatory effects that are completely separate from its antimicrobial action (Gabler & Creamer, 1991). A toxic side effect of Tet is the causing of microvesicular steatosis in the liver, which occurs dose dependent through inhibition of mitochondrial ß-oxidation of fatty acids and cholesterol biosynthesis (Fréneaux et al., 1988). Hepatic microvesicular steatosis can have severe consequences in some people (Westphal, Vetter & Brogard, 1994). Known molecular mechanisms include the inhibition of mitochondrial β-oxidation and peroxisome proliferator receptors (PPARs), and, in high doses, protein synthesis. Other genes affected play roles in cell proliferation, nucleoside metabolism and signal transduction. Additionally, Tet inhibits the induction of IL-1-converting enzyme and reduces cyclooxygenase-2 expression and prostaglandin $E_2$ production. Also the Poly(ADP-ribose) polymerase-1 (PARP-1), which promotes both cell death and inflammation when activated by DNA damage, is inhibited (Yin et al., 2006). The clear dose and time dependent mode of action enables us to examine if the same biological interpretations following Tet treatment can be inferred from different platforms.

# 3 RESULTS AND DISCUSSION

## 3.1.1 Results of the platform comparison study

### 3.1.1.1 Experimental layout

*Technical comparison (Figure 25A)*

RNA was isolated from a male Wistar rat and the titration series was performed with dilution steps of initially 10% and for the later steps 20% resulting in 7 samples, ranging from pure liver to pure kidney RNA (100%:0%, 90%:10%, 70%:30%, 50%:50%, 30%:70%, 10%:90%, 0%:100%; Liver:Kidney). Each sample was hybridized in technical triplicates on both platforms. The combination of biological differences in gene expression and the known inverse titration of both organs allow the assessment of the relative accuracy of each platform based on differentially detected genes and dilution effects.

*Biological comparison (Figure 25B)*

Liver samples from rats treated with low (50 mg/kg) or high (150 mg/kg) doses of Tet or a vehicle control were taken 6 h; 1 d or 3 d after treatment. RNA extraction was conducted as already described (see chapter 2 for details).

To obtain the *in vitro* samples, livers of male Wistar rats were perfused, primary hepatocytes isolated and cultured in SW format. Cells were treated with either vehicle control (0.5% DMSO) or Tet (low dose 40 µM or high dose 200 µM) twice, 72 h and 120 h after seeding. Cells were collected 6 h, 24 h and 72 h after the initial treatment. All samples were split, labelled according to the manufacturers' manuals and hybridized to either the Illumina RatRef-12 array or the Affymetrix Rat Genome 230 v2.0 array.

# 3 RESULTS AND DISCUSSION

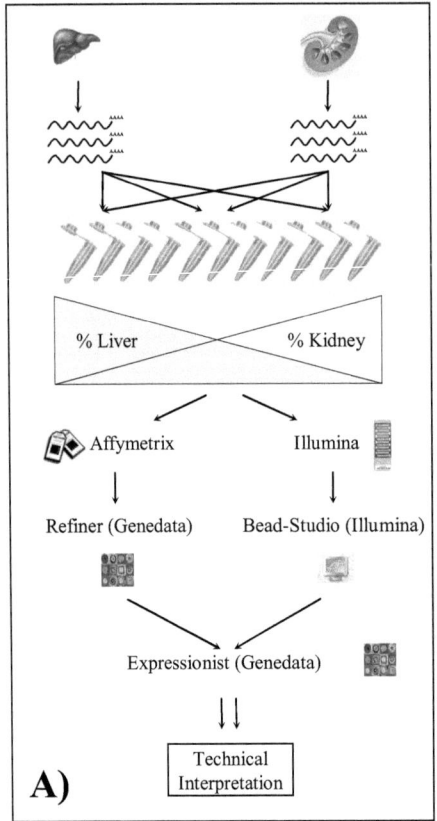
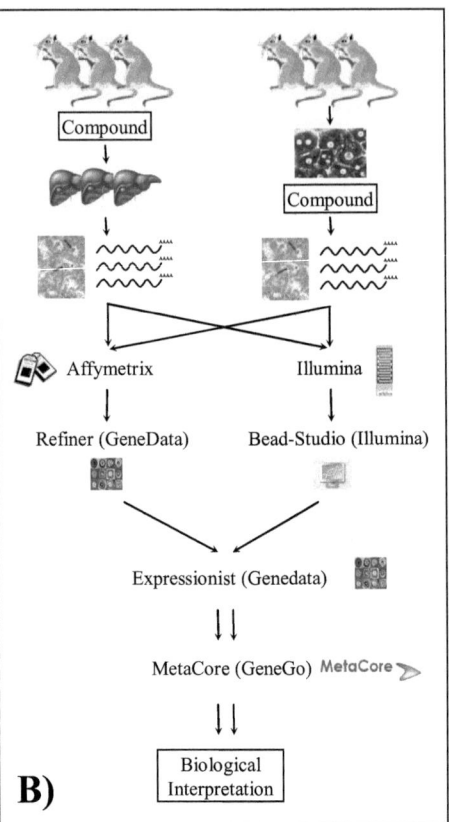

Figure 25: Experimental layouts of the studies conducted for comparing Affymetrix and Illumina global gene expression platforms. A) Technical comparison, a titration series between total RNA isolated from liver and kidney (100%:0%, 90%:10%, 70%:30%, 50%:50%, 30%:70%, 10%:90%, 0%:100%; liver:kidney). B) Biological comparison, an in vivo and an in vitro toxicogenomics studies were compared. Three biological replicates of either animals or hepatocytes in SW culture were treated with Tet at two doses.

*Data extraction and probe mapping*

Affymetrix data was extracted by the GCOS-Software, normalized with the RMA method and checked for quality parameters within the Expressionist®- Refiner software. Illumina data was processed and checked for quality in BeadStudio (Illumina). Data was imported into separate sessions of Expressionist®Analyst (Genedata), Illumina data was normalized with the LOESS-method, and both datasets were analyses in an analogous manner.

## 3 RESULTS AND DISCUSSION

Because of their differences in probe design and the fact that they are based on different versions of sequence databases, it is necessary to map the probe sequences contained on both chips to a common database version. This step was required because gene identifiers can change between different versions of the database due to new knowledge about specific genes or splice variants. There is a need to assure the identifiers of both platforms to characterize the same gene. Therefore, probe sequences from each platform were mapped to transcript sequences from RefSeq Release 19 (downloaded from ftp://ftp.ncbi.nih.gov/refseq/R_norvegicus/mRNA_Prot). A probe was defined as valid if it perfectly matched a transcript sequence and did not perfectly match any other transcript sequence with a different gene symbol. For Affymetrix probe sets, individual probes were determined to be valid by applying the definition above. Then probe sets were defined as valid if at least 80% of the probes within the set were valid. This procedure resulted in a gene list of 7,271 valid probes common on both platforms which was used in subsequent studies.

### 3.1.1.2  Intraplatform comparability

Due to technical differences the data produced by Illumina and Affymetrix contrast strongly in their intensity values. Therefore, the intraplatform comparability was examined by comparing the coefficients of variance (CV). The CV was used instead of the standard deviation because it is a dimensionless number and independent from the mean. CVs were calculated for each of the 7,271 valid genes using the 3 technical replicates for all samples of the titration series as well as the 3 biological replicates of the toxicogenomic dataset. The distribution of the replicate CV values of both platforms is shown as a series of box plots in Figure 26. The technical variance is directly compared to the biological variance arising from the individual differences of the animals used.

# 3 RESULTS AND DISCUSSION

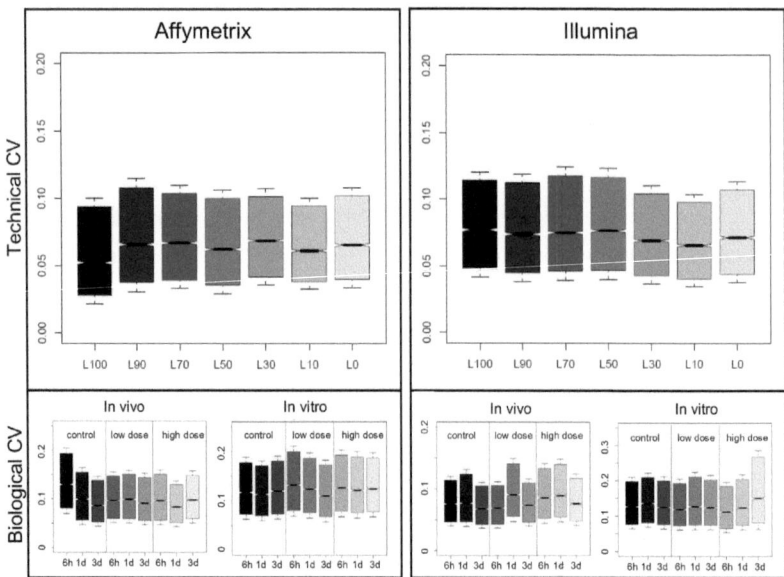

Figure 26: Box plots showing the distribution of the coefficients of variance (CV) for the 7,271 identically detected genes for the technical and biological replicates. The constriction of the bars denotes the median CV, the bars themselves include 50% of all CV values and the whiskers an additional 10%. The x-axis indicates the samples, the amount of liver RNA in the titration sample (L100 to L0) for the technical comparison and the time points of control, low and high dose for the biological comparison.

The median value of the technical variance for three replicates demonstrated analogous rates for both platforms. For Illumina, the CV was, with 7.3%, slightly higher than for Affymetrix (6.3%). The distribution of the CV values was also comparable and showed an asymmetrical shape. Thereby, the nature of the sample (Liver or Kidney) seems to have no effect on the result.

The median value for the biological variance ranged from 6.7% to 13.6%. For the *in vitro* samples measured with Illumina, it was only slightly higher than the median of the technical variance (7.8%). In contrast to this, the distribution of the CV values per gene was broader. Although the median of CV values is higher for *in vivo* samples measured with Affymetrix (9.8 %), their distribution is in the same range as for Illumina. The *in vitro* samples showed slightly, but not significantly, increased median CV values compared with the *in vivo* samples for both platforms (12.1% for Affymetrix and 12.7% for Illumina). The Isolation of hepatocytes and the time of incubation seem to be an additional factor that

# 3 RESULTS AND DISCUSSION

introduces variability into the gene expression data, although it is still within acceptable limits.

These findings correlate well with the results of the MAQC consortium (Shi et al., 2006; Klebanov & Yakovlev, 2007), where 5% to 15% of variance was reported for different global gene expression platforms (Affymetrix and Illumina were both below 10%).

Several reasons are responsible for these differences in the signal detection. Affymetrix and Illumina have fundamental differences in probe design and number of probes. Whereas Affymetrix uses a set of eleven 25mer oligonucleotides probes with perfect match and mismatch controls, Illumina instead uses 50mer oligonucleotides as probes in 30-fold redundancy. Sequence variations in the probe sets that target the same gene at different locations, the GC content, sequence length, intraplatform cross-match opportunities and the location of the probe sequence in relation to the 3'-end of the target gene might additionally cause different strengths of binding and therefore contribute to different levels of signal intensity. It has been shown that probes with complete sequence matches yield concordant results across platforms. There is a direct correlation between probe sequences and signal intensities for probes that target the same gene on different platforms (Pusztai, 2006).

## 3.1.1.3  Interplatform comparability

The interplatform comparison could only be performed indirectly. Due to their differences in probe sequences, labeling and hybridizing techniques, the resulting intensity values are fundamentally different. To overcome this problem, relative expression values between the titration samples and the 100% liver sample were calculated and compared. The relative expression values from the 7,271 commonly detected were collectively imported into Expressionist®Analyst and analyzed for common changes. Genes which had a more than 2-fold expression difference between liver and kidney samples and a pValue lower than 0.05 (ANOVA) were grouped according to their profile over the titration series with the help of SOM clustering (see chapter 2.2.5).

Six groups of genes were identified by SOM clustering (Figure 27). Groups E and F showed genes with a medium level expression in both tissues and a rising or falling expression profile with each dilution step and a close to linear slope in both platforms Groups A and B were similar but showed higher expressed genes reaching the saturation of intensity measurement. This results in a nonlinear increase of intensity.

# 3 RESULTS AND DISCUSSION

A subset of genes, contained in groups C and D, had showed no correlated or contradicting expression between both platforms. The intensity values of many (but not all) of those genes were close to the background level. Small variations in intensity therefore result in large fold change values and no clear concentration dependency can be detected.

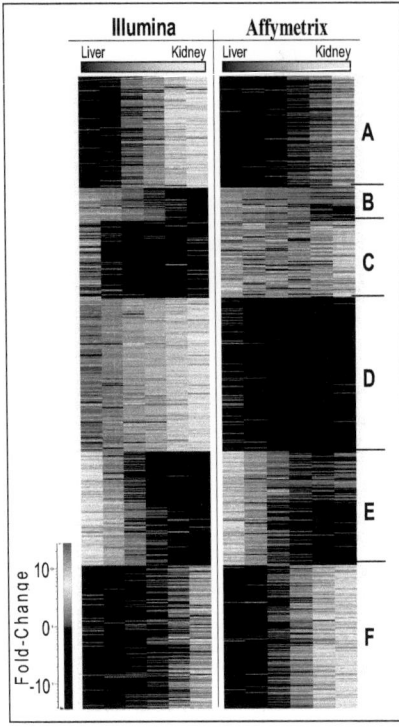

Figure 27: HeatMap generated by SOM-clustering of genes according to their fold change profile relative to the liver. The 7,271 commonly detected genes were filtered by a fold change ≥ 2 and a pValue of ≤0.05 between liver and kidney samples to retain only genes with a linear dependency. Clusters A, B, E and F contain genes shown to have equal tendencies across both Platforms, clusters C and D are a subset of genes with either no clear or contradictory tendency between both platforms.

The histogram shown in Figure 28 depicts the distribution of CVs of the titration experiment for both platforms. The value 1 indicates a perfect correlation and that the intensity values of the genes demonstrated the same behavior in the samples measured, -1 resembles negative correlation which means an inverse behavior. For Affymetrix, about 75% of the genes have a correlation of 1 to 0.9 and -1 to -0.9, for Illumina this value is 69%. The genes in between have lower linear dependency to the titration samples.

# 3 RESULTS AND DISCUSSION

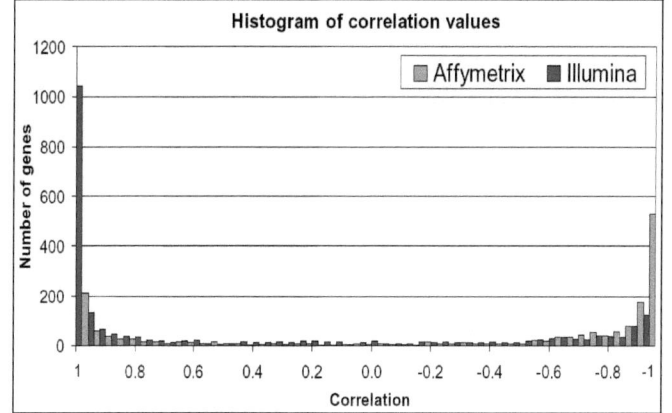

Figure 28: Histogram of the correlation coefficients of genes to the titration curve. The number of genes, found to have a more than 2 fold different expression levels in both tissues was plotted against their correlation values.

To further explore and validate these findings, the rat Tet toxicogenomics dataset was analyzed. Fold change values and pValues of this dataset were calculated for both platforms and each dose, time point and experiment type (*in vivo* or *in vitro*) relative to the time matched vehicle controls. The resulting gene lists were ranked either by the pValue (Figure 29A) or by the fold change (Figure 29B). The comparability between the gene lists was quantified using the "OrderedList" functionality of the Bioconductor R software (Lottaz et al., 2006).

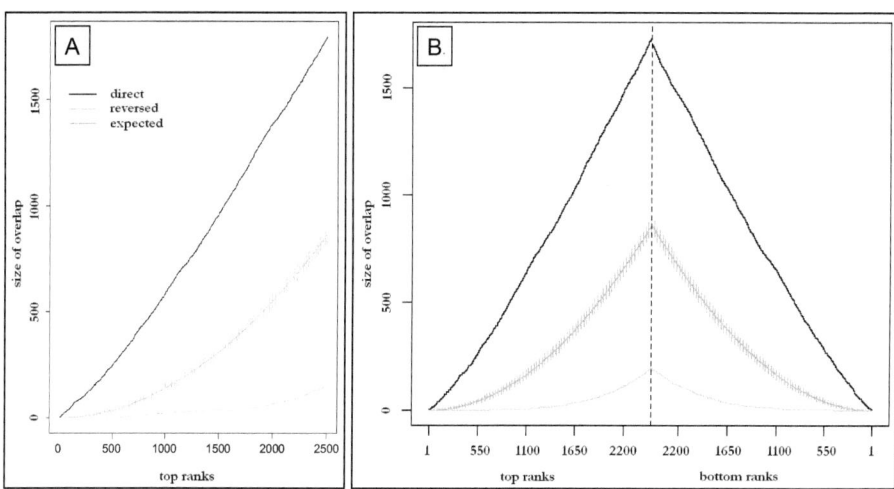

Figure 29: Gene list comparison (example shown for *in vitro*, high dose, 24 h). Genes have been ranked according to the p-Value (A) and to the extent of the fold change (B). The size of overlap of the top 500, 1000, 1500 etc. (labeling of the axis) genes of these lists were computed and compared to an overlap expected just by chance (middle line) and to the result obtained by reversing one of the two lists (lower line).

## 3 RESULTS AND DISCUSSION

Ranked gene lists were searched from the top (pValue ranked lists) or from both sides simultaneously (fold change ranked lists) for commonly occurring genes. The background of genes overlapping just by chance was calculated by comparing randomly perturbed gene lists 1,000 times. The negative control was obtained by inverting one of the two gene lists and comparing the top of one list with the bottom of the other.

The p-Values for the possibility to derive the obtained results just by chance were calculated (Appendix 2 and Appendix 13). The results show that the lists of top-ranked genes are highly saturated with genes detected by both platforms. Differences in the score indicating the overlap between the gene lists were detected and are plotted in Figure 30. The degree of overlap is strongly influenced by the nature of the samples. Gene lists of samples treated with low doses of Tet generally showed a lower analogy than others treated with high doses. In addition, time effects were seen *in vivo* and *in vitro*. The overlap of gene lists from both platforms is small 72 h after dosing compared to earlier time points. This can be explained by time dependent effects of Tet. The differences in scores between high and low doses of Tet *in vivo* or *in vitro* generally showed the same trend.

The highest overlap between the platforms for lists of genes was detected *in vivo* 6 h and *in vivo* and *in vitro* 24 h after high dose treatment. These are exactly the time points were the highest effect of the treatment was expected and are therefore best suited to analyze the effect of the compound on gene expression. Initial changes (6 h after dosing) leading to a high gene list overlap might be due to acute inflammatory effects. This would explain the discrepancy between *vivo* and *in vitro*. The latter is missing non parenchymal liver cell types, e.g. Kupffer cells, which are important for the induction and maintenance of inflammatory mechanisms.

# 3 RESULTS AND DISCUSSION

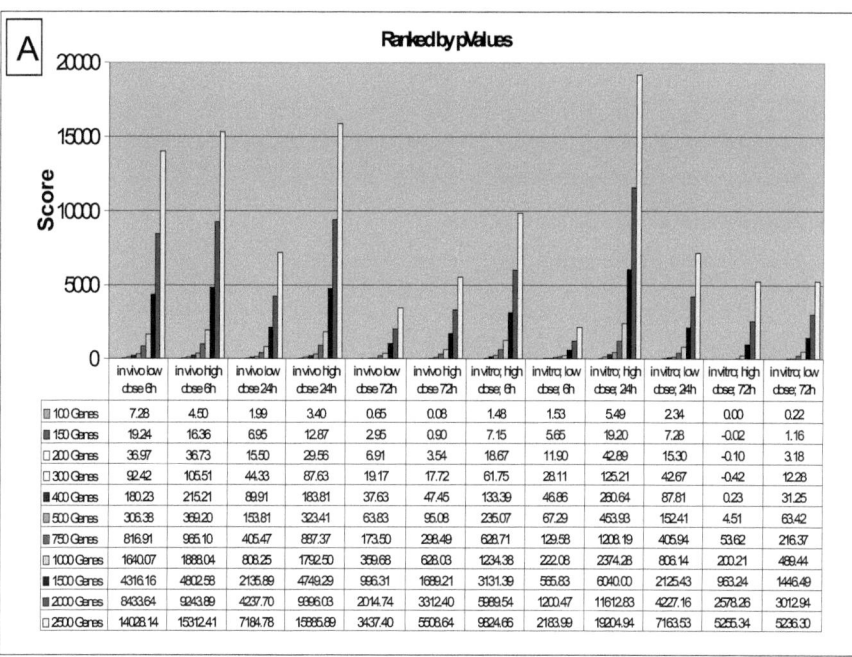

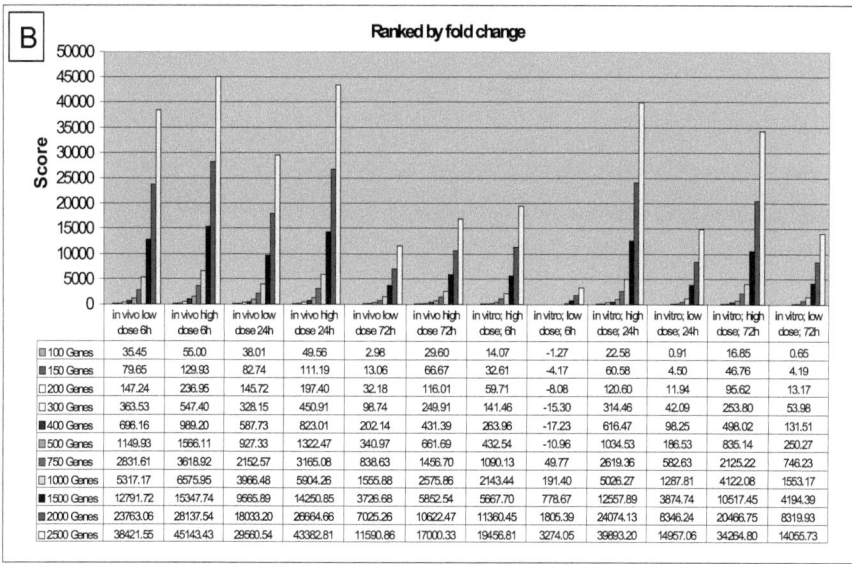

Figure 30: The difference of the scores calculated by the gene list overlap and the negative control were plotted for all the experiments. Scores were computed on the basis on the number of overlapping genes and reflect in principle a weighted sum of these values. A) Genes have been ranked by pValue; B) Genes have been ranked by fold change.

## 3 RESULTS AND DISCUSSION

These results were confirmed by a correlation analysis (
Figure 31). Both platforms showed a high concordance, with high correlation coefficients, between each other. There were only minor differences in the correlation coefficients compared to the vehicle control for the 72 h time point and the 24 h time point (low dose). Significantly lower correlation coefficients were detected 6 h after treatment for both doses and 24 h after treatment with the high dose.

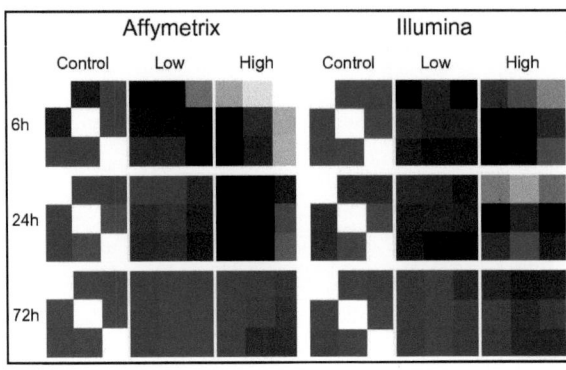

Figure 31: Correlation map of *in vivo* samples of tetracycline treated cells. Each square resembles one experiment; grey represents a high correlation, black represents medium correlation and white represents a low correlation.

Genes found to be changed in expression after treatment with Tet *in vivo* and *in vitro* (≥2-fold, pV≤0.05) were common within both platforms. Lowering the fold change value to 1.5 lowered the platform concordance to 88.2%. In most cases not only the direction but also the extent of deregulations was very analogous between both platforms.

These results show that the variance across technical replicates is in a satisfactory range and even the individual differences of biological replicates caused only a slight increase. Conducting biological replicates instead of technical replicates helps to increase the statistical significance and therefore the match between the results of Illumina and Affymetrix.

### 3.1.1.4  Biological interpretation

Whereas the histopathological analysis of the *in vivo* samples showed no abnormality (data not shown, see Zidek et al., 2007, the morphological analysis of Tet treated primary rat hepatocytes showed a clear accumulation of lipid droplets over time (Figure 32) Cells treated with high doses of Tet were more affected and showed additional signs of cellular damage. This proved that the mechanisms leading to microvesicular steatosis *in vivo* are also present *in vitro* and that the sandwich culture model therefore is a qualified tool to analyze the mechanistic basis of the toxic effects of Tet.

# 3 RESULTS AND DISCUSSION

The effect of treatment on gene expression can largely be seen 6 h after dosing *in vivo* and 24 h after dosing *in vivo* and *in vitro*. Whereas the effects endure *in vitro*, a recovery of the animals can be seen *in vivo*. Further analyses were accomplished within the Expressionist®Analyst software from Genedata and the biological interpretation was supported with MetaCore™ pathway analysis tools from GeneGo.

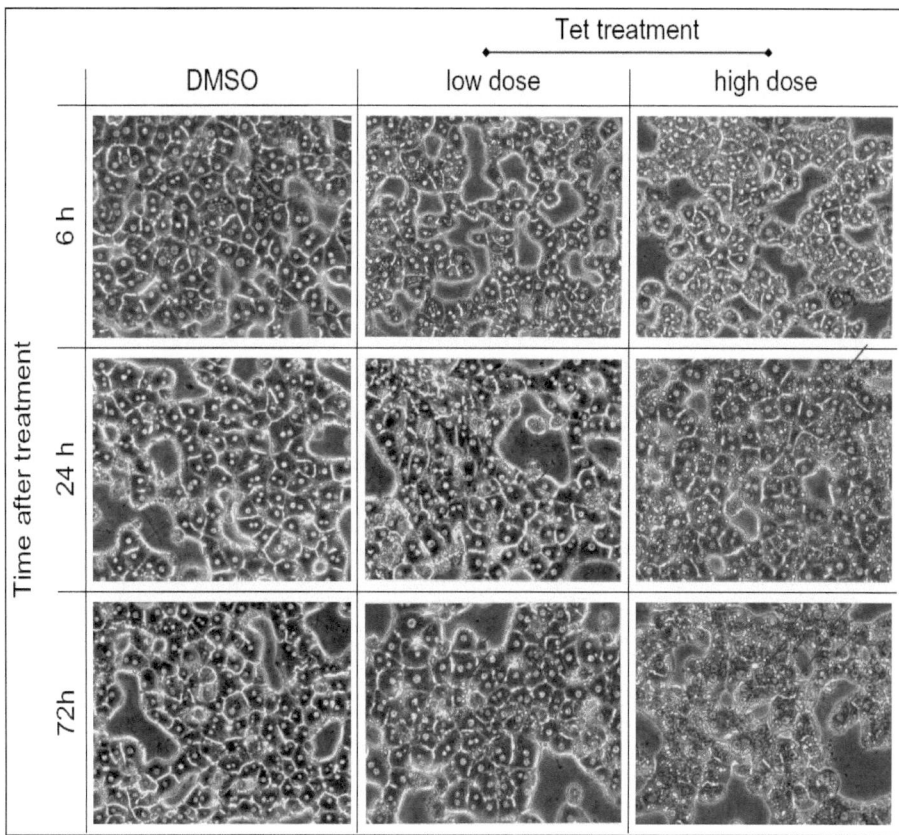

Figure 32: Primary rat hepatocytes treated with either DMSO (vehicle control) or low and high doses of Tet for 6/24/72 h. Cells were pre-cultured in sandwich culture for two days to acclimatise to the culture conditions and subsequently dosed with either 40µM or 200µM Tet. Both doses caused an accumulation of lipid droplets inside the cells and this effect was more pronounced in the high dose.

# 3 RESULTS AND DISCUSSION

Figure 33 shows a PCA which separated samples from both platforms of the *in vivo* (A and B) and *in vitro* (C and D) experiments. The PCA analysis shows the basic tendencies within the data, which resembles the biological effects of treatment.

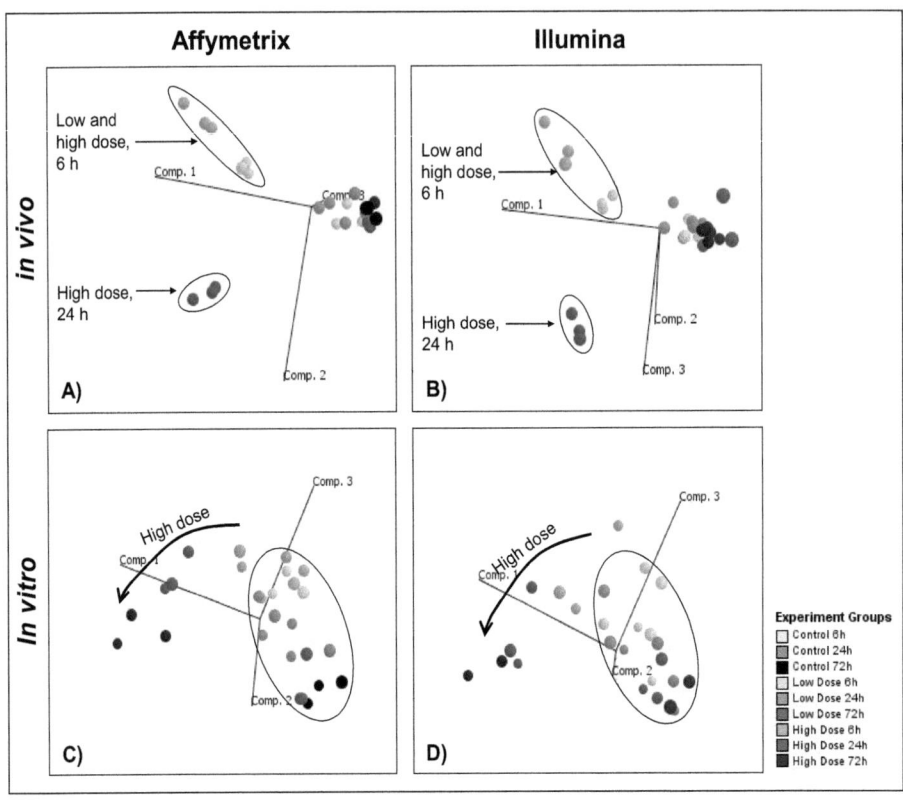

Figure 33: Principal components analysis (PCA) of the same datasets measured with Affymetrix Rat Genome 230 2.0 Array (A and C) and Illumina RatRef-12 Expression BeadChip arrays (B and D). Each point resembles the principal expression characteristics of all 7,271 common genes. The Tet *in vivo* study shows a clear separation of the experiments from the control group for both doses after 6 h and the high dose 24 h after treatment. *In vitro*, the separation is less clear after 6 h but high doses also separate at later time points.

The time and dose dependent effects were observed *in vivo* and *in vitro*. Vehicle controls, low dose treatment groups 24 h and 72 h after treatment and high dose group 72 h after treatment clustered closely together *in vivo*. Two separate clouds, one containing both dosing groups 6 h after treatment and the other with the high dose experiments 24 h after treatment, indicate a change in gene expression in these animals. Whereas both treatment

# 3 RESULTS AND DISCUSSION

groups caused similar gene expression changes after 6 h the gene expression of the low dose animals returned to the control level after 24 h. The high dose group after 24 h separated from all groups indicating more severe effects. After 72 h even high dose animals appeared to have returned to normal animal gene expression levels. This can be explained with the single dose treatment of the animals and the reversible effect of Tet.

*In vitro* (Figure 33 C and D) experiments showed related, but not identical, results to the *in vivo* samples. Due to the study design, where hepatocytes were dosed a second time 48 h after the first treatment, no regeneration effects were seen at 72 h. In fact, at 72 h even stronger effects were observed, indicating an increasing degeneration of these hepatocytes. The low dose experiments were not clearly separated from the controls, although they showed a tendency into the direction of the high dose experiments, indicating only a weak response to treatment.

The data from both *in vivo* and *in vitro* experiments are consistent across both platforms, which showed a high concordance of the 7,271 common genes. The high similarity between the PCAs show that not only the basal level but also any changes in gene expression after treatment were detected reliably by both Affymetrix and Illumina. The extent of these changes can be explained by the expected toxicity of Tet. The initial treatment caused an acute immune response in the animals, which was over in the low dose animals by 24 h. *In vitro*, the initial effects were less pronounced but subsequently, analogous tendencies were observed.

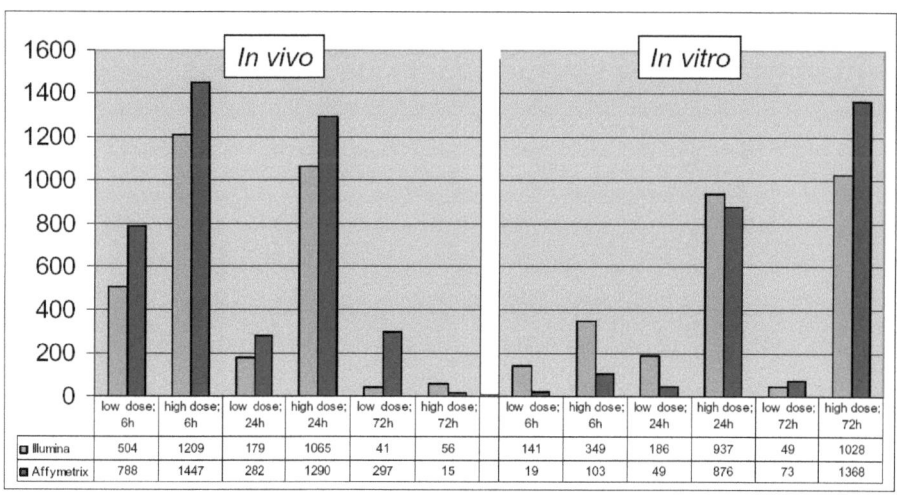

Figure 34: Number of genes significantly deregulated by treatment with Tet in either *in vivo* or *in vitro* experiments

# 3 RESULTS AND DISCUSSION

The findings of the previous analysis were reflected by the number of genes deregulated after treatment (Figure 34). In vivo, already 6 h after treatment a substantial number of genes were deregulated and the high dose had a greater impact than the low dose. 24 h After treatment, the high dose still showed strong deregulations in vivo whereas the low dose showed only minor alterations. After 72 h only slight disturbances in gene expression were observed.

The number of significantly deregulated genes in vitro rose only in the cells treated with high dose Tet over time. Cells treated with low doses were not noticeably affected. The early time point showed no substantial deregulation, indicating technical differences between in vivo and in vitro mechanisms. 24 h After the initial treatment, the number of genes deregulated rose to 937 (Illumina) and 876 (Affymetrix) and after 72 h a maximum of 1028/1368 deregulated genes was reached.

To get insights into the molecular mechanisms of Tet activity, the significantly deregulated genes (fold change > 1.5 and pValue < 0.05), measured with Affymetrix and Illumina, were analyzed using the MetaCore™ pathway analysis tool (GeneGo). To account for time as well as dose dependency, two different time points, 6 h and 24 h, and both doses were analyzed for the in vitro samples and 24 h and 72 h time points were analyzed for the in vivo experiments. Results were examined for biological affects and platforms compared

Gene expression changes caused by Tet treatment were involved in a variety of cellular processes (Table 9). The most affected pathways were associated with lipid metabolism followed by genes involved in signal transduction and cation homeostasis, inflammation, nucleotide and nucleic acid metabolism, protein and amino acid metabolism and cell cycle. Whereas no severe morphological effects could be detected 6 h after treatment, more than 500 genes were significantly deregulated more than 1.5-fold. Listed in Table 9 are the top seven up and down regulated pathway maps and GO processes. Already at this early stage, cholesterol, lipid and energy metabolism were inhibited by high dose treatment of Tet. At the same time, inflammatory processes, such as the JAK/STAT signalling, the immune response and the metabolism of nucleic acids were activated. Altogether, this suggests early perturbations may lead to the accumulation of fatty acids and triglycerides in the cell and to a loss of energy production. Early responses to cellular stress combined with an up regulation of nucleotide, RNA and protein synthetic process was also observed. The latter might be a compensatory process due to the inhibition of protein synthesis by high doses of Tet on the level of translation. The fact that the inflammatory response is

## 3 RESULTS AND DISCUSSION

mainly mediated by hepatic macrophages, the Kupffer cells, explains the lack of an early inflammatory response *in vitro*.

| Down regulated | | Up regulated | |
|---|---|---|---|
| GeneGo „maps" | GO processes | GeneGo „maps" | GO processes |
| Cholesterol Biosynthesis | Lipid metabolic process | PDGF signalling via STATs and NF-kB | Nucleotide and nucleic acid metabolic process |
| Regulation of lipid metabolism via LXR, NF-Y and SREBP | Cellular lipid metabolic process | Histamine H1 receptor signalling, immune response | RNA metabolic process |
| Regulation of fatty acid synthase activity | Positive regulation of chondrocyte differentiation | Immune response_IL1 signalling pathway | Biopolymer metabolic process |
| Triacylglycerol metabolism | Organic acid metabolic process | TPO signalling via JAK-STAT pathway | Primary metabolic process |
| Role of CDK5 in cell adhesion | Alcohol metabolic process | MIF-mediated glucocorticoid regulation | Macromolecule metabolic process |
| Glycolysis and gluconeogenesis | Steroid metabolic process | Apoptosis and survival TNFR1 signalling pathway | Regulation of cellular metabolic process |
| Unsaturated fatty acid biosynthesis | Carboxylic acid metabolic process | Leptin signalling via intracellular cascades | Cellular metabolic process |

Table 9: Top 7 "maps" and GO processes significantly affected 6 h after treatment *in vivo* (only results from Affymetrix are shown, Illumina generally delivered resembling results). Thresholds: Fold change≥1.5; P-value≥0.05.

24 h After treatment, Tet caused concordant changes in gene expression *in vivo* and *in vitro*. Table 10 shows the top ranked commonly affected maps and GO processes for both conditions. Besides the already consistent down regulation of lipid metabolism, amino acid metabolism was also affected. When there is a lack of energy in the cells, amino acids are used for energy production (Woolfson, 1983) and, because of the relationship between energy and nitrogen metabolism, an increase of urea synthesis. Accordingly, genes involved in protein catabolic pathways, such as proteosomal subunits, were activated and amino acid anabolic processes were inhibited.

Many intracellular signaling cascades were up regulated 24 h after dosing leading to large changes in gene expression (Table 10). The WNT signalling pathway is known to play multiple roles in hepatocytes, influencing the cytoskeletal composition, liver zonation and metabolism. Radisavljevic and González-Flecha showed in 2004 that oxidative stress

## 3 RESULTS AND DISCUSSION

activates signalling cascades essential for cell proliferation via sequential induction of mitogenic signalling genes, like phosphatidylinositol-3-kinase (PI3K), Akt and Ran (Radisavljevic & González-Flecha, 2004). Ran is a small GTPase that is essential for the translocation of RNA and proteins through the nuclear pore complex during interphase and has regulatory capabilities of mitotic spindle formation.

Also noticeable is the collective increase of several aminoacyl-tRNA synthetases and proteins involved in RNA processing and ribosomal biogenesis. This can be considered as a cellular reaction to the inhibition of protein synthesis.

Altogether, *in vivo* as well as *in vitro*, severe impairments of cellular metabolism, energy homeostasis and translation were detected and was consistent across both microarray platforms.

| Down regulated | | Up regulated | |
|---|---|---|---|
| GeneGo „maps" | GO processes | GeneGo „maps" | GO processes |
| Tryptophan metabolism | Carboxylic acid metabolic process | TGF, WNT and cytoskeletal remodelling | Nucleotide and nucleic acid metabolic process |
| Regulation of lipid metabolism via PPAR, RXR and VDR | Organic acid metabolic process | Signalling via PI3K/AKT and MAPK cascades | RNA processing |
| Peroxisomal branched chain fatty acid oxidation | Monocarboxylic acid metabolic process | RAN regulation pathway | tRNA metabolic process |
| Cholesterol biosynthesis | Lipid metabolic process | Cytoskeleton remodelling | Cellular metabolic process |
| PPAR regulation of lipid metabolism | Cellular lipid metabolic process | Signal transduction, AKT signalling | Ribosome biogenesis and assembly |
| Mitochondrial long chain fatty acid beta-oxidation | Fatty acid metabolic process | Chemokines and adhesion | Smooth endoplasmic reticulum calcium ion homeostasis |
| Leucine, isoleucine and valine metabolism | Nitrogen compound metabolic process | Aminoacyl-tRNA biosynthesis in cytoplasm | Endoplasmic reticulum calcium ion homeostasis |

Table 10: Top seven "maps" and GO processes significantly affected *in vivo* and *in vitro* 24 h after treatment with Tet. (Only the results from Affymetrix are shown, Illumina generally delivered resembling results) Thresholds: Fold change≥1.5; P-value≥0.05.

Hepatocytes were dosed a second time and therefore, no signs of recovery as seen in the animals from the *in vivo* experiments, were expected. Again, the top ranked pathways and

# 3 RESULTS AND DISCUSSION

GO processes illustrate the heavy impact of Tet on lipid and energy metabolism. The up regulation of ribosomal RNA production in the cells increases the need for new synthesized nucleotides indicated by the increased expression of genes involved in their synthesis (Table 11).

| Down regulated | | Up regulated | |
|---|---|---|---|
| GeneGo „maps" | GO processes | GeneGo „maps" | GO processes |
| Cholesterol Biosynthesis | Lipid metabolic process | Aminoacyl-tRNA biosynthesis in cytoplasm | RNA processing |
| Cytoskeleton remodelling | Cellular lipid metabolic process | Cell cycle_Role of SUMO in p53 regulation | Primary metabolic process |
| Cell adhesion_Plasmin signalling | Carboxylic acid metabolic process | Signal transduction_AKT signalling | Cellular metabolic process |
| Chemokines and adhesion | Organic acid metabolic process | GTP-XTP metabolism | Metabolic process |
| TGF, WNT and cytoskeletal remodelling | Monocarboxylic acid metabolic process | ATM/ATR regulation of G1/S checkpoint | Biosynthetic process |
| Propionate metabolism | Fatty acid metabolic process | CTP/UTP metabolism | tRNA metabolic process |
| Integrin outside-in signalling | Carbohydrate metabolic process | ATP/ITP metabolism | Cellular biosynthetic process |

Table 11: Top seven Maps and GO processes significantly affected *in vitro* 72 h after treatment with tetracycline. Thresholds: Fold change≥1.5; P-value≥0.05. (Again, only the results from Affymetrix are shown, Illumina generally delivered resembling results).

Both microarray platforms detected deregulations of genes involved in the cholesterol biosynthesis pathway. Although some of the genes could not be detected in all experiments, the biological interpretation from each was consistent. Cholesterol biosynthesis is closely associated with the metabolism of lipids. It is an extremely important biological molecule that has roles in membrane structure as well as being a precursor for the synthesis of steroid hormones and bile acids. The rate limiting step of this process is the conversion of acetyl-CoA to 3-hydroxy-3-methyl glutaryl-CoA by HMG-CoA synthase. This gene has a complex regulation and was found, together with other key-genes in this pathway, to be down regulated at multiple time points. One source for the acetyl-CoA molecules needed for the synthesis of cholesterol is the mitochondrial β-oxidation of fatty acids (Figure 35). Massive interruption of this process was observed by

# 3 RESULTS AND DISCUSSION

both platforms, which may be one trigger that caused the deposition of fatty acids and triglycerides in the cell. Fatty acid binding protein (FABP) was one of the few genes that were affected differentially *in vitro* and *in vivo*. Whereas it was down regulated *in vitro*, a strong induction *in vivo* was detected. *In vivo*, the regulation of FABP is closely connected to cholesterol biosynthesis and the cholesterol level in the cells (Montoudis et al., 2008). Even though this important protein was oppositely regulated, an accumulation of lipid droplets in cultured hepatocytes was taking place.

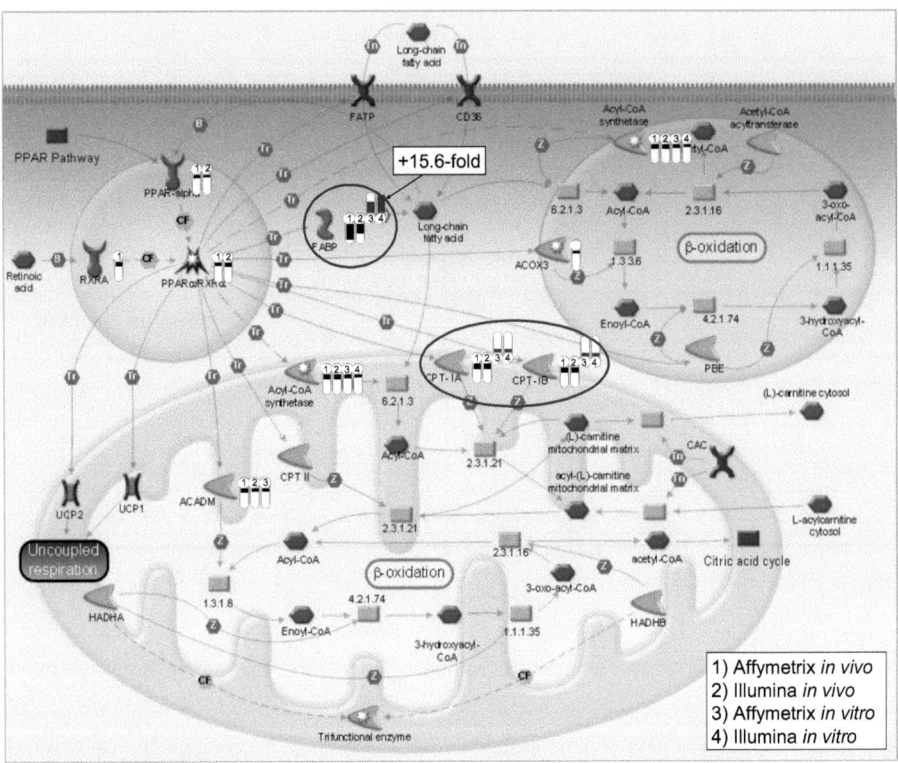

Figure 35: Transcriptional regulation of lipid metabolism by PPARα. The expression of several genes involved in this pathway was repressed. Deregulation is indicated by either rising or falling bars. The relative height resembles the extent of deregulation (modified from Metacore, GeneGO).

Perturbations in intracellular signalling are also connected with microvesicular steatosis. One of the top ranked pathways found to be affected was the Janus kinase-signal transducers and activators of transcription (JAK-STAT) signalling pathway. It plays an

# 3 RESULTS AND DISCUSSION

important role in the regulation of cellular development, growth and homeostasis and enables the cell to detect extracellular signals like cytokines, hormones, transporting them into the nucleus, consequently modulating gene expression by directly binding to promoter regions of genes. Waxman and his coworkers showed that cytochrome P450 enzymes, mainly Cyp2c11, are transcriptionally regulated by inhibition of this pathway (Waxman, 1999). Both, the deregulation of the JAK-STAT pathway, as well as the inhibition of xenobiotic metabolism, could be shown in this study with both microarray platforms.

Another consequence of activating the JAK-STAT cascade is the initiation of inflammatory processes and proliferation of the hepatocytes. Downstream genes of JAK-STAT signalling are important transcription factors, like c-Myc and NF-κB, which were also found to be activated by Tet treatment. c-Myc is, amongst many other functions, capable of driving cell proliferation by activating the expression of cyclins and inhibiting p21 expression. Gamma amino butyric acid (GABA), a neurotransmitter which also plays an important role in the regulation and inhibition of hepatocyte proliferation, was found to be consistently down regulated. Inflammatory processes were, analogous to the previous results, mainly seen 6 h after treatment and predominantly *in vivo*.

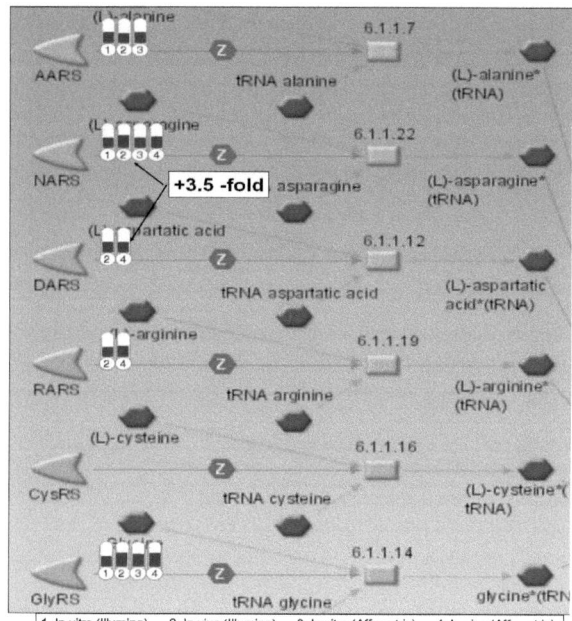

Figure 36: Induction of several aminoacyl-t-RNA synthetases (modified from Metacore, GeneGO).

# 3 RESULTS AND DISCUSSION

STAT has a very important role in cellular growth and differentiation mechanisms and is responsible for the up regulation of ribosomal RNA synthesis. Tet preferentially binds to 70S ribosomes of bacteria inhibiting protein synthesis, but, with a lower affinity, they also inhibit the functionality of the 80S ribosome of eukaryotic cells (Ogata et al., 2000). In fact, a massive change in protein synthesis and related processes was detected.

Several aminoacyl-t-RNA synthases, responsible for the generation of aminoacyl-t-RNA, were induced, both *in vivo* and *in vitro* (Figure 36).

Additionally, the induction of rRNA producing enzymes was observed, e.g. the induction of Polymerase I. tRNA synthetic processes and the generation of nucleoside triphosphates by the nucleoside diphosphate kinase (NDPK) (Figure 37A). At the same time, polymerase II, responsible for the transcription of mRNA, was repressed and genes belonging to the exosome complex, which is the key player in RNA degradation, were induced. Also downstream events of RNA-metabolic processes were affected. Furthermore, the initiation of translation- and elongation factors, such as eIF3 or eIE2B, was clearly induced. Rack1, eIF2 and eIF4E were only detected as significantly deregulated *in vivo* (Figure 37B). All these changes lead to an imbalance in RNA homeostasis and can be interpreted as a compensatory reaction of the cells to overcome the reduction of protein synthesis by the binding of Tet.

# 3 RESULTS AND DISCUSSION

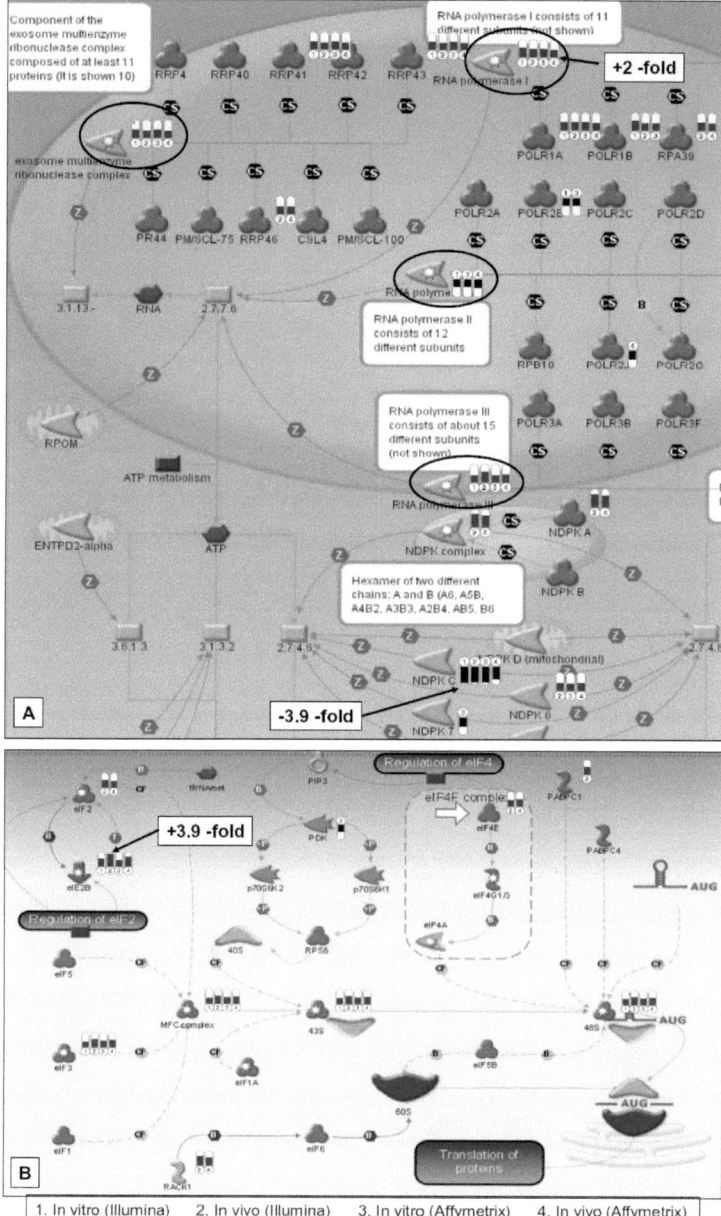

Figure 37: Perturbations in RNA metabolism. A) Details of the RNA and nucleotide homeostasis in cells. The RNA-polymerase I and the exosome were heavily induced whereas the RNA polymerase II was repressed (circles). B) Translation initiation, deregulation is indicated by either rising or falling bars. The relative height resembles the extent of deregulation (modified from Metacore, GeneGO).

# 3 RESULTS AND DISCUSSION

All the effects described above were detected as deregulated *in vivo* as well as *in vitro*. Both platforms yielded comparable results, with regard to the number of deregulated genes, the dimension of deregulation and therefore the biological interpretation was identical.

Besides the common effects of Tet on hepatocytes *in vivo* and *in vitro*, differences in cellular reactions were detected. The changes in gene expression 24 h after treatment were analyzed for mechanisms specifically affected only *in vitro* or only *in vivo*. Using the network building capability of MetaCore™, several networks, enriched with genes specific to either one of the two experiments, were generated and ranked by pValue (Table 12).

| Unique for Tet *in vitro* | | Unique for Tet *in vivo* | |
|---|---|---|---|
| Network | pValue | Network | pValue |
| protein transport (21.4%), establishment of protein localization (21.4%), regulation of JAK-STAT cascade (7.1%) | 3.41E-79 | DNA repair (25.0%), response to DNA damage stimulus (27.5%), DNA metabolic process (32.5%) | 1.69E-45 |
| cell cycle process (48.7%), cell cycle (48.7%), regulation of progression through cell cycle (41.0%) | 2.32E-33 | cell cycle phase (39.0%), cell cycle process (48.8%), mitotic cell cycle (36.6%) | 9.27E-22 |
| vitamin metabolic process (36.8%), ventricular cardiac muscle cell differentiation (28.9%), cardiac muscle cell differentiation (28.9%) | 1.87E-24 | intracellular signalling cascade (65.9%), protein kinase cascade (47.7%), signal transduction (79.5%) | 1.21E-11 |

Table 12: Top ranked networks based on genes detected only *in vivo* or *in vitro*.

Networks built from genes affected only *in vitro* were involved in the transport of proteins, parts of the JAK-STAT pathway, progression through cell cycle and induction of mitosis. Also mechanisms of cell adhesion and cellular reorganization were more pronounced than *in vivo*. On the other hand, mechanisms only affected *in vivo* were involved in DNA repair, inflammatory response and intra cellular signalling. The fact that both lists contained networks concerning cell cycle progression and other overlapping mechanisms indicate that the same underlying mechanisms were induced by Tet and that there might be different possibilities for the cell to fine-tune the exact regulation of gene expression.

# 3 RESULTS AND DISCUSSION

## 3.1.2 Conclusions of the platform comparison study

Eventhough major difference exists between the paltforms, a high degree of similarity and comparability of the results was found. In this study, two large datasets were analyzed to elucidate the intra- and inter-platform comparability of two commercially available global gene expression platforms, the RatRef-12 Expression BeadChip (Illumina) and the Gene Chip® Rat Genome 230 2.0 Array (Affymetrix). Both platforms have fundamental differences in design and layout. They are based on different versions of the RefSeq sequence database and use different algorithms to design their probes. A mapping of the probe sequences of both platforms to the actual RefSeq Release 19 allowed the comparison of genes perfectly matched by both platforms. This mapping reduced the number of valid genes to 7,271 which were used in subsequent studies. The substantial size of the study provided the possibility to assess the characteristics of intra- and inter-platform differences with great statistical significance and to analyze the dataset in several different ways.

The technical variation of the data, shown by the CV values, was lower than 10% showing a good repeatability of both techniques. The interplatform comparison was more susceptible to variances. Due to the complexity of producing these types of platforms, concentration variations of reagents during reverse transcription, the effect of time and performance and the personal factor contribute to this variability. One should be aware that only a few of these basic causes can be eliminated. Microarray techniques are very sensitive to deviations and need a high level of standardization to minimize extraneous influences

The titration experiment demonstrated the sensitivity of both platforms. The measurement of a linear increase of intensity values was possible for medium expressed genes, whereas saturation effects for highly expressed genes were visible. However, a set of genes showed no correlation between the platforms. Due to the identical samples measured on both platforms, there are mechanisms which may be causative for this observation. Most importantly, the location of the probe (-set) on the target cRNA sequence contributes to the variability of expression results. Stafford and Brun (2007) showed a correlation between the probe distance and measured results. Additionally, longer probe sequences, as used by Illumina (50mers), are less sensitive to degraded cRNA and possess different binding efficiencies. Differences in condensing algorithms, the data extraction and the multiple possibilities to analyze of the data also had great influence on the platform performance. Finally, a greater amount of genes showed no linear

## 3 RESULTS AND DISCUSSION

dependency if measured with Illumina suggesting saturation effects for the high expressed genes.

Ranking genes by fold change gave more reliable results than pValue ranked lists. Fold changes were calculated by comparing the measured intensity values directly whereas the pValue incorporates the signal to noise ratio. Combining the fold change based approach with the statistical significance (pValue) additionally increased the overlap.

The robustness of both microarray platforms was tested by applying a "real life" toxicogenomic test study. The implementation of biological replicates increased the variance in gene expression. Nevertheless, the concordance of ranked gene lists generated by pValue or fold change showed a large overlap. The size of this overlap was heavily dependent on the biological context of the samples and increased together with the number of genes deregulated by compound treatment. The data from the *in vitro* experiments seem to be more variable, the medians of the CVs tended to be higher than from the *in vivo* experiments. One possible explanation for this is the cellular stress caused by the perfusion and subsequent cell culture. Many changes in gene expression are caused during the perfusion procedure and related to the switching of hepatocytes from $G_0$-phase of the cell cycle back into $G_1$-phase (Papeleu et al., 2006). Additionally, it is also associated with various other effects like cytoskeletal perturbation (Baker et al., 2001; Chapman et al., 1973), dedifferentiation (Bayad et al., 1991), activation of immune response (Li et al., 2001), induction of apoptosis (Zvibel, Smets & Soriano, 2002; Czaja, 2002), the loss of polarization (LeCluyse, Audus & Hochman, 1994; Luttringer et al., 2002) and the activation of several intracellular signalling pathways (De Smet et al., 1998; Elaut et al., 2006a; 2006b; Boess et al., 2003).

A strong effect of time in culture on the variability between biological replicates may help explain the increased CV. However, this was not observed and it can be assumed that the effects of isolating the cells and culturing them in sandwich culture are only a minor reason for the increased CV. The fact that for the *in vivo* study a different rat strain (Sprague-Dawley) was used than for the *in vitro* study (Wistar) may be a significant cause for the variance observed.

This conformity of detection was also seen in the Tet toxicogenomic study. The data from both platforms, analyzed separately, led to the same biological conclusions. Although there might be a bias introduced by probe mapping and selection in terms of biological content, both platforms clearly showed the proposed mechanisms of action of Tet. Inhibition of the mitochondrial β-oxidation together with impaired intracellular RNA and protein homeostasis are mechanisms leading to the accumulation of lipids and

# 3 RESULTS AND DISCUSSION

triglycerides in the cells, which *in vivo* leads to the toxic endpoint, microvesicular steatosis. Contributing to this toxicity might be the increased protein catabolism causing the liberation of nitrogen, which is normally removed from the cell through urea production or is reused through the citric acid cycle. Both pathways were also affected by treatment with Tet and are therefore contributing to its mechanism of toxicity.

The results of this study clearly show that both global gene expression techniques can be considered equally qualified and can be used for further toxicogenomic studies. Additionally, new details of the mechanisms of action of Tet were elucidated. Interestingly, these mechanisms were detected with high concordance not only *in vivo*, but also *in vitro*. The combination of an *in vitro* cell culture model with global gene expression approaches will facilitate the process of investigating mechanisms of action and in the prediction of possible toxic risk factors earlier then currently possible.

# 3 RESULTS AND DISCUSSION

## 3.2 Establishment of a longer term cell culture of primary rat and human hepatocytes

A recent report on the root causes of failed drugs over the last 10 years stated that hepatotoxicity and cardiovascular toxicity are the main reasons (Schuster, Laggner & Langer, 2005). Hepatotoxicity in humans has the poorest correlation to regulatory animal testing with only half of the cases of human hepatotoxicity found in clinical trials being confirmed with concordant signals in animal toxicity studies (Olson et al., 2000). The development of new, more predictive models for hepatotoxicity screening is therefore crucial for the improvement of the drug developmental process. The replacement of animal tests by *in vitro* methods allows the combination of early screening and mechanistic studies and the realisation of the 3R principle. Currently, there are several *in vitro* models used for screening for hepatotoxicity, each of these models with its own advantages and drawbacks with regards to availability, throughput, viability of the cells over time and the opportunity to analyse multiple of parameters (chapter 1.5). The process of dedifferentiation of hepatocytes leading to a loss of liver specific functions, as well as the complexity of other models that do not allow their use in a higher throughput, are two of the main limitations restricting hepatocyte use in toxicological screening or basic research. At the same time, the possibility to perform experiments under strictly controlled and standardized laboratory conditions is favourable. The refinement of the existing primary hepatocyte cultures, allowing their use for longer term toxicity testing, will be a step towards the acceptance of these techniques as standard screening methods and will help to reduce animal testing. The opportunity to increase incubation times allows one to study long-term effects and also to apply pharmacologically relevant concentrations of the test compound. Since the number of cells needed for the analysis of a specific parameter is usually low, multiple experiments can be conducted with one batch of cells at the same time, making it possible to obtain various data from the same source.

The careful selection of endpoints, with respect to the relevance to the *in vivo* systems, is of great importance. One has to be aware that cells are always in contact with their surrounding tissue, other cell types and receive multiple signals from the entire organism under *in vivo* conditions and that these complex networks are not present *in vitro*. All results from isolated hepatocytes, as a mono-factorial model, have to be analyzed against this background.

# 3 RESULTS AND DISCUSSION

Hepatocytes cultured in monolayer (ML) not only loose 75% of their total CYP450 during the first 24h after isolation, but also other liver specific functions and differentiation markers (Gómez-Lechón et al., 2004; Davila & Morris, 1999; Farkas & Tannenbaum, 2005a). Several attempts to optimize the culture conditions have been reported, including the use of extracellular matrix (ECM) material, such as matrigel overlay (Schuetz et al., 1988) or collagen in a sandwich conformation (LeCluyse et al., 1994), the use of optimized culture medium (Enat et al., 1984), medium supplements (Sidhu & Omiecinski, 1995) and co-culture with other cell types (epithelial cells, sinusoidal cells or Kupffer cells) (Begue et al., 1994; Donato, Castell & Gómez-Lechón, 1994). These improvements allow the hepatocytes to regain cellular morphology, polarisation and to maintain physiological rates of albumin secretion (Dunn et al., 1991). Whereas the classically used monolayer culture is not suited for longer time culture of hepatocytes, the sandwich culture has proven to maintain some liver specific features for longer times, at levels comparable to *in vivo* conditions (Kern et al., 1997; Dunn et al., 1989) and to slow down the process of dedifferentiation (Tuschl & Müller, 2006).

## 3.2.1 Morphological and functional characterization of primary rat hepatocytes

Hepatocytes were isolated from male Wistar rats using a modification of the two-step perfusion method described by Seglen (Seglen, 1976). Cell viability was assessed by trypan blue dye exclusion and hepatocytes with >85% viability were plated as described previously. After seeding, cells appeared rounded and distinct from each other. In our laboratory, the SW culture was established using collagen I as an extracellular matrix environment, a serum free, amino-acid rich media composition (DMEM-F12) and dexamethasone and ITS as supplements (chapter 2.2.1). This culture was compared to rat hepatocytes cultured in ML culture with and without the addition of serum and SW culture with the addition of serum.

### 3.2.1.1 Morphological examinations

Cells were examined for morphological changes after seeding every day for up to two weeks. Already 4h after seeding, when media was changed from seeding media to culture media, a morphological distinction was seen between ML and SW cultures. Cells in ML had already regained their polygonal shape and started to establish extensive cell-cell

## 3 RESULTS AND DISCUSSION

contacts, whereas SW-cultured cells remained spherical and isolated for a longer period of time, probably resulting from the cells´ immersion in the three dimensional ECM environment of the collagen gel (Figure 38). Cells in monolayer spread out and had a more flattened morphology, mainly due to their attempt to establish contact with the ECM, whereas cells cultured in SW, after an initial delay, remained polygonal in shape. Initially, the cytoplasm appeared clear and membranes were smooth in both culture systems.

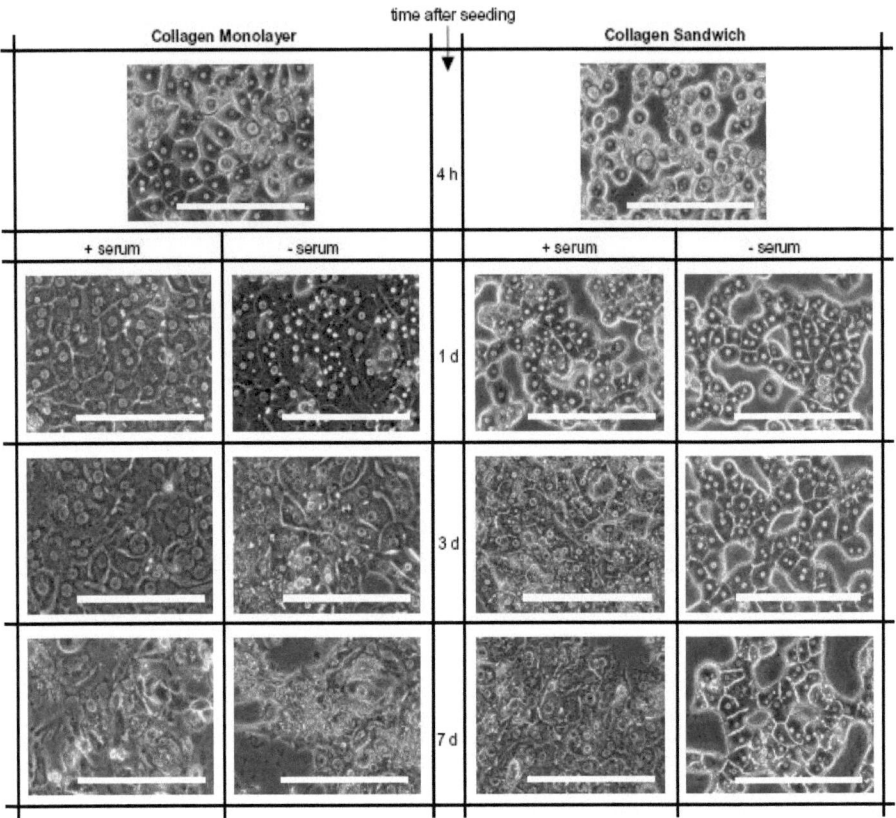

Figure 38: Effect of ECM environment and media formulation on morphological development and structural integrity of primary rat hepatocyte cultures. Cells were cultured for the indicated times on collagen monolayer or in a collagen gel sandwich with serum-free or serum-containing medium. Arrows indicate bile canaliculi-like structures. The white scale bar in the bottom right of each image corresponds to 200 µm.

One day after seeding, cells in all types of culture had made contact with each other and started to build structures which are described as bile canaliculi (Gautam, Ng & Boyer;

# 3 RESULTS AND DISCUSSION

1987; LeCluyse et al., 1994). The number and distinctiveness of these structures increased in cells cultured without serum, which is consistent with the findings of Terry and Gallin, who reported an inhibitory effect of serum on the formation of bile canaliculi (Terry & Gallin, 1994). Over time, cells in monolayer spread out until confluency and therefore had a flattened appearance, accompanied by an increase in the size of the nucleus. There were no longer well-delineated plasma membrane borders and bile canaliculi-like structures disappeared almost entirely. They moved towards each other and built clusters of cells. This was accompanied by the a more fibroblast-like morphology. Together, this depicts the dedifferentiation process in ML with and without serum. The cytoplasm of cells cultured with serum appeared granulated and inclusion bodies were first detected on day 3. In contrast to this, cells cultured in SW without serum displayed a stabile polygonal morphology with extensive bile canaliculi networks and a clear cytoplasm. This was true up to 14 days of culture. Cellular mobility and re-entry into the cell cycle was observed for cells cultured with serum and cells cultured in ML which started detaching from the culture plate surface. All these findings are in accordance with previously reported effects of serum, the overlay of cells with ECM-material and media supplementation (Dunn et al. 1989; Musat et al., 1993; LeCluyse et al., 1994; Tuschl & Müller, 2006).

It has been reported that changes induced by perfusion, morphological changes and intracellular energy and redox homeostasis are related to the dedifferentiation processes of hepatocytes (Greetje et al., 2006). However, the restoration of cell polarity combined with the regeneration of bile canaliculi and gap junctions leads to an increased expression of liver specific genes and a preservation of liver functions (Wilkinson & Dickson, 2001; Hamilton, Westmorel & George, 2001; LeCluyse et al., 1994). Since hepatocyte differentiation, drug metabolism and toxicity are inherently linked, the liver specific metabolic capability should ideally be maintained on *in vivo* level for as long as possible.

To acquire deeper insights into the functionality of the cultured hepatocytes, several cell type specific functions were examined. One of the most important features of hepatocytes is their ability to metabolise xenobiotics (chapter 1.3). The concentration of the specific CYP isoforms, regulated in multiple ways, has a major impact on the cells metabolic activity. Several transcription factors are responsible for the differential expression (Table 13), but a high degree of cross talk and interactive regulation has been reported (Yan & Caldwell, 2001; Guengerich, 2003; Dickins, 2004).

# 3 RESULTS AND DISCUSSION

| Enzyme | Transcription factor | Inducer | Substrates | Percentage of total CYP-enzyme in liver |
|---|---|---|---|---|
| CYP 1A1 | AhR | BNF | Polycyclic aromatic hydrocarbons | 1.2 |
| CYP 2b | CAR | PB | Cyclophosphamide, Nicotine | 1.9 |
| CYP 2C | GH/CAR/PXR | PB | Retinoids | 65 |
| CYP 3A | PXR/CAR/GR | Dex | various substrates | 14.6 |

Table 13: List of CYP isoforms tested in this study with appropriate transcription factors, potent inducers, typical substrates and their overall abundance in liver.

### 3.2.1.2 CYP inducibility

During this study, the inducibility of the CYP 1A, 2B, 2C and 3A isoforms was used as a sign of cell viability and differentiation status. Cells were cultured in ML and SW culture as previously described and dosed at 0 h, 3 d and 9 d with the appropriate inducer for 48 h. CYP 1A1 was induced with β-naphthoflavone (BNF; 10µM), CYP 2B and 2C with phenobarbital (PB; 500µM) and CYP 3A with dexamethasone (Dex; 50µM). The expression of specific CYP mRNAs was determined by TaqMan-PCR and the relative enzyme activity was measured using specific spectrophotometric methods (results were generated as part of a joint work with Gregor Tuschl, PhD-student).

Figure 39 shows that at early time points, the cells were still responsive to CYP induction. CYP 1A was heavily induced on the mRNA level in ML (160-fold) whereas in SW-culture the induction was only about 55-fold. Interestingly, on the enzyme activity level the activity of CYP 1A in SW culture superimposed the activity in ML. On the mRNA level, the inducibility of CYP 1A was consistent over time. In contrast, the induction of enzyme activity decreased over time in both culture systems. After 3 days, the activity of CYP 1A was 6 fold higher than the controls in ML and still 32-fold higher in SW. After 9 d in culture, CYP 1A could no longer be induced in ML but still reached 18-fold induction in SW culture. In general, cells remained much more responsive to CYP 1A induction in SW culture, where after 9 d in culture marked increase of enzyme activity was still detected.

# 3 RESULTS AND DISCUSSION

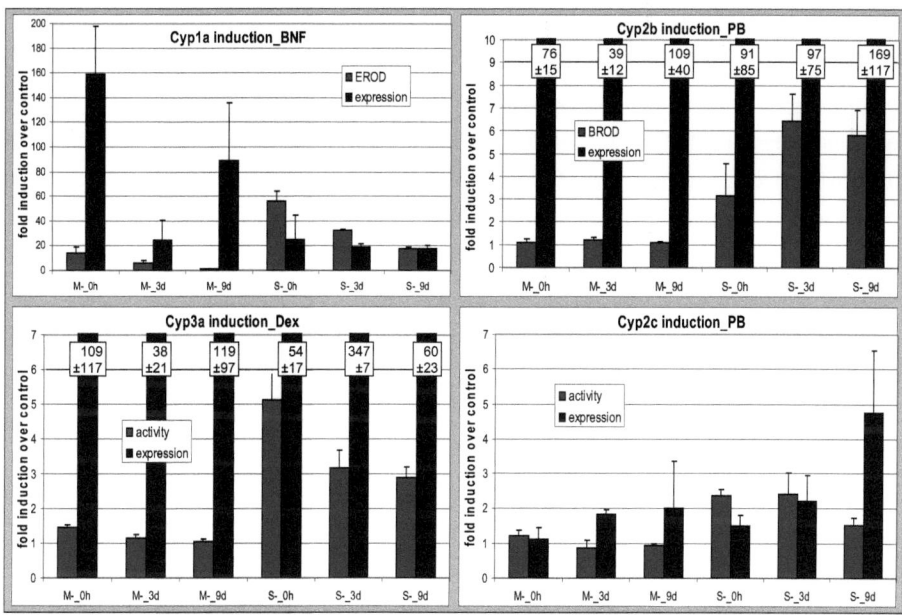

Figure 39: Relative induction of enzyme activity and mRNA expression for CYP1A, 2B, 3A and 2C. Depicted are the results of two cell cultures, ML and SW without serum. Cells were induced with either 10 µM BNF, 50 µM PB or 500 µM Dex on days 0, 3 or 9 of culture and samples were taken 48h after induction. Bars illustrate changes in enzyme activity (light bars) or mRNA expression (dark bars) relative to time matched vehicle controls. Bars illustrate mean values of fold induction from triplicate measurements with standard deviation.

The responsiveness of cells to PB and Dex mediated CYP 2B and CYP 3A induction was stable over time in both types of culture. The mRNA levels of CYP 2B and CYP 3A were about 50-100 times higher than in the uninduced control. Differences between both culture conditions were again detected on the enzyme activity level. Whereas no induction in enzyme activity was detected for ML culture, both enzymes were induced in SW culture at all time points. The activity level was 3-7 times above the control level and inducibility was retained until the end of the culture period.

Unlike the other CYPs, CYP 2C was neither inducible on the mRNA nor on the enzyme activity level in ML culture at the 0 h time point. Over time no increase was detected on the activity level, but mRNA expression was two fold induced at later time points. In SW culture, a small increase (about 2-fold) was initially detected for activity and expression. The inducibility of CYP 2C mRNA expression increased over time up to 5 fold after nine days of culture. In contrast the enzyme activity inducibility remained stable over time.

## 3 RESULTS AND DISCUSSION

Additional western blot analyses showed good correlations with the previous results of gene expression and protein activity tests. Isolated protein was separated by SDS-PAGE, proteins were blotted and subsequently CYP isoforms were detected with specific antibodies. Figure 40 shows examples of the results for CYP 1A1, 2B and 3A1. The determined signals were detected at a molecular weight between 50 – 60 kDa and are therefore in good agreement with the calculated molecular weights of the CYP isoforms at 59 kDa, 56 kDa and 57 kDa, respectively.

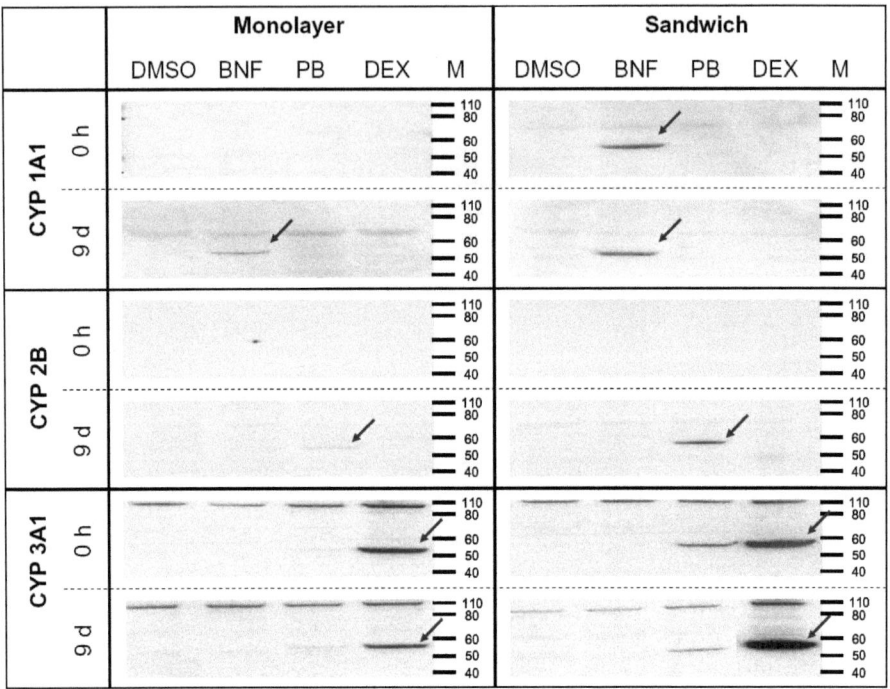

Figure 40: Protein extracts of induced hepatocytes were separated by SDS-PAGE and CYP isoforms were subsequently detected by western blot analysis as described. The arrows highlight the induced CYP-isoforms.

CYP 1A1 was unchanged at 0 h but was weakly induced on protein level after 9 d in ML-FCS culture by BNF. In contrast to this, CYP 1A1 already was induced at the early time point in SW-FCS culture and inducibility endured over the time of culturing. The CYP 2B isoform could not be induced at the starting point in either culture but after 9 d, PB caused a slight increase in both cultures which was more pronounced in SW-FCS culture. The CYP 3A1 isoform was induced in both types of cell culture at all time points by DEX.

# 3 RESULTS AND DISCUSSION

Whereas the decreasing signal intensity over time for ML-FCS cultured cells implicates a decreasing inducibility, SW-FCS cultured cells showed exactly the opposite effect. Additionally, cells cultured in SW-FCS exhibited an increased level of CYP 3A1 after treatment with PB, which could also be seen on the activity level (data not shown) and which was not true for cells cultured in ML-FCS conformation.

In general, the enzyme activity and the inducibility on mRNA and protein level of the CYP isoforms tested was higher and more stable over time in SW culture. This is an indication of a higher capability and a more differentiated status of these cells.

### 3.2.1.3 Canalicular transport

The reestablishment of cell-polarity, the formation of bile canaliculi together with the expression of genes encoding for the transport of xenobiotics are a prerequisite for functional transport processes in cultured hepatocytes. It was previously demonstrated that SW-cultured hepatocytes re-established functional polarity and form bile canaliculi at their contact sites (LeCluyse et al., 1994; Talamini, Kappus & Hubbard, 1997). The ATP-dependent canalicular anion transporter Mrp2 (Multidrug resistance-associated protein 2) is responsible for the transport of multivalent organic anions, including glutathione and glucuronide conjugates (Akerboom et al., 1991; Elferink et al., 1995). As canalicular efflux may be the rate limiting step in biliary excretion of xenobiotics, the influence of culture conditions on the functionality of according transporters was examined. Cells were incubated with carboxy-DCFDA, a fluorescent substrate for Mrp2, and therefore the dye efflux from hepatocytes cultured in either ML or SW culture into the bile canaliculi was determined over time.

At the beginning of the culture, on day 0, no canalicular structures were seen and consequently, no transport was detected. Together with the reestablishment of cellular polarity, canalicular structures developed at the contact site of cells with longer times. As previously stated, these structures were more pronounced in cells cultured without the addition of serum and were more stable in SW culture. The fluorescent substrate accumulated in cells without contact to other cells. It was transported out of the cells only if the canalicular structures in between the cells were established (Figure 41).

After 3 days in culture, only cells cultured in SW culture without serum showed pronounced canalicular networks which remained active until the end of culture on day 9. As expected, other culture methods were unable to to obtain transport activity of the substrate. After 3 days in ML culture, some cells appeared to have integrated the

## 3 RESULTS AND DISCUSSION

fluorescent substrate into granular structures of the cell (Figure 41, arrow 1). This could be caused by Mrp2 molecules being accumulated in intra-hepatocytic vesicles. Previous studies showed the storage of hepatic transporters inside the cell where they are delivered to the canalicular domain following increased physiological demand (Wakabayashi, Kipp & Arias, 2006; Kipp & Arias, 2002). The lack of cellular polarization and canalicular structures may cause an accumulation of these vesicles.

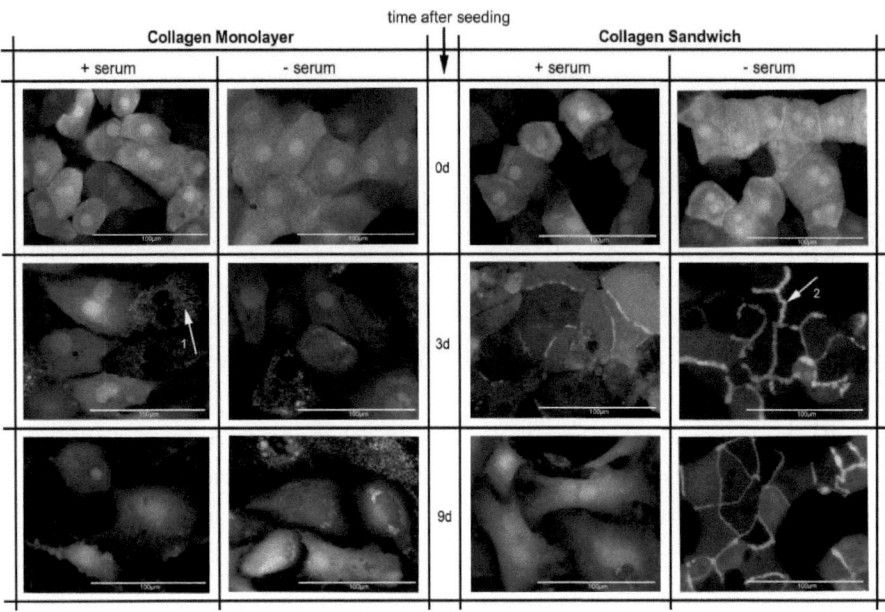

Figure 41: Microscopic pictures of hepatocytes cultured in ML and SW with and without serum. To visualize canalicular transport processes, they were incubated with carboxy-DCFDA and cells were cultured for up to 9 d. Arrows indicate 1) the accumulation of the dye in granular structures and 2) the accumulation of the dye in canalicular structures.

### 3.2.1.4 Conclusions of the morphological and functional data

Primary hepatocytes are a widely used model to study acute toxic effects or drug metabolism. Primary cultures of isolated hepatocytes, as a mono-factorial model, display most of the metabolic liver functions and are therefore well suited for this purpose.

The use of strict standardization, higher throughput and consistent capabilities of primary cells for toxicological issues are major advantages of *in vitro* systems. A lot of work has been undertaken to establish and optimize a culture method for primary hepatocytes that

## 3 RESULTS AND DISCUSSION

overcomes the disadvantages of dedifferentiation. The study described above showed clearly that the environment of an *in vitro* culture has a critical impact on liver specific functionality of primary hepatocytes, including morphology, gene and protein expression, as well as the loss of other cell type specific attributes. The beneficial effects of ECM overlay in SW culture showed an ability to retain a differentiated status and some important liver specific functions, like albumin secretion, biliary transport processes or metabolism (Dunn et al., 1989; LeCluyse et al., 2000; LeCluyse et al., 1994). The time of culture could thus be prolonged up to several weeks without severe morphological changes (suggesting reduced dedifferentiation). By optimizing the media composition and a careful selection of media supplementation, the formation of functionally active bile canaliculi was promoted. In this chapter, the beneficial effects of ECM overlay on the survival rate, on cell morphology and several essential functional aspects of hepatocytes were clearly shown. Already the morphological examination of primary hepatocytes over time showed distinct differences in cellular behavior in different cell cultures. Cells cultured in SW-FCS were organized in acinar structures characteristic of the tissue of origin (Farkas & Tannenbaum, 2005b; LeCluyse et al., 2000). Further details of improved structural components have been previously described by Davila (Davila & Morris, 1999).

In addition to the polygonal shape, the three dimensional environment has positive effects on gene expression. The SW-FCS culture showed not only the preservation of morphological properties but also an increased inducibility of several CYP isoenzymes, both on the level of gene, on protein expression and on the enzymatic activity. These results are in agreement with other researchers, who also reported improved viability and phase 1 metabolism (LeCluyse et al., 1994; Dunn et al. 1989; Tuschl & Müller, 2006; Gebhardt et al., 2003; Hamilton et al., 2001), even when other media compositions or Matrigel was used. The key signal for this improvement therefore seems to be the introduction of a third dimension by plating the cells into a gel and giving them the possibility to retain their physiological form instead of a flattened morphology as for ML cultures.

These results support the applicability of long-term hepatocyte cultures for CYP-induction studies. It has even been suggested that serum-free collagen sandwich cultures can be used to examine CYP induction of several test compounds consecutively in one culture with recovery phases between treatment stages (PRIMACYT Cell Culture Technology GmbH, personal communication). This would be a step towards higher throughput and also help to further reduce animal usage in preclinical drug development. A recently published report explicitly promoted the addition of several CYP inducers into the culture media to keep the cells induced and to maintain elevated levels of metabolic enzymes throughout the culture (Kienhuis et al., 2007). The ability of this system to obtain results physiologically relevant results has still to be proven.

The reorganization of canalicular structures could be enhanced by serum free media and the addition of Dex. These structures were stable and functionally active over the whole time of SW culture, shown by the transport experiments with carboxy-DCFDA. The lack of transport activity at early time points of culture may be caused by endocytotic processes removing Mrp2 from the cell surface during the process of perfusion, which is only reversed by the reestablishment of cellular polarity (Graf & Boyer, 1990). The fact that canaliculi-like structures are stable over time makes these cultures especially valuable for transport studies. An additional effect of Dex is the inhibition of spontaneous apoptosis by inhibiting caspase-8 activation and increasing anti-apoptotic signals like Bcl-2 and Bcl-$x_L$ (Bailly-Maitre et al., 2002).

Altogether, these results show that hepatocytes cultured in serum-free collagen sandwich conformation partly recover from stress during liver perfusion, adapt to the cell culture conditions and stay morphologically unchanged for several weeks. They regain their functionally important cell polarity, rebuild cell borders (tight junctions, bile canaliculi) and retain several aspects of their functionality over time in culture offering the ability to investigate alterations in cellular structures induced by chemical treatment with classic light microscopy. Furthermore, the increased use of human cells will add additional value to the results.

## 3.3 Global expression studies with different human and rat cell culture systems

The utility of *in vitro* cultured hepatocytes for toxicological studies is highly dependent on the preservation of biochemical and metabolic functionalities.

The application of novel "-omics" techniques allows the design of new strategies and is expected to be applicable in early screening and mechanism-based risk assessment in toxicology (Stubberfield & Page, 1999; Suter, Babiss & Wheeldon, 2004; Pennie et al., 2000). Recent studies showed the principal applicability of *in vitro* systems in combination with "-omics" technologies to generate valid and useful data concerning hepatotoxicity (Farkas & Tannenbaum, 2005b; Groneberg et al., 2002). However, there is still a need for improving the culturing conditions to increase predictivity and significance of these *in vitro*

# 3 RESULTS AND DISCUSSION

models (Beigel et al., 2008). The possibility of getting insight into the mechanisms affected by a compound after treatment has to be analyzed against the background of basal gene expression. Additionally, the knowledge of the underlying mechanisms of toxicity is expected to facilitate species extrapolation and to help predict possible risk factors.

Currently, rodent *in vivo* systems are the experimental models of choice, but *in vitro* systems such as primary hepatocytes in SW culture, are now being established and used as replacement or at least as an early screening. For the application of *in vitro* toxicity studies and the interpretation of data generated by toxicogenomic studies *in vitro*, new aspects have to be considered. As cells are cultured in an artificial environment, it is crucial to be familiar with the basal gene expression for each culture method. Several factors have been suggested to contribute to the phenotype of mature hepatocytes *in vivo*. The concentration gradient of a large number of hormones and other signals, like metabolites and oxygen, transported with the blood flow, allow the cells to detect and respond to the actual physiological status of the body (Sell, 2001; Püschel & Jungermann, 1994). In addition, the tissue architecture and composition (Bedossa & Paradis, 2003; Reid et al., 1992), paracrine signalling and the direct communication with other cell types of the liver (González et al., 2002) affect the metabolic state of hepatocytes. The temporal loss of liver specific functions, the main obstacle of using primary hepatocytes, could be due to the loss of external signals.

In the case of longer-term culture of hepatocytes, the adaptation to the cell culture conditions and the change of gene expression over time has to be carefully considered before starting toxicological studies. The procedure of isolating the hepatocytes has an influence on cellular gene expression and induces inflammatory and dedifferentiation processes (De Smet et al., 1998; Bayad et al., 1991). Further alterations may be introduced by adaptation processes to the culture conditions and by the duration of culture and are highly dependent on the type of culture. Morphological changes over time in culture, as observed in ML culture, are inherently connected to fundamental changes in gene expression.

This study was conducted to gain a better understanding of how varying culture conditions affect gene expression in primary human and rat hepatocytes, to examine the principal applicability for toxicological studies and to select a system of choice for subsequent studies. Functional differences between the different cell cultures relative to the liver were revealed as important for data interpretation. Special emphasis was put on initial changes introduced by the preparation and plating of the cells, the changes over the time in culture and the influence of the overlay with collagen to generate a three dimensional ECM

# 3 RESULTS AND DISCUSSION

environment. Generally, two types of cell culture, short-term cultures and longer-term cultures, have to be discriminated (Figure 42, Details see Chapter 1.5). Culture methods used for short-term toxicity testing were liver slices and cell suspensions. Whereas the latter is used for metabolic studies for only a few hours (Gebhardt et al., 2003; Cross & Bayliss, 2000), liver slices have been characterized for up to 48 h in culture (Lupp, Danz & Müller, 2001). In contrast to isolated hepatocytes, liver slices contain all cell types of the liver and therefore gene expression data will be different to hepatocytes alone. To account for this factor, the whole liver was used as the reference system for liver slices.

Hepatocytes in ML culture and in SW culture were cultured for up to 9 d as already described. In the rat experiments, cells were incubated with (ML+/SW+), or without (ML-/SW-) the addition of serum, human hepatocytes were only cultured without serum. Additionally, the gene expression of an established cell line (for rat FaO cells, for human HepG2 cells) was analyzed. As a new and promising approach, the HepaRG cell line was analyzed. For all isolated cell culture methods, freshly isolated hepatocytes were used as a reference for the change of gene expression over time. Samples were taken and hybridized to either an Illumina RatRef-8 or a HumanRef-6 BeadChip array. All culture conditions and time points were measured in biological triplicates. Data was uploaded into Expressionist®Analyst (Genedata), normalized with the LOESS algorithm and analyzed for each culture type separately. Results of the subsequent pathway analyses in MetaCore™ (GeneGo) were compared across different cultures and time points. Gene expression changes of 45 genes were confirmed with TaqMan RT-PCR.

# 3 RESULTS AND DISCUSSION

## short term | long term

| rat | 0h | 2h | 4h | 6h | 1d | 2d | 4d | 6d | 10d |
|---|---|---|---|---|---|---|---|---|---|
| | Liver | | | | SW | SW | SW | SW | SW |
| | | | | | ML | ML | ML | ML | ML |
| | Slices | Slices | | Slices | Slices | Slices | | | |
| | Fresh cells | Susp. | Susp. | Susp. | Susp. | | | | |

time ⟶

| human | 0h | 2h | 4h | 6h | 1d | 2d | 3d | 4d | 5d | 7d | 11d |
|---|---|---|---|---|---|---|---|---|---|---|---|
| | Liver | | | | | SW | SW | SW | SW | SW | SW |
| | | | | | | ML | ML | ML | ML | ML | ML |
| | HepaRG | | | | | HepaRG | HepaRG | | HepaRG | HepaRG | |
| | Fresh cells | Susp | Susp | Susp | Susp | | | | | | |

Figure 42: Overview of the different cell culture models used in this study. The time intervals where samples have been taken are specified.

The main goal of all clustering algorithms is to order experiments according to their intercluster difference and thereby gaining a logical overview of their relationship to each other. Figure 43 shows a hierarchical clustering of the different culture types conducted with rat and human hepatocytes. It is clear that the gene expression profiles of short term cultures (liver slices and suspension culture) are relatively similar to the liver and freshly isolated cells. Interestingly, the liver slices separated from this cluster already after 6 h. For the long-term rat hepatocyte cultures, a separate cluster was built, which split into three subclusters. The first one contains early time points of ML as well as SW cultures. The later time points (4 d until the end of culture) built the second sub-tree of this cluster which in turn can also be subdivided into SW and ML cultures cultured without serum. The third sub-cluster, clearly separated from the other two, was built up from cells cultured with the addition of serum. Two small groups completely separated from all other experiments, cells cultured in ML with serum and the hepatoma cell line (FaO).

# 3 RESULTS AND DISCUSSION

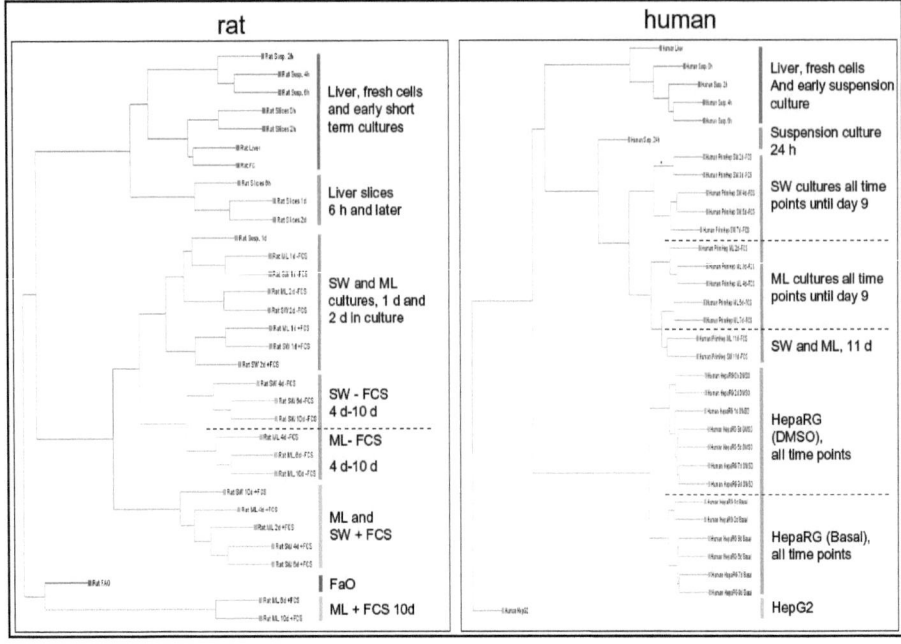

Figure 43: Hierarchical cluster analysis of the different culture types conducted with rat and human hepatocytes. Groups of experiments for each time point and culture type were pooled and are shown here as one data point. The cluster height reflects the inter-cluster difference and the tree-segments indicate groups of experiments with high concordance in gene expression.

The cluster analysis of human gene expression resulted in slightly different results from the rat analysis. Short-term experiments clustered together with the FC and liver for the initial period of culture and separated after one day in culture. The ML and SW cultures separated from the other conditions, but as two distinct sub-clusters. As human hepatocytes showed better stability in gene expression, all time points were grouped together, even after 11 d in culture. The outlier group was built from data of the HepG2 cell line. All time points and both culture conditions of HepaRG cells formed one large cluster with two separated sub-clusters, which was much closer to primary hepatocytes than to the other cell line used in these experiments (HepG2).

Given the immense amount of data and the large number of genes found to be deregulated in all of the cell cultures, only general trends are discussed in this chapter. Gene expression changes caused by the different types of cell culture, mechanisms and pathways important for toxicological studies and the liver specific character of hepatocytes will be highlighted.

## 3.3.1 Initial changes introduced by the process of perfusion

### 3.3.1.1 Primary rat hepatocytes

Changes in gene expression related to the perfusion itself were analysed by a comparison of freshly isolated hepatocytes (FC) with the liver. 535 Genes were found to be significantly (pValue < 0.01) deregulated more than two-fold, 403 of these were decreased and the expression of the other 132 genes was increased (Appendix 7 and Appendix 8). The higher number of genes being reduced is already an indication for the causative process, as the change of mRNA abundance may reflect more the lack of other cell types with different gene expression than a change of gene expression in hepatocytes themselves. To confirm this hypothesis, these two groups of genes, and the affected pathways and processes, were analyzed (Table 14). Genes found to be down regulated were involved in inflammatory processes, like antigen presentation or interferon signalling, cell-matrix interactions, blood coagulation or angiogenesis. These mechanisms are, at least partially, the task of the other cell types in the liver.

Kupffer cells are resident tissue macrophages, which play a key role in inflammatory processes in the liver. They are able to produce a variety of cytokines, which act in a paracrine manner on hepatocytes (Ramadori & Armbrust, 2001) by binding to highly specific cell-surface receptors. This binding may activate a vast number of intracellular signalling cascades, with clear changes on gene expression. Interleukin 18 (IL18), for example, which was found to be decreased after perfusion, has the potential to activate inflammatory responses and to activate the release of atopic effector molecules, such as histamine, in mast cells and basophiles. IL-18 and IL-12 act synergistically to stimulate natural killer cells to produce IFN-gamma, an immunomodulatory cytokine (Gracie, Robertson & McInnes, 2003). Therefore, endogenous IL-18 plays a major role in induction of some types of liver injuries in mice and human (Tsutsui et al., 2003). Other inflammation related genes and genes involved in antigen presentation and leukocyte trans-endothelial migration were found to be less abundant after perfusion, indicating the loss of Kupffer cells. Endothelial cells are reported to be actively involved in inflammatory processes (antigen presentation), which was also found to be reduced.

The ECM environment of the liver is important not only for cellular attachment but also for intra- and intercellular signalling. *In vivo*, signalling occurs via several molecules produced by the different cell types. Decorin is a small proteoglycan that is able to regulate cell proliferation, migration and different growth factors' activities. It has been reported to be

## 3 RESULTS AND DISCUSSION

produced by Ito and endothelial cells, but not in hepatocytes and Kupffer cells and to be induced during acute liver damage (Gallai et al., 1996). Here, it was found to be less abundant after perfusion (-7.8-fold). Additionally Type I, Type III and Type IV procollagen expression was found to be reduced, which normally takes place predominantly in nonparenchymal cells (Milani et al., 1989), indicating the absence of cell types producing these collagens.

| Down regulated | Up regulated |
| --- | --- |
| Cell adhesion; Cell-matrix interactions | Cell cycle; G1-S Interleukin regulation |
| Proteolysis; ECM remodelling | Reproduction; FSH-beta signalling pathway |
| Blood coagulation | Signal transduction; ERBB-family signalling |
| Proteolysis; Connective tissue degradation | Cell cycle; G1-S Growth factor regulation |
| Cell adhesion; Platelet-endothelium-leucocyte interactions | Signal transduction; Leptin signalling |
| Development; Blood vessel morphogenesis | Reproduction; GnRH signalling pathway |
| Apoptosis; Apoptosis mediated by external signals | Inflammation; IL-6 signalling |
| Proliferation; Negative regulation of cell proliferation | DNA damage-Checkpoint |
| Inflammation; Interferon signalling | Signal transduction; ESR1-nuclear pathway |
| Development; Regulation of angiogenesis | Inflammation; Histamine signalling |

Table 14: Top 10 ranked GO processes found to be deregulated in relation to the liver after isolation of rat hepatocytes.

Nevertheless, processes such as cell cycle, intracellular signalling pathways or inflammatory processes (e.g. IL-6 and histamine signalling) were found to be induced (Table 14). It is known that hepatocytes are primed for proliferation during isolation (Etienne et al., 1988; Loyer et al., 1996), which could clearly be reflected in this data. Although IL6 was not directly deregulated, pathways and processes induced by IL6 were observed to be induced. IL6 together with IL1 activate the MAPK (mitogen-activated protein kinase) cascades and the JAK/STAT pathway (Heinrich et al., 2003). The activated MAPK pathway is linked to cell cycle progression. Activating the JAK/STAT pathway results in multiple changes in gene expression, as it is involved in the immune response, principal cell fate decisions, regulating the processes of cell proliferation, differentiation and apoptosis.

Altogether, these results show the effective elimination of nonparenchymal cell types. It is important to note that inflammatory processes mediated by these cells will only take place in a limited manner in culture. Although the time from perfusion to sampling was relatively short for rat, some early inflammatory processes could already be detected. This may have been initialized during the perfusion of the liver (via signalling of the still existing nonparenchymal cells). Intracellular signalling pathways connected to inflammation and cell cycle processes were activated in FC, indicated by the up-regulation c-Jun, ATF and Gadd45 d. Changes in cytoskeletal structure and processes concerning ECM remodelling are inherent to the perfusion procedure and can not be overcome.

Liver slices, which were not perfused, retain their original architectural structure and the inherent liver cell heterogeneity with their cell-cell interactions, were directly compared to the liver. At the beginning of culturing (0 h) 1,074 genes were found to be deregulated, 452 were up, 622 down regulated. These genes represented inflammatory responses, response to wounding and several intracellular signalling pathways. Noticeable was the induction of translational processes, but also genes correlated to DNA-damage and signal transduction (related to stress response) were up regulated.

### 3.3.1.2 Primary human hepatocytes

It is well known that species-specific differences in gene expression and metabolic activity can cause completely different behaviour of the cells in culture (Hengstler et al., 2000; O'Brien, Chan & Silber, 2004; Richert et al., 2002). For a direct comparison, human hepatocytes were observed under the same conditions so that results of global gene expression data were analyzed with regard to similarities and differences to the processes taking place in rat hepatocytes.

Primary human hepatocytes were prepared from pieces of liver obtained from partial lobectomy. The time from operative intervention in the hospital to isolation of the hepatocytes was longer than the "in lab" procedure of rat liver perfusion. Kupffer cells secrete signalling molecules, like TNF$\alpha$ and other cytokines, thereby activating an inflammatory response in hepatocytes. This fact was reflected by additional differences in gene expression.

# 3 RESULTS AND DISCUSSION

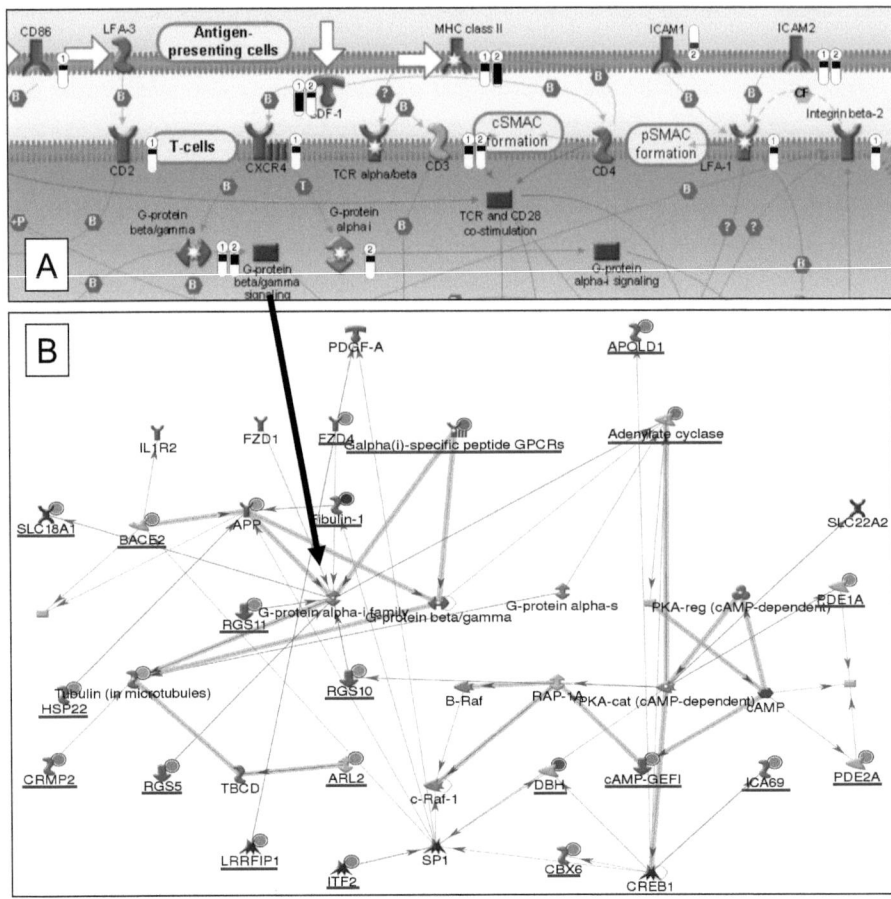

Figure 44: Cellular surface receptors and their connection to cellular signalling. A) Cell-surface related genes and their expression values in freshly isolated hepatocytes in relation to the liver. The fold change is shown as bars (1= rat orthologue; 2= human), rising or falling bars indicate induction or repression of transcription. B) Network of G protein signalling and cAMP associated genes deregulated after perfusion of liver. The underlined genes were found to be reduced in freshly isolated cells.

As expected, the major changes in gene expression between liver and FC resulted from the removal of other hepatic cell types. In particular adhesion molecules, like integrins and cell surface markers, or ECM related genes were found to be significantly reduced. T-cells, for example make brief contact with antigen-presenting cells (APCs) facilitated by chemokines and adhesion molecules, including integrins. The TCR-CD3 (T-cell receptor complex) recognizes the peptide-major histocompatibility complex MHC class II. Integrins

## 3 RESULTS AND DISCUSSION

like Itgb2 (Integrin beta2) are then dynamically redistributed to the site of contact. Cd2, a cell surface antigen involved in T lymphocyte activation and proliferation was reduced, as was Cxcr4, a $G_i$ protein-coupled receptor for the chemokine Sdf-1 (stromal cell-derived factor-1) (Wettschureck & Offermanns, 2005) (Figure 44). Downstream processes of these $G_i$ proteins are coupled via phosphoinositide-specific phospholipase C (PLC-gamma1) (Illenberger et al., 2003) and PI3K (Brock et al., 2003) to intracellular second messenger mechanisms, mediating the immune response and a variety of other intra cellular processes. As an example, a network was built from the down regulated genes, integrating G-protein signalling, cAMP-mediated signalling and the regulation of adenylate cyclase activity, which in turn regulates multiple processes.

Many genes involved in the functional reorganization and biogenesis of the cytoskeleton and ECM remodelling processes were lost. Genes involved in xenobiotic metabolism related processes were also affected.

In contrast to the rat hepatocytes, cell cycle related processes were not found to be induced to a large extent, indicating that no proliverative mechanisms were taking place at this early time point in human hepatocytes. Additionally, stress induced processes were detected resulting in a rise of genes involved in the inflammatory response (Complement system of inflammation). Another difference to the situation in rat was that many genes involved in translational and transcriptional processes were induced, reflecting the reaction of human hepatocytes to an increased need to produce proteins and maybe the longer time to react to the external signals caused by the extended time from dissection to cell isolation. In rats, these processes were found to be deregulated only to a minor degree. Correspondingly, there was an induction of several enzymes responsible for amino acid and energy metabolism, indicating a raised need for energy in the cells.

Interestingly, several major hepatic pathways were induced, including steroid inactivation, the hydroxylation by CYP enzymes and conjugation with glucuronide and sulphate. The induction of steroid biotransformation enzymes is partly mediated as a feedback loop through a group of nuclear receptors, including the glucocorticoid receptor (GR), the constitutive androstane receptor (CAR), the pregnane X receptor (PXR), and the peroxisome proliferator activated receptors (PPARs) (You, 2004). These transcription factors also have important roles in regulation of liver specific gene expression and xenobiotic metabolism. Additionally, GR activation has immunosuppressive abilities by preventing the transcription of immune related genes and leads to increased plasma amino acids (Hayashi et al., 2004).

# 3 RESULTS AND DISCUSSION

| Down regulated | Up regulated |
|---|---|
| Cell adhesion; Cell-matrix interactions | Translation initiation |
| Cell adhesion; Platelet-endothelium-leucocyte interactions | Proteolysis; Ubiquitin-proteosomal proteolysis |
| Cytoskeleton; Actin filaments | Response to hypoxia and oxidative stress |
| Cytoskeleton; Regulation of rearrangement | Proteolysis in cell cycle and apoptosis |
| Development; Neurogenesis: Axonal guidance | Translation in mitochondria |
| Proteolysis; ECM remodelling | Inflammation; Complement system |
| Proteolysis; Connective tissue degradation | Translation; Elongation-termination |
| Cell adhesion; Leucocyte chemotaxis | Transcription; mRNA processing |
| Inflammation; Histamine signalling | Transport; Iron transport |
| Cell adhesion; Integrin-mediated cell-matrix adhesion | Transport; Manganese transport |

Table 15: Top 10 ranked GO processes found to be deregulated in relation to the liver after isolation of human hepatocytes

## 3.3.2 Temporal changes in global gene expression

For a full characterization of the impact of culture conditions on the behavior and functionality of hepatocytes over time, transcriptional changes were analyzed globally across the complete dataset. Therefore, fold-changes and statistically significance were calculated in relation to the particular starting points of the culture, which was defined as the reference sample (Appendix 3 and Appendix 4). For the short term culture methods, such as liver slices and suspension cultures, reference samples were defined as the 0 h time point after isolation, which means freshly cut liver slices or freshly isolated hepatocytes, respectively. The latter was used to eliminate the background of gene expression changes due to the lack of other cell types.

As previously described, the process of isolating hepatocytes caused a large number of gene expression changes which, at least in part, can be considered as common and therefore are present in all types of cultures. Consequently, the 1 d time point after plating was defined as the starting point for the longer term culture methods. The initial changes were thereby excluded from the analysis and evaluated separately. Due to the fact that the human hepatocytes were prepared and plated in France, the first time point analyzed, 2 d after perfusion, was used as the reference sample.

# 3 RESULTS AND DISCUSSION

Short term cultures generally showed a high correlation to their reference experiments (Figure 45). This is true not only for the liver slices, which still contain all liver-typical cells, but also for the hepatocyte suspension cultures. Major effects were first detected after 6 h for liver slices and suspension cultures and after 1 day in culture, clear differences were seen. After one day, the gene expression in both cultures was measurably different to controls correlating with the decline in viability observed for these cells.

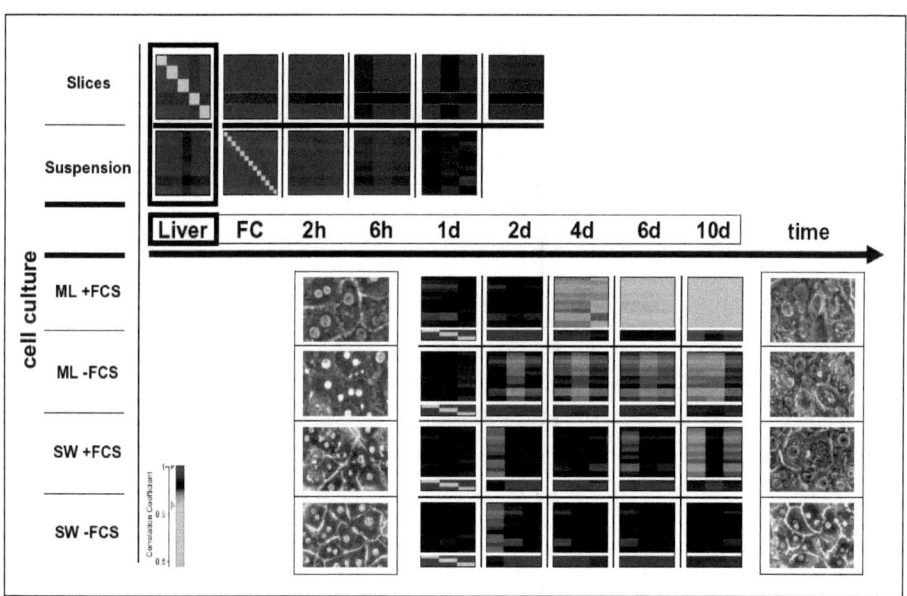

Figure 45: Heat maps of the correlation coefficients of rat cell culture experiments compared to the reference system over time. Each square in a column or line represents the gene expression correlation of a given sample at a certain time point (arrow) relative to the reference experiments. The intensity-changes in global gene expression were used as the basis for the calculation of the correlation. Long-term experiments were split: the upper part of the square shows the correlation of the experiments to freshly isolated cells, the lower part indicates the correlation to the 1 d sample, which was defined as the reference experiment for later analyses. Dark squares indicate high correlation (>0.9), whereas light indicates a low correlation. The pictures show cells of each longer-term culture at day one (left) and day 10 (right) of culture.

The longer term cultures were compared to FC as well as to cells in culture for one day. Shown in the lower part of Figure 45 are the heat maps visualizing the correlations between each time point and FC (above white line in each square) and day one of culture (below white line in each square). A reduction of the correlation coefficient, visualized by a shift from dark to black to light, indicates significant changes in global gene expression in

## 3 RESULTS AND DISCUSSION

comparison to the references. For all cultures, by day one a reduced correlation was seen, although it was most pronounced in ML+FCS. As shown in the previous chapter, the initial changes introduced by the elimination of other cell types and the initial adaptation processes are likely to cause similar changes in all types of cultures.

The correlation coefficient of ML+FCS cultured cells decreased over time when compared with gene expression in FC and with cells one day in culture, reflecting the advancing dedifferentiation processes. This result perfectly correlates to the morphological analyzes described before with no stabilization of gene expression detected.

The removal of FCS from the culture media and the addition of Dex improved the correlations. The extent of initial changes was reduced and processes moving the cells away from hepatocyte-like gene expression were significantly slowed down, at least globally, after two days in culture. Until the end of culture, the gene expression of these cells showed more stability. As the aim of toxicogenomics is the detection of gene expression changes caused by compound treatment, it is important, especially *for in vitro* models, to reduce the background of genes changing due to other factors, such as the culturing, to a minimum.

Cells cultured in SW in the presence of serum showed the initial changes which were less pronounced compared to ML+FCS. Globally, the cells remained in this state until day four. Afterwards, a reduction of the gene expression correlation coefficient was detected. This process was intensified at later time points indicating the onset of dedifferentiation in these cells.

In SW culture without serum the addition of Dex had additionally positive effects on global gene expression. The gene expression changes due to the isolation process and adaptation to the culture environment, although still quite high, were least pronounced and global gene expression over time was most stable of all cultures tested. From two days in culture until the end of the culture, an increase in correlation to FC was observed suggesting some regenerative processes were taking place in these cells.

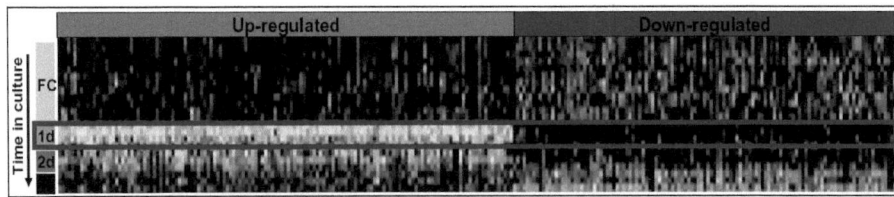

Figure 46: Heat map of genes transiently deregulated one day after perfusion in sandwich culture without serum.

# 3 RESULTS AND DISCUSSION

Genes found to be transiently deregulated after one day in culture and returning to their original expression level (Figure 46) were mainly genes known to be involved in early stress response, inflammatory mechanisms and intracellular signalling. Networks built from these specifically deregulated genes (confidence of 95% to be only deregulated at 1 d in SW-FCS) confirmed these findings but also showed a link to the regulation of fatty acid biosynthetic processes (Table 16). The expression of the PPARs was reduced 1.8-fold. This transcription factor is known for its ability to induce gluconeogenesis and to reduce fatty acid β-oxidation.

| Processes | Size | Target | p-Value |
|---|---|---|---|
| immune system process (40.0%), V(D)J recombination (7.5%), nitric oxide transport (5.0%) | 50 | 10 | 1.05e-21 |
| protein kinase cascade (44.0%), stress-activated protein kinase signaling pathway (26.0%), protein amino acid phosphorylation (44.0%) | 50 | 10 | 1.64e-21 |
| fatty acid biosynthetic process (23.1%), carboxylic acid biosynthetic process (23.1%), organic acid biosynthetic process (23.1%) | 50 | 8 | 8.45e-18 |
| regulation of biosynthetic process (20.6%), regulation of cellular biosynthetic process (20.6%), biological regulation (79.4%) | 50 | 9 | 2.35e-19 |
| response to stress (65.1%), positive regulation of cellular metabolic process (46.5%), positive regulation of metabolic process (46.5%) | 50 | 8 | 7.23e-17 |

Table 16: Top five networks highly enriched with genes found to be deregulated only at day one in SW-FCS cultured hepatocytes. "Size" refers to the number of network objects contained and "Target" is the number of affected objects contained in these networks.

Figure 47 shows the correlation of global gene expression for the different human cell cultures tested. Again, the short term suspension culture retained liver specific gene expression only for a short time. After 6 h, global gene expression was still hepatocyte-like, but after this time point a rapid change was detected.

# 3 RESULTS AND DISCUSSION

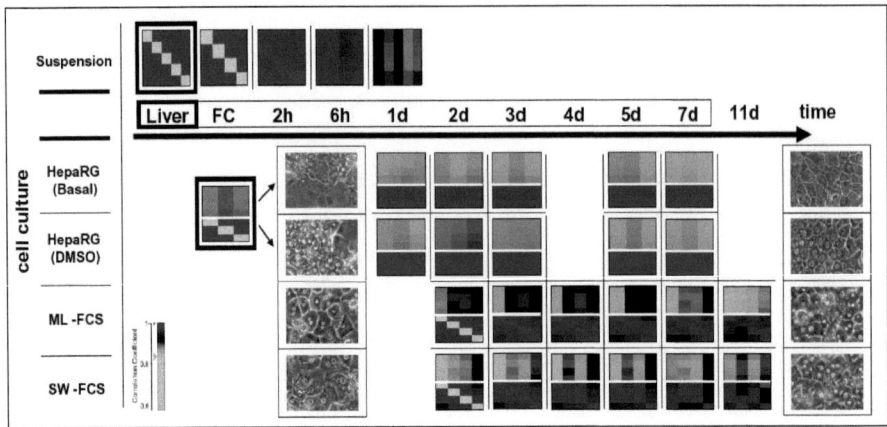

Figure 47: Heat maps of the correlation coefficients of human cell culture experiments to their reference systems over time. Experiments were ordered according to the time scale (big arrow) and separated into short- and long-term experiments. The intensity-changes in global gene expression were used as the basis for the calculation of the correlation. Long-term experiments are split up; the upper part of the square shows the correlation of the experiments to freshly isolated cells, the lower part indicates the correlation to the status 1 d after plating which was defined as the reference experiment for later analyses. Dark squares indicate high correlation, light indicate low correlation. The pictures show cells of each longer-term culture at day one (left) and day 10 (right) of culture.

The results of the long term cultures displayed differences from the results gained with rat hepatocytes. Due to technical reasons, the 2 d time point was the first sample to be taken and therefore this was defined as a second reference, together with FC. For ML and SW cultures, a distinctly worse correlation was detected at the initial time points. This change of gene expression was less pronounced in ML culture indicating a greater stability of these cells. Over time, both cultures demonstrated only minor changes pointing to a generally better stability of gene expression in human cells compared with the situation in rat. Another source of variance when working with primary human cells is the large inter-individual donor difference. Both the basal gene expression and the individual reactions of the cells can be remarkably different. This was confirmed by our data. Four different donors were clearly differentiated, based on their gene expression and the extent of gene expression changes over time (Figure 47 ML and SW). The correlation "in-between" donors at a certain time point was 0.97 for primary cultured human hepatocytes. For the suspension culture, the level of correlation between different time points was in the same range (0.95). Therefore, genes found to be differentially deregulated may be influenced more by donor specificity than by time in culture.

# 3 RESULTS AND DISCUSSION

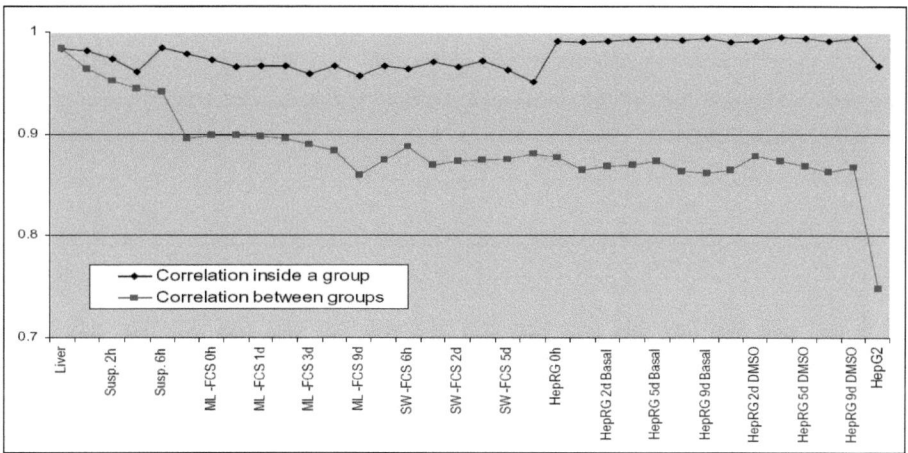

Figure 48: Plot of intra group and inter group correlation coefficients of human hepatocyte cultures.

Experiments with primary human hepatocytes should be carefully analyzed with respect to donor specific gene expression. If possible, more than three biological replicates should be included to ensure that general biological trends are visible above any individual variances.

For both rat and human, the established cell lines (FaO and HepG2, respectively) were found to vary greatly from primary cells, showing many differences in global gene expression. Another cell line, the recently established HepaRG, showed a high stability of gene expression over time. Additionally, the gene expression was closer to that of primary human hepatocytes than that of HepG2 cells (Figure 48). Large differences were detected compared to FC, maybe due to the lack of inter-individual differences and the increased stability of gene expression over time in culture. These cells may therefore be a suitable experimental system for toxicogenomics studies. Further analyses have to be conducted, including the monitoring of the existence of certain metabolic enzymes, which allows liver-like metabolism in these cells (chapter 3.3.6.4).

### 3.3.3 Analysis of protein expression with SELDI-TOF

Proteins, as the effector-molecules in cells, are dependent not only on the amount of transcribed mRNA but also on multiple post-transcriptional and translational mechanisms. It is well known that the amount of a protein is not necessarily correlated with the gene

# 3 RESULTS AND DISCUSSION

expression (Gygi et al., 1999; Chen et al., 2002). To study if gene expression changes during culture of primary hepatocytes translated into differences in protein expression studies were conducted using the SELDI technology. The abundance of certain protein masses in ML-FCS and SW-FCS cultured primary rat hepatocytes were measured and analyzed (Figure 49).

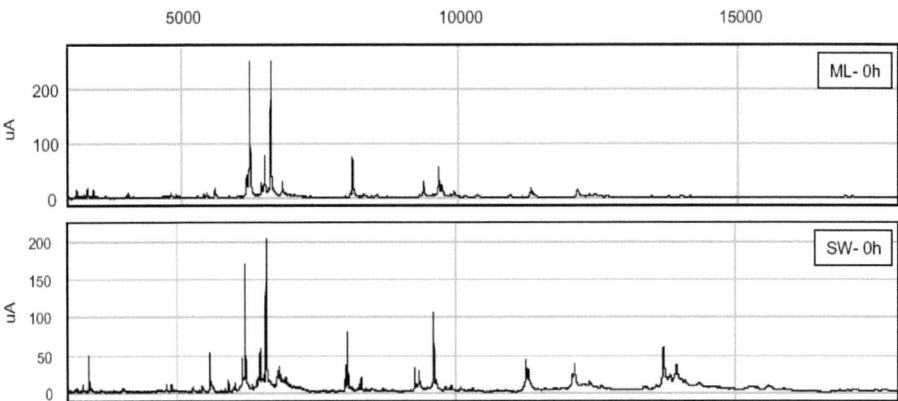

Figure 49: Representative SELDI-spectra detected by analysis of protein samples of either ML-FCS (upper spectrum) or SW-FCS (lower spectrum) cultured rat hepatocytes. Four biological replicates were measured per time point and culture condition and subsequently analyzed for changes over time.

The ProteinChip CM10 array was used to bind and detect positively charged proteins. A hierarchical clustering based on significant mass-ion-peaks detected within the spectra showed a clear separation of early (0 h – 1 d) and late (3 d – 9 d) time points for both culture types. Inside both clusters, individual time points were partially separated. To improve discrimination, only mass-ion-peaks which were significant in all spectra of all animals were identified and chosen as the basis for further analysis. This resulted in 33 mass-ion-peaks for ML-FCS cultured cells, and 26 for SW-FCS. Time points were analyzed for changes in peak intensity separately and compared to the protein profile of freshly isolated cells. Although the resulting heat map representing the correlation of the protein expression to the reference (Figure 50A) shows no clear separation of ML-FCS and SW-FCS, more severe changes in protein expression were detected in ML-FCS indicated by the stronger colours representing positive or negative changes in correlation.

# 3 RESULTS AND DISCUSSION

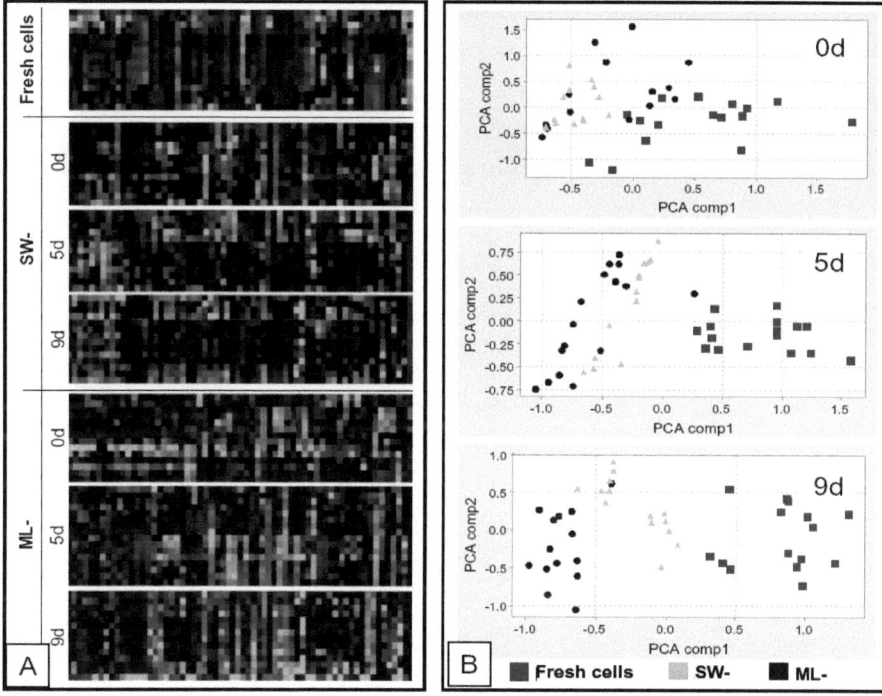

Figure 50: A) Correlation map of 59 mass-ion-peaks detected in samples of ML-FCS and SW-FCS cultured cells. Light resembles a low and dark a high correlation to the reference spectrum. B) Two-dimensional PCAs computed by using the SELDI-Spectra analysis of technical replicate measurements of four biological replicates.

Shown in Figure 50B are two-dimensional PCAs, demonstrating the spread of the data within each experiment. At early time points, differences between cell cultures and freshly isolated cells were less pronounced and therefore the data clouds overlapped. FC were only slightly separated and ML-FCS cultures tended to be located closer to FC than SW-FCS cultures, although this result was not statistically significant. At later time points, clouds separated as individual groups. After 5 d in culture, the protein expression of SW-FCS cultured cells was closer to FC than ML-FCS cultured cells. This effect was enforced after 9 d in culture, protein expression of SW-FCS cultured cells was detected to be less changed and therefore to be more hepatocyte like than the continuously changing protein expression of ML-FCS cultured cells.

Although protein profiling does not allow an exact identification of the proteins underlying the 59 mass-ion-peaks, these results fit well with the results of gene expression, which

# 3 RESULTS AND DISCUSSION

indicated changes at early time points in culture and a greater stability of SW-FCS cultured cells. Improvements of the SELDI technology, to allow identification of single peaks and to improve the sensitivity of peak detection, will further enhance the usability and utility of this technique for identifying protein patterns. By combining both genomic and proteomic approaches, possibilities to further elucidate mechanisms of toxicity using cultured primary hepatocytes will be improved.

### 3.3.4 Gene expression in established cell lines used as reference

The gene expression in established cell lines was compared to FC. FaO is a rat hepatoma cell line with a hepatocyte like phenotype. Some liver-specific enzymes and liver-enriched transcription factors were found to be expressed, although in lower abundance (Clayton, Weiss & Darnell, 1985) than *in vivo*. It has been used for mechanistic analyses for PPARalpha target genes and the induction of apoptosis (König & Eder, 2006; Coyle et al., 2003), lipid metabolism (Latruffe et al., 2000) or CYP expression studies (Hakkola, Hu & Sundberg, 2003).

In comparison to FC, substantial differences in gene expression were detected, 4952 genes were differentially expressed in this cell line. Of the 2951 down regulated genes, many were involved in the regulation of lipid metabolism, MAPK signalling, metabolism of xenobiotics by cytochrome P450 and several important metabolic pathways. Additionally, cellular adhesion was found to be impaired, implying that the cells are less responsive to extracellular stimuli. It's not surprising that many of the higher expressed genes were involved in cell cycle progression and DNA replication, but also several intracellular signalling cascades, like the ERK, Wnt, Insulin and ErbB pathways, showed increased expression.

# 3 RESULTS AND DISCUSSION

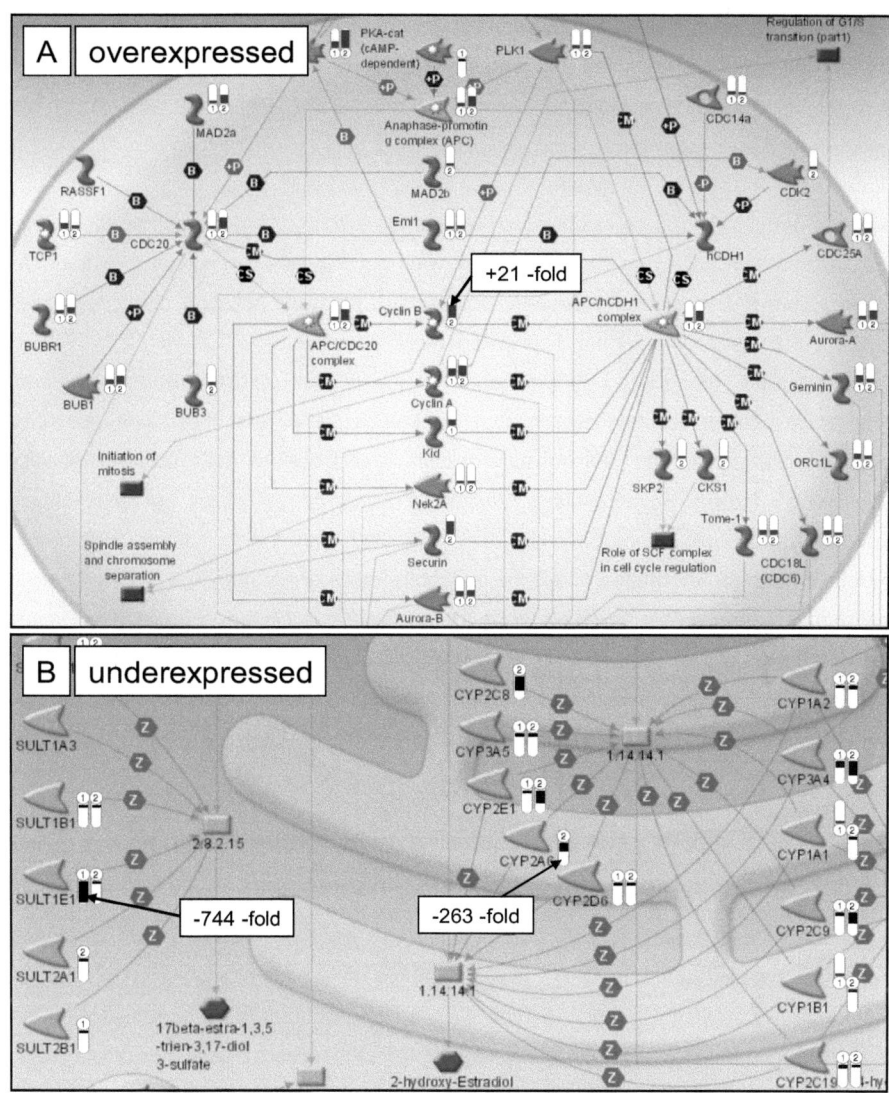

Figure 51: Example of canonical pathway maps showing over and underexpressed genes in the stable cell lines FaO (rat) or HepG2 (human). A) Detail of the anaphase promoting complex (APC). B) Detail of the estradiol metabolism pathway (modified from Metacore, GeneGO).

The human hepatoma derived HepG2 cell line, analogous to the FaO cells, is often used for mechanistic studies, although there is only poor predictivity to the *in vivo* situation (Brandon et al., 2003; Knasmüller et al., 2004). Some differences in gene expression to

## 3 RESULTS AND DISCUSSION

FaO cells (rat) were detected, however the predominant tendencies were found to be similar. Cell cycle related genes and adhesion molecules were overexpressed and genes involved in cellular differentiation, especially intracellular signalling and xenobiotic metabolism, were deregulated.

Figure 51A shows the anaphase promoting complex (APC), which is an important regulator of cell cycle progression, which targets the mitotic cyclins for degradation. This, and several other cell cycle related proteins, was found to be overexpressed in both cell types. Figure 51B depicts the estrogen metabolism pathway including many repressed genes, which also play important roles in xenobiotic metabolism.

Taken together, pronounced differences in many of the cellular mechanisms were detected in both established cell lines. It must be assumed that these changes have severe consequences on cellular mechanisms and therefore also on liver specific functionality. Toxicity experiments conducted in either one of these cell lines should therefore be carefully planned and the data generated treated with caution. Additionally, there is a need for knowledge about the metabolism of any test compound. Extrapolation to the *in vivo* situation has to be performed very carefully to circumvent misinterpretation. These cell lines should be used only for special toxicological questions and results should be interpreted against the background of reduced metabolic activity and altered intracellular signalling leading to non-physiological reactions.

### 3.3.5 Changes of gene expression early in culture - Cellular adaptation processes in primary hepatocytes

It has been shown that the most dramatic change in gene expression occurs during the first day of culturing (our data, Beigel et al., 2008). To review this processes taking place in cultured hepatocytes, the initial changes of gene expression on the first day after plating were studied separately. The gene expression of freshly isolated cells was compared to the gene expression of cells cultured for one day in either SW or ML culture with or without the addition of serum. To obtain relevant results, commonly affected genes were selected and processes taking place in all types of culture were analyzed.

As can be seen in Table 17, more than 50% (1,838) of genes were commonly deregulated in all four types of cell culture. This remarkably high percentage indicates common processes which are ongoing and are probably due to the isolation of cells and general adaptation processes to the new environment. Many of these processes are of course independent from the culture conditions.

# 3 RESULTS AND DISCUSSION

| Culture system | Overall | Down regulated | Up regulated |
|---|---|---|---|
| ML culture + FCS | 3780 | 1681 | 2099 |
| ML culture - FCS | 3025 | 1612 | 1413 |
| SW culture + FCS | 3112 | 1650 | 1462 |
| SW culture - FCS | 3621 | 1920 | 1701 |

Venn diagram:
- ML -FCS: 1187
- ML +FCS: 1942
- SW +FCS: 1274
- SW -FCS: 1783
- Common overlap: 1838

Table 17: Number of genes deregulated after one day in culture. The Venn-diagram on the right side shows the overlap of the overall-gene lists. 1,838 Genes were commonly deregulated and used for further analyses.

To further analyze these common mechanisms and highlight any differences in the adaptation processes between different culture conditions, genes differentially expressed compared to FC in any of the cultures were chosen. Table 18 shows the top 10 canonical pathways affected by the adaptation process.

Among the most affected pathways, amino acid and energy metabolism were ranked at the top, indicating a reduction of amino acid synthesis. Two processes may contribute to this effect. First, hepatocytes are very metabolically active cells *in vivo*, with a large number of proteins produced and secreted into the system. The lack of external signalling may lead to a reduction in these processes, thereby slowing down the synthesis rate and therefore the high need for the production of amino acids is reduced. Second, at least parts of these pathways were induced by the perfusion process and their reduction after 1 d in culture can therefore be seen as a recovery process by returning to their original (lower) expression levels.

The top ranked down-regulated pathway was the regulation of lipid metabolism via several transcription factors. This is of importance because the lipid metabolism is not only closely related to xenobiotic metabolism, but also these transcription factors are responsible for the induction of several enzymes involved in metabolism, cell cycle and inhibition of apoptosis (Latruffe et al., 2000; Kersten et al., 2001; Kliewer et al., 1999). Additionally, fatty acids themselves have the ability to bind to transcription factors and therefore influence the overall gene expression of the cells (Wolfrum & Spener, 2000; Wolfrum et al., 2001; Sampath & Ntambi, 2004). Other processes found to be negatively affected were inflammation-related, such as parts of the complement system, the kallikrein-kinin system, both of which depend on blood circulating proteins and therefore were expected to be reduced.

# 3 RESULTS AND DISCUSSION

| Down regulated | Up regulated |
|---|---|
| Regulation of lipid metabolism via PPAR, RXR and VDR | Cytoskeleton remodelling |
| Glycine, serine, cysteine and threonine metabolism | Cell adhesion; Integrin mediated cell adhesion |
| Leucine, isoleucine and valine metabolism | Role of tetraspanins in the integrin-mediated cell adhesion |
| Alanine, cysteine and L-methionine metabolism | TGF, Wnt and cytoskeletal remodelling |
| Oxidative phosphorylation | Endothelial cell contacts by non junctional mechanisms |
| Peroxisomal branched chain fatty acid metabolism | Signal transduction; Akt signalling |
| Propionate metabolism | Regulation of actin cytoskeleton by Rho GTPases |
| Tryptophan metabolism | Transcription; Role of Akt in hypoxia induced HIF1 activation |
| Mitochondrial ketone bodies biosynthesis and metabolism | Fibronectin-binding integrins in cell motility |
| Immune response; Lectin induced complement pathway | Translation; Insulin regulation of protein synthesis |

Table 18: Top 10 canonical pathways affected by genes commonly deregulated as part of the adaptation process to cell culture.

The pathways found to be heavily induced were involved in cellular adhesion, cytoskeletal remodelling and the corresponding intracellular signalling dependent on these processes. After perfusion, the cells have to adhere to the surface of the culture dishes and to rebuild cellular contacts. Along with this, the reestablishment of their polarization and their polygonal shape is going on. All these processes require cytoskeletal remodelling and are known to influence gene expression, especially integrins. These transmembrane molecules are not only connected to the cytoskeleton but also to intracellular signalling mechanisms, again directly influencing gene expression (Stupack, 2007; Giancotti & Ruoslahti, 1999; Giancotti & Tarone, 2003; Häussinger, Reinehr & Schliess 2006). AKT signalling, for example, is downstream of integrin mediated signalling and influences cell adhesion and intracellular structural protein formation. Figure 52 shows the induction of several genes involved in this pathway.

Interestingly, several inflammatory pathways were induced indicating that hepatocytes themselves are partially capable of initiating an inflammatory response alone. The Jak-Stat pathway is known to be initiated through certain cytokines, like IL-6, which is one of the most important mediators of the acute phase response. Although the initial signal, IL-6, is secreted by macrophages; downstream receptor mediated events take place in other cell types.

# 3 RESULTS AND DISCUSSION

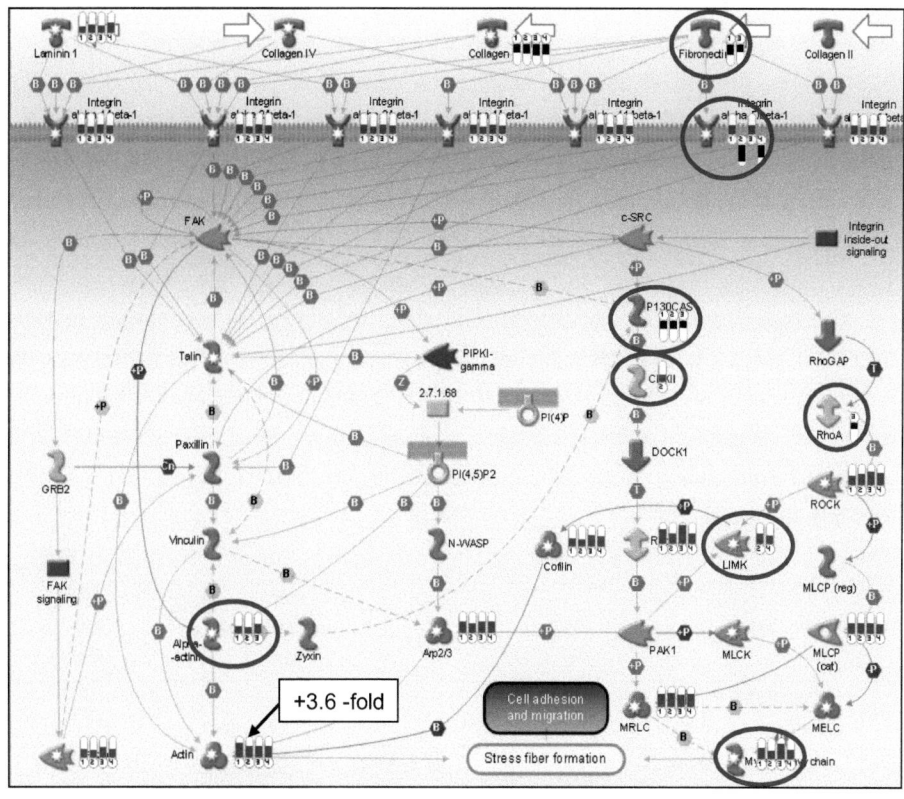

Figure 52: Canonical pathway map showing the changes in the expression of genes involved in signal transduction by AKT signalling. Rising bars indicate induction, decreasing bars the repression of gene expression. Circles indicate genes found to vary in expression between the different types of culturing on day one (modified from Metacore, GeneGO).

The previous results reported in this work showed that the SW culture without the addition of serum both, morphologically and in terms of global gene expression, conserved best the *in vivo* situation of the liver. At this early time point (1 d), the differences between the cell cultures were only minor with none of the top ranked pathways or processes being affected in one and not in the other cell cultures. The differences were restricted to the degree of expression changes of a gene between the cultures and to single genes found in only one sample. This may be explained by the cut-off values selected, which filtered genes expressed just below in one sample whereas they pass in other samples.

# 3 RESULTS AND DISCUSSION

Therefore, the initial processes can be considered as common to all cultures, only the extent can be influenced by the type of cell culture.

About 46% of genes found to be more than 1.5 fold deregulated in either ML-FCS or SW-FCS cultures, (pValue <0.05) were found to be deregulated just below this level in the other cultures (Table 19). These results illustrate a central problem in the analysis of global gene expression. The setting of cut-off values is always correlated with a loss of information, which in turn may be biologically important. Different approaches have been proposed to overcome this drawback (Guo et al., 2006; Chen et al., 2007).

These specifically filtered genes play important roles in cellular fate. Mbtps1, a serine protease that cleaves ER membrane-bound sterol regulatory element-binding proteins (SREBPs), plays a central role in the regulation of lipid metabolism. This transcriptionally active fragment of SREBP is released from the membrane for translocation to the nucleus. Hsbp1 may be involved in the stabilization or repair of cytoskeletal elements and Bcl2l11 and Bcl2l2 both belong to the BCL-2 protein family, the first promoting and the latter inhibiting apoptosis.

| Name | Description | pValue SW-FCS | Fold-Change SW-FCS | pValue ML-FCS | Fold-Change ML-FCS |
|---|---|---|---|---|---|
| Mbtps1 | Membrane-bound transcription factor protease | 3.84E-04 | -2.19 | 4.64E-02 | -1.47 |
| Ca3 | Carbonic anhydrase 3 | 2.52E-02 | -1.34 | 8.16E-04 | -1.61 |
| Ilkap | Integrin-linked kinase-associated serine/threonine phosphatase 2C | 9.73E-05 | -1.51 | 1.24E-03 | -1.33 |
| Hsbp1 | Heat shock factor binding protein 1 | 7.86E-07 | -1.86 | 5.48E-04 | -1.39 |
| Mt3 | Metallothionein 3 | 3.81E-06 | 1.63 | 1.57E-03 | 1.42 |
| Ikbkap | Inhibitor of kappa light polypeptide enhancer in B-cells, kinase complex-associated protein | 6.55E-03 | 1.39 | 9.51E-05 | 1.74 |
| Arnt | Aryl hydrocarbon receptor nuclear translocator | 6.17E-06 | 2.38 | 4.73E-03 | 1.34 |
| Tsg101 | Tumor susceptibility gene 101 | 2.59E-03 | 1.42 | 1.55E-04 | 1.60 |
| Edn1 | Endothelin 1 | 2.57E-03 | 1.30 | 6.18E-05 | 1.57 |
| Creb1 | cAMP responsive element binding protein 1 | 6.15E-05 | 1.48 | 3.23E-06 | 1.61 |
| Bcl2l11 | BCL2-like 11 (apoptosis facilitator) | 5.52E-07 | 1.59 | 8.07E-09 | 1.48 |
| Bcl2l2 | Bcl2-like 2 | 2.75E-07 | 1.75 | 2.42E-03 | 1.47 |

Table 19: Selection of genes found to be filtered out in either SW –FCS or ML –FCS due to just one value not fulfilling the cut off values.

## 3 RESULTS AND DISCUSSION

### 3.3.5.1  Liver slices

When analyzing the gene expression changes over time in relation to the reference experiment, the 6 h time point showed especially striking results in liver slices. Whereas in all other culture systems the number of deregulated genes increased continuously over time, the maximum of 1824 genes was deregulated at 6 h in liver slices (

Figure 53). After this peak, the number of deregulated genes significantly declined, implicating a transient mechanism only active for the first few hours in culture. The 790 genes affected only at this certain time point (Figure 53) were filtered out and analyzed for mechanistic function.

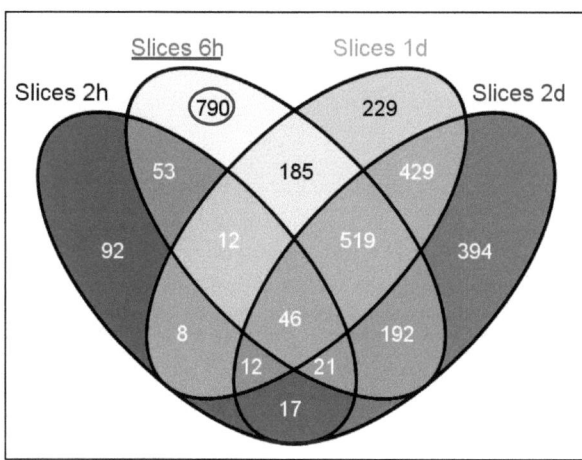

Figure 53: Venn-diagram of deregulated genes at certain time points. The number of genes in each overlapping segment indicates genes commonly deregulated in these experiments. The circle indicates the number of genes only deregulated 6 h after culturing.

Many of the genes induced were involved in chemotaxis, inflammatory response, cell adhesion and downstream signalling. These are processes which normally take place because of wounding, cellular stress or other pro-inflammatory stimuli activating cytokine signalling. Indeed, several cytokines were found to be heavily up regulated indicating a strong influence of activated Kupffer cells on gene expression.

Table 20 shows the top ranked networks built with genes commonly deregulated in liver slices with the percentage of certain cellular processes indicated in parentheses. Networks showing mostly down-regulated genes showed affects on several mechanisms concerning cellular biosynthetic processes, metabolism and replication. Interestingly, an apoptotic

## 3 RESULTS AND DISCUSSION

mechanism, the activation of caspase via cytochrome c, was reduced which contradicts the general trend of induced cellular stress. This indicates the delicate balance of regulation of apoptotic processes in cells with several pro- and anti-apoptotic mechanisms taking place simultaneously.

| common down regulated | p-Value | common up regulated | p-Value |
|---|---|---|---|
| neurotransmitter metabolic process (13.6%), nitrogen compound metabolic process (27.3%), ketone body biosynthetic process (4.5%) | 2.54E-32 | small GTPase mediated signal transduction (29.5%), cell morphogenesis (40.9%), cellular structure morphogenesis (40.9%) | 6.65E-08 |
| response to chemical stimulus (36.8%), protein export from nucleus (10.5%), male somatic sex determination (5.3%) | 9.87E-26 | cell-matrix adhesion (18.4%), cell-substrate adhesion (18.4%), cell adhesion (28.9%) | 8.7E-30 |
| caspase activation via cytochrome c (13.3%), apoptotic program (23.3%), complement activation (16.7%) | 1.15E-26 | response to stress (44.7%), biological regulation (74.5%), response to external stimulus (29.8%) | 2.64E-26 |
| phosphoinositide-mediated signalling (25.0%), G-protein signalling, coupled to IP3 second messenger (phospholipase C activating) (21.4%), positive regulation of protein kinase activity (25.0%) | 5.6E-18 | wound healing (20.5%), blood coagulation (15.9%), coagulation (15.9%) | 2.49E-22 |
| chromatin silencing at telomere (8.0%), telomeric heterochromatin formation (8.0%), chromatin silencing at rDNA (8.0%) | 8.19E-20 | chemotaxis (37.5%), taxis (37.5%), locomotory behavior (39.6%) | 1.57E-14 |

Table 20: Cellular mechanisms affected by time induced gene expression changes in liver slices.

Building the networks based on the 790 genes specifically deregulated after 6 h principally confirmed the results of the time course analysis with the induction of inflammatory response, stress-activated protein kinase signalling and the induction of the cell cycle as a signal for the start of early regenerative processes taking place. Simultaneously, the expression of genes involved in nucleic and amino acid metabolism was clearly reduced which may be a consequence of oxidative stress. This is a major cause of liver damage that can be initiated by ischemia/reperfusion due to missing blood flow, thus generating an oxygen deficit in the inner layers of the slices. The main sources of reactive oxygen species (ROS) for hepatocytes are internal CYPs, Kupffer cells and neutrophils, with the latter two being missing in isolated hepatocyte cultures. It has been shown that an imbalance between the generation of ROS and the antioxidant defence capacity of the cell affects major cellular mechanisms, including the metabolism of lipids, proteins and DNA

(Cesaratto et al., 2004). ROS can also influence gene expression profiles by affecting intracellular signal transduction pathways (Cesaratto et al., 2004). Signalling by activated Kupffer cells, involving TGF beta and other cytokines, leads to stimulated proteoglycan synthesis, proliferation, and transformation into myofibroblast-like cells.

Several chemo-attractant genes, like cytokines, were up regulated indicating an activation of hepatic macrophages and an ongoing immune response were de-regulated (Figure 54). At the same time, anti-inflammatory processes were induced, indicated by thioredoxin reductase 1 (Txnrd1), which was 3-fold induced exclusively at 6 h and is a critical antioxidant enzyme for the protection against oxidative stress. Stefin A2 (Stfa2), the expression of which was induced 17.8-fold, acts as a cysteine protease inhibitor, amongst which the caspases are an important group.

| Unique for down regulated Slices 0 h/6 h | p-Value | Unique for up regulated Slices 0 h/6 h | p-Value |
|---|---|---|---|
| amino acid transport (12.0%), L-amino acid transport (8.0%), amine transport (12.0%) | 2.63E-60 | intracellular signalling cascade (46.7%), cell development (55.6%), cellular component organization and biogenesis (62.2%) | 9.16E-11 |
| DNA metabolic process (50.0%), DNA repair (33.3%), response to DNA damage stimulus (35.7%) | 1.8E-28 | response to stimulus (62.8%), response to stress (44.2%), stress-activated protein kinase signalling pathway (14.0%) | 8.42E-17 |
| transcription from RNA polymerase II promoter (41.7%), macromolecule metabolic process (80.6%), cellular metabolic process (86.1%) | 1.76E-24 | regulation of progression through cell cycle (31.2%), regulation of cell cycle (31.2%), insulin receptor signalling pathway (12.5%) | 4.29E-15 |

Table 21: Cellular mechanisms affected by gene expression changes exclusively in liver slices after 6 h in culture

The changes in gene expression in liver slices in general were characterized by a very intense immune response at all time points. This is potentially a large disadvantage and thus it has to be questioned whether their use in global gene expression studies makes sense against the advantage of retaining the liver specific architecture, cellular composition and therefore liver specific responses. The immune cells of the liver are already activated by the process of generating the slices. Additionally, the lack of blood flow drives the hypoxia in the inner layers of the slice leading to multiple reactions and increased effects on gene expression in these cells. These processes lead to a transient

# 3 RESULTS AND DISCUSSION

induction of inflammatory processes in slices after 6 h in culture (Table 21 and Figure 54). These processes may potentially overlay any additional effects caused by compound treatment. However, for the analysis of direct toxicity that affects non-parenchymal cells, liver slices are one of the few *in vitro* system options available.

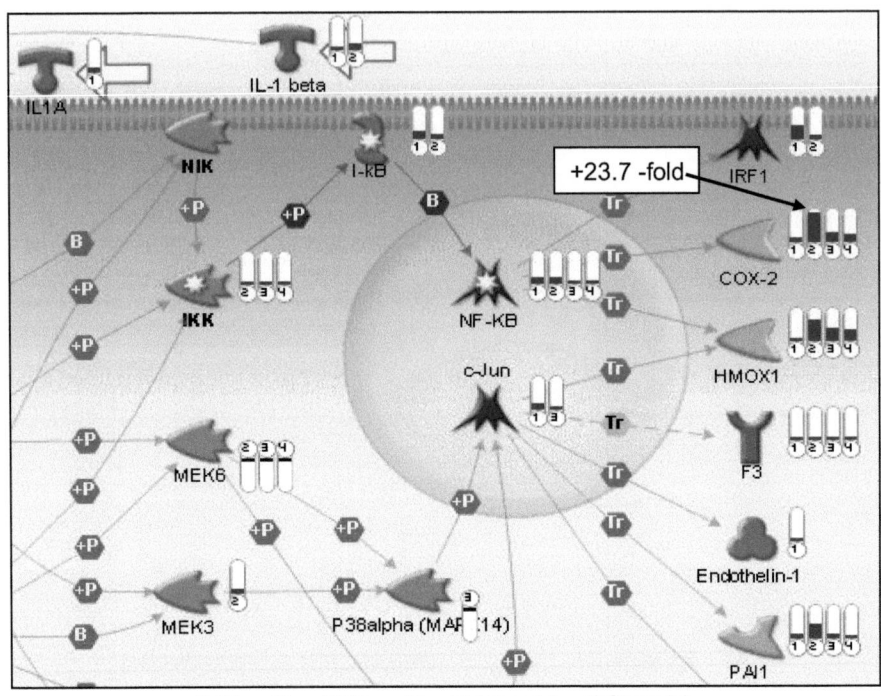

1) Slices 2h   2) Slices 6h   3) Slices 1d   4) Slices 2d

Figure 54: Time course of gene expression changes in liver slices. Shown is a part of the IL1 signalling pathway indicating a strong activation at early time points with the return to moderate expression levels by day 2. Rising bars indicate induction, decreasing bars the repression of gene expression (modified from Metacore, GeneGO).

## 3.3.6 Molecular mechanisms affected over time in culture

### 3.3.6.1 Overview of the affected mechanisms in rat hepatocytes

In order to investigate the differences in gene expression taking place during culturing, with a special emphasis on the differences in the experimental systems used, genes were grouped according to gene ontology in several functional categories and further analyzed (Figure 55). This approach was chosen to reduce the number of genes, which introduced a

# 3 RESULTS AND DISCUSSION

high background noise into the data when taken as a whole. Additionally, it has the advantage of filtering the data while minimizing the loss of important and specific information.

The gene expression of short-term cultures (liver slices and suspension culture) shared a high correlation to the reference (freshly isolated hepatocytes) indicating the advantage of short term culturing. As early as 6 h after the isolation of the cells, larger changes in gene expression were seen, which increased over time.

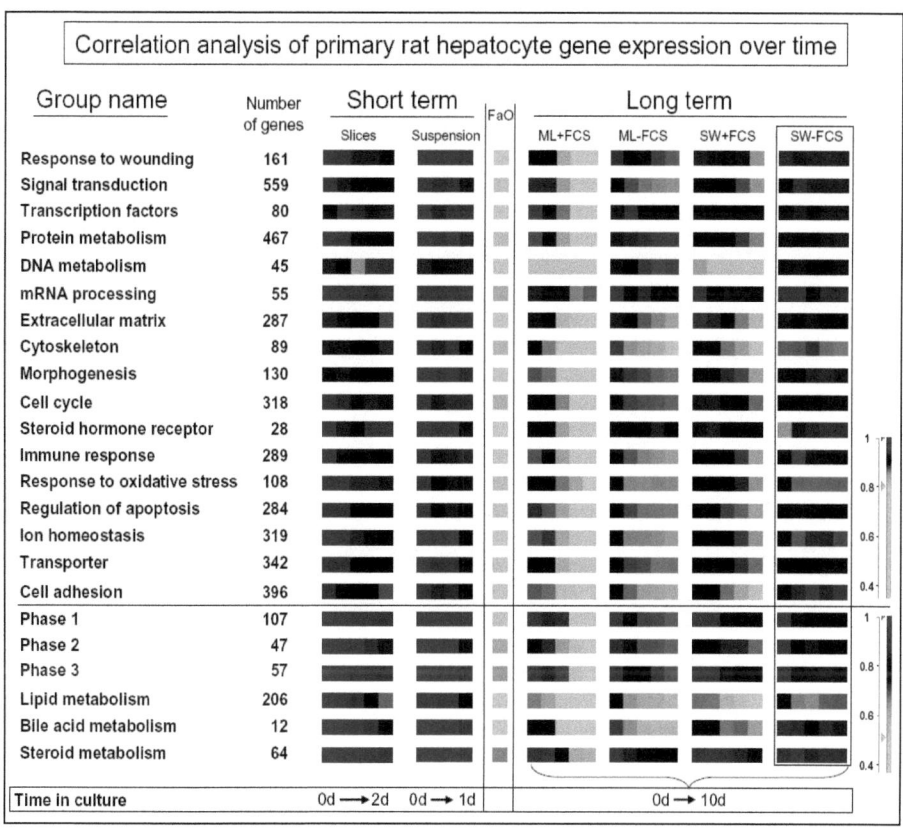

Figure 55: Temporal correlation plots of functional gene groups representing important cellular and liver specific mechanisms for different primary rat hepatocyte culture methods. Changes in the correlation of gene expression in comparison to the reference experiments (FC) are indicated by a change of colour. The calibration bars on the right side indicate the colour scheme which was chosen for an optimal visualization.

## 3 RESULTS AND DISCUSSION

The long-term cultures all failed to preserve this high level of correlation to fresh hepatocytes over time. Generally, hepatocytes cultured with the addition of FCS tended to show changes in gene expression after 2 – 5 d, in all gene groups, indicating a strong dedifferentiation processes. The same effect was seen in cells cultured in ML culture, where initial gene expression changed rapidly, followed by a more gradual change over time. The gene expression of cells cultured in SW culture without FCS was more stable over time. In this culture system initial changes did take place indicating an adaptation process to the culture conditions. For the later time points, the gene expression stabilized or even recovered, indicated by an increasing correlation, for example for protein metabolism, mRNA processing or lipid metabolism when compared to the starting point of the culture.

The functional classification of genes revealed the involvement of several biological processes as well as clear differences between the culture systems used. It is not intended here to describe all changes in gene expression taking place during culturing, instead, by discussing few, discriminating genes, the differences between the culture systems are discussed and general tendencies of gene expression changes elucidated.

### 3.3.6.2 Response to wounding, oxidative stress and immune response

Genes which are known to code for markers of hepatotoxicity or cellular stress, such as heme oxigenase1 (Hmox1), paraoxonase1 (Pon1) and several cytokines, were amongst the genes found to be differentially deregulated between the cultures (Table 22). Hmox1 is an essential enzyme in heme catabolism which has also a protective role against cellular stress, especially during inflammatory processes and oxidative stress (Wunder & Potter, 2003). It is induced by cytokines, hypoxia or ROS and is hypothesized to contribute to the decrease of CYP activity in culture (Kutty et al., 1988). This gene was induced initially in all cultures but reduced in expression over time in FCS-free long term cultures.

Already in short-term cultures a transient induction of cytokines and pro-inflammatory genes was detected. The chemokine ligand 1 (Cxcl1) acts as a neutrophil chemoattractant and was heavily induced during early stages of culture. In longer time cultures, especially in SW-, the expression of Cxcl1 was reduced again to an expression close to the control. Other cytokines, like Interleukin1 (Il1a), which is involved in various immune responses and inflammatory processes, are normally expressed in macrophages and monocytes and are therefore likely to be reduced in hepatocyte cultures. The alpha-2-macroglobulin (A2m), a protease inhibitor and cytokine transporter is a classic marker for activated

# 3 RESULTS AND DISCUSSION

immune responses in the liver (Kurokawa et al., 1987). It was induced during suspension culture, in ML-FCS culture and in early stages of SW-FCS.

The inflammatory process of hydrolyzing oxidized phospholipids to generate free oxidized fatty acids is mediated by platelet-activating factor acetylhydrolase (Pla2g7), which was induced in suspension and long term cultures with FCS. Hydroxisteroid (11-beta) dehydroxigenase1 (Hsd11b1) was reduced in all long term cultures with the exception of SW-FCS. This enzyme catalyzes the conversion of the stress hormone cortisol to the inactive metabolite cortisone.

| Symbol | Accession-Nr. | Susp 1 d | Slice 1 d | ML+FCS 1 d | 6 d | 10 d | ML-FCS 1 d | 6 d | 10 d | SW+FCS 1 d | 6 d | 10 d | SW-FCS 1 d | 6 d | 10 d |
|---|---|---|---|---|---|---|---|---|---|---|---|---|---|---|---|
| A2m | NM_012488 | 3.8 | | | 2.5 | | 43.8 | 9.9 | 12.3 | | 2.9 | 51.4 | | | |
| Ccnd1 | NM_171992 | | -3.0 | | 2.6 | 5.4 | -8.8 | -2.3 | | | 2.6 | -10.3 | -4.8 | -4.1 | |
| Cpb2 | NM_053617 | | -2.4 | | -6.1 | -11.1 | | -3.3 | -3.4 | -2.1 | | | -2.8 | -2.4 | |
| Crp | NM_017096 | -5.3 | -4.2 | -40.9 | -31.4 | | -5.2 | -3.2 | | -3.4 | -3.5 | | | | |
| Cxcl1 | NM_030845 | 22.9 | 15.1 | 39.3 | 15.1 | 13.5 | 13.7 | 6.5 | 6.2 | 46.1 | 15.2 | 15.6 | 12.8 | 3.4 | 2.7 |
| Cxcl2 | NM_053647 | 4.1 | 3.3 | 22.6 | 8.5 | 3.9 | 4.7 | 4.4 | 4.2 | 18.6 | | 2.2 | 6.8 | | |
| F10 | NM_017143 | -3.6 | -2.4 | -3.1 | -36.9 | -46.7 | -2.3 | -9.3 | -10.4 | | -4.0 | -3.7 | | -3.6 | -2.6 |
| Hmox1 | NM_012580 | 8.4 | 4.8 | 11.3 | 4.3 | 7.0 | 7.3 | | | 22.9 | 4.1 | 7.9 | 17.0 | | |
| Hrmt1l2 | NM_024363 | 4.0 | 2.5 | 2.2 | 4.5 | 4.2 | | 2.0 | 2.3 | 2.0 | 2.4 | 2.5 | | | |
| Hsd11b1 | NM_017080 | | | -47.2 | -24.8 | | -2.5 | -2.5 | | -8.5 | -7.6 | | | | |
| Il1a | NM_017019 | -4.1 | -2.7 | | | -4.6 | -6.7 | -5.5 | -2.9 | | -5.3 | -5.2 | -5.6 | -5.7 | |
| Il1b | NM_031512 | | | | -2.3 | -3.0 | -3.0 | | | | -2.3 | -2.4 | -2.5 | -2.8 | |
| Ndst1 | NM_024361 | | | | -3.4 | -4.1 | | -2.79 | -3.2 | | -2.0 | -2.5 | | | |
| Pla2g7 | NM_001009353 | 3.5 | | | 2.3 | 9.8 | | | | | 3.0 | | | | |
| Pon1 | NM_032077 | | | -97.6 | -110.5 | | -13.4 | -14.7 | | -3.4 | -5.4 | | -4.1 | -3.9 | -8.5 |
| Proc | NM_012803 | | | -4.5 | -20.0 | -25.1 | -2.4 | -8.0 | -6.5 | -2.6 | -5.5 | -5.3 | -2.2 | -3.5 | -2.5 |
| Saa4 | NM_001009478 | | -2.2 | -105.3 | -59.1 | | -2.6 | -2.5 | | -2.2 | -2.2 | | | | |
| Serpind1 | NM_024382 | -3.9 | -13.3 | -14.7 | -220.9 | -226.4 | -12.3 | -110.9 | -125.2 | -13.7 | -8.7 | -9.8 | -10.2 | -69.1 | -97.8 |
| Txn2 | NM_053331 | | | -2.2 | -2.7 | -2.6 | | -2.0 | -2.2 | | | | | | |
| Tp53 | NM_030989 | 2.4 | 2.6 | 4.0 | | | 2.3 | 2.3 | 2.5 | 2.7 | 2.4 | | | | |

Table 22: Fold change values of several genes concerning the response to wounding, oxidative stress and the immune response. Genes selected were at least 2-fold deregulated at multiple time points and had a significance level of lower than 0.05 in at least one of the cultures.

Another gene indicating an increase of oxidative stress was the reduction of thioredoxin (Txn) expression in ML cultures. Txn is a small, di-thiol containing protein and a key player in maintaining cellular redox status and redox-controlled cell functions by transferring

## 3 RESULTS AND DISCUSSION

reducing-equivalents to disulfide groups (Burke-Gaffney, Callister & Nakamura, 2005). Besides this, several transcription factors, like p53, NFκB, AP1 and the glucocorticoid receptor, are known to possess thiol groups and to be partly regulated by Txn, thereby altering various essential cellular processes.

It is known that hepatocytes are primed to re-enter the cell cycle during hepatocyte isolation, a process known to be triggered by inflammation and to underlie the dedifferentiation process of cultured hepatocytes (Papeleu et al., 2006). For cell cycle progression, additional growth factors, like EGF (Epidermal Growth Factor) or HGF (Hepatocyte Growth Factor) are required. The expression of Cyclin D1 (Ccnd1), found to be induced in hepatocytes cultured with FCS, separates the cells from these signals and initiates the proliferation.

Another process affected was the regulation of blood coagulation. Under normal conditions, hepatocytes are triggered to increase the synthesis of coagulant and complement factors and protease inhibitors by proinflammatory cytokines, as a response to wounding (Dhainaut et al., 2001). In culture, the expression of serpin peptidase inhibitor (Serpind1), which rapidly inhibits thrombin, carboxypeptidase B2 (Cpb2), which down regulates fibrinolysis, and protein C (Proc), a zymogen that catalyzes the inactivation of blood coagulation cofactors like coagulation factor X (F10), are clearly repressed in all types of culture. This can be seen as a physiological response to wounding and induction of wound healing processes due to the isolation procedure itself.

### 3.3.6.3 ECM, cytoskeleton and tissue remodelling

Large differences were also detected in the gene expression of ECM components, cell adhesion and cytoskeletal related genes (Table 23). The cellular morphology and formation of cell-to-cell and cell-to-matrix- contacts have proven to be of essential importance for cellular survival and functionality (Dunn et al. 1989; Richert et al., 2002; Hamilton et al., 2001) and are one of the key differences distinguishing the cell cultures from each other.

Collagens are the main constituent of the ECM. Collagen 1a1 and 3a1 (Col1a2 and Col3a1) were heavily down regulated during the perfusion, indicating the loss of several collagen expressing cell types. Especially Col3a1 is known to be expressed in connective tissues and blood vessels. Whereas the collagen expression in cultures without FCS remained stable, although at a low level in freshly isolated hepatocytes, the expression rose again over time when cultured with FCS. This may be a sign of the progressive

## 3 RESULTS AND DISCUSSION

dedifferentiation of hepatocytes towards a fibroblast like cell type and the induction of proliferation.

| Symbol | Accession-Nr. | Susp 1 d | Slice 1 d | ML+FCS 1 d | ML+FCS 6 d | ML+FCS 10 d | ML-FCS 1 d | ML-FCS 6 d | ML-FCS 10 d | SW+FCS 1 d | SW+FCS 6 d | SW+FCS 10 d | SW-FCS 1 d | SW-FCS 6 d | SW-FCS 10 d |
|---|---|---|---|---|---|---|---|---|---|---|---|---|---|---|---|
| Actb | NM_031144 | | | 3.0 | 2.8 | 3.0 | 2.8 | 2.7 | 2.7 | 3.7 | | | 2.8 | | |
| Actn1 | NM_031005 | | | 2.2 | 4.9 | 5.1 | | 4.0 | 4.3 | | 2.8 | 2.1 | | | |
| Cfl1 | NM_017147 | | | 2.5 | 2.6 | 2.5 | 2.3 | 2.6 | 2.5 | | 2.2 | 2.2 | | | |
| Col1a2 | NM_053356 | -2.1 | -15.5 | -37.9 | | 4.3 | -33.6 | -15.0 | -3.0 | -27.0 | | 5.0 | -31.6 | -28.1 | -9.9 |
| Col3a1 | NM_032085.1 | -2.7 | -11.2 | -14.4 | -8.0 | | -14.1 | -13.5 | -9.0 | -13.9 | -9.0 | | -14.6 | -14.5 | -13.6 |
| Defb1 | NM_031810 | | | 6.3 | | | 28.9 | 17.7 | 11.4 | 2.3 | | | 23.8 | 32.2 | 20.9 |
| Gja1 | NM_012567 | | -4.5 | -10.1 | 11.5 | 12.2 | -10.8 | -9.2 | -3.9 | -9.0 | | 6.6 | -12.5 | -11.9 | -5.8 |
| Lamc1 | XM_341133 | 2.4 | | 2.2 | 2.5 | | 2.8 | 2.7 | 3.1 | | | 2.3 | | | |
| Mgp | NM_012862 | | -8.5 | -12.9 | -3.2 | | -12.5 | -12.3 | -5.8 | -9.9 | -2.3 | | -12.6 | -12.4 | -9.7 |
| Mmp12 | NM_053963 | 24.5 | | | 116.1 | 226.1 | | | | | 43.5 | 104.1 | | | |
| Msn | NM_030863 | | | | 5.6 | 14.8 | | 3.6 | 4.6 | | 3.1 | 3.9 | | | |
| Myh10 | NM_031520 | | | 3.1 | 5.2 | 5.2 | | 2.5 | 2.9 | 2.2 | 3.0 | 3.0 | | | |
| Nexn | NM_139231 | | | | 4.6 | 3.5 | | 2.4 | 2.6 | | | | | | |
| Pfn2 | NM_030873 | | | | 4.3 | 4.9 | | 2.7 | 3.8 | | 2.3 | 2.5 | | | 2.2 |
| Spp1 | NM_012881 | 18.6 | | | 100.6 | 199.4 | | | | | 22.6 | 78.7 | | | |
| Timp1 | NM_053819 | 7.5 | -2.96 | 2.3 | 11.2 | 13.4 | | | 2.6 | | 4.9 | 7.3 | | -2.4 | -2.4 |
| Tpm1 | NM_019131 | | | | 6.3 | 5.8 | | 2.3 | 2.2 | | 3.2 | 3.0 | | | |

Table 23: ECM, adhesion or cytoskeletal related genes distinguishing the different cell cultures from each other.

The influence of FCS on inflammatory processes in isolated primary hepatocytes is demonstrated by matrix metalloproteinase12 (Mmp12), which is also called macrophage elastase and is involved in the breakdown of extracellular matrix in physiological as well as inflammatory processes (Mohammed et al., 2005). This enzyme is normally found in epithelial tissue and contributes to wound healing, but is also found in hepatoma cells triggering neovascularisation (Lyu & Joo, 2005). Mmp12 was found to be induced only in suspension and in late time points of ML and SW culture when cultured with FCS. The endogenous metalloproteinase inhibitor (Timp-1) was induced in all cultures except for SW-FCS, indicating changes in the reorganisation of the ECM environment as a reaction to cellular damage and inflammation or growth which may help explaining the change in cell morphology.

The cytoskeleton and their contact to the ECM by cell adhesion molecules and external signalling are connected to intracellular signalling cascades and mediate specific and

## 3 RESULTS AND DISCUSSION

important cellular processes. The reestablishment of these contacts, together with the reestablishment of cellular polarity and the stability of the actin cytoskeleton, are crucial requirements for hepatotypic functionality and for reducing the cellular stress (Page et al., 2007). The Gap junction protein alpha (Gja1) was reduced at early time points in culture but induced later on, except for SW– cultured cells. Gja1 is associated with endothelial cells and immature hepatocytes, again indicating the dedifferentiation processes in culture after addition of FCS (large induction ML+FCS 124-fold induced and SW+, 59-fold) (González et al., 2002).

The contact between ECM and the reorganisation of the actin cytoskeleton in response to external signals is mediated by profilins (Pfn 2), tropomyosin 1 (Tpm1) and moiesin (Msn), which were all induced in long term cultures, except for SW-. Actin itself (Actb) was mainly induced in ML cultured cells reflecting the need to reorganize the cytoskeleton due to their flattened shape. Finally, myosin heavy polypeptide 10 (Myh10) and secreted phosphoprotein 1 are physiologically expressed in immature smooth muscle cells and endothelial cells (Hiroi et al., 1996) and were induced by ML culturing and after the addition of FCS.

### 3.3.6.4 Metabolic competence

The metabolic competence of hepatocytes is one of the key elements defining their usability for toxicological studies. Besides the inducibility of CYP enzymes, which has been discussed extensively in chapter 3.2, there are several other genes involved in phase 1, phase 2 and phase 3 metabolisms. Previous studies have demonstrated predominantly a down regulation of phase 1 metabolism in cultures already over night as well as in later stages of culture (Baker et al., 2001; Lupp et al., 2001; Richert et al., 2002). These findings were generally corroborated by our studies, but in SW-FCS cultured cells the decrease was less pronounced and they displayed a more stable gene expression over time.

Table 24 shows genes involved in phase 1 metabolism, which were differentially deregulated in primary rat hepatocyte cultures. The gene expression of several CYP isoforms was strongly repressed, however the extent of deregulation differed greatly. For example Cyp8b1 was repressed in all cultures, but whereas the expression was reduced up to 171-fold in ML+FCS, 21-fold in ML-FCS and 14-fold in SW+FCS on day 10 in culture, it was reduced only 2.3-fold in SW-FCS cultures. Other CYPs, like Cyp2c and Cyp3a1, were inhibited by the addition of FCS to the culture media but not in DEX containing, FCS free cultures. The three dimensional environment of SW culture had a

# 3 RESULTS AND DISCUSSION

positive effect on Cyp2a1 expression, Cyp1a2 however was unaffected and its expression was reduced equally in all cultures.

| Symbol | Accession- Nr. | Susp 1 d | Slice 1 d | ML+FCS 1 d | ML+FCS 6 d | ML+FCS 10 d | ML-FCS 1 d | ML-FCS 6 d | ML-FCS 10 d | SW+FCS 1 d | SW+FCS 6 d | SW+FCS 10 d | SW-FCS 1 d | SW-FCS 6 d | SW-FCS 10 d |
|---|---|---|---|---|---|---|---|---|---|---|---|---|---|---|---|
| Adh1 | NM_019286 | | | -18.8 | -67.4 | -46.9 | | -2.5 | -2.9 | -7.7 | | | | | |
| Adh4 | NM_017270 | | | -3.0 | -5.5 | -6.1 | -2.5 | -2.6 | -2.8 | -3.1 | -3.0 | -3.4 | -2.9 | | |
| Adhfe1_predicted | XM_342794 | -17.1 | -8.6 | -6.5 | 123.3 | 104.0 | -4.0 | -33.3 | -22.6 | -6.5 | -25.0 | -40.0 | -3.9 | -4.7 | -2.6 |
| Cyp1a1 | NM_012540 | | | | 3.1 | 3.8 | | 2.6 | 5.1 | | | | | 4.0 | 11.9 |
| Cyp1a2 | NM_012541 | | | -5.4 | 138.7 | 100.4 | -3.5 | 103.5 | -70.8 | -8.4 | -92.6 | -83.9 | -4.3 | -64.7 | -69.2 |
| Cyp2a1 | NM_012692 | -8.0 | -5.1 | -8.9 | -55.7 | -50.6 | -4.6 | -18.8 | -18.3 | -4.3 | -4.0 | -4.2 | -3.9 | -3.0 | -2.4 |
| Cyp2c | NM_019184 | -3.7 | -4.7 | -2.6 | 276.3 | 188.6 | -2.5 | -4.7 | -7.0 | -2.8 | -36.8 | 119.5 | -2.4 | -3.0 | -2.4 |
| Cyp2e1 | NM_031543 | -2.5 | -3.6 | | 360.9 | 336.4 | | 216.4 | 262.4 | | 170.1 | 267.7 | | 100.1 | -91.5 |
| Cyp3a1 | NM_173144 | -2.9 | -2.7 | -2.1 | 403.2 | 397.8 | | -2.0 | -2.0 | -2.2 | -42.6 | 100.0 | | | |
| Cyp3a3 | NM_013105 | -5.4 | -3.7 | -2.4 | 278.7 | 233.4 | | | | -2.4 | -47.1 | -78.9 | | | |
| Cyp8b1 | NM_031241 | -43.4 | -9.1 | -66.0 | 222.0 | 171.4 | -46.2 | -46.8 | -20.8 | -39.7 | -56.4 | -13.9 | -39.8 | -4.6 | -2.3 |
| Fmo1 | NM_012792 | -22.2 | -19.1 | -4.3 | -59.1 | -57.3 | -16.7 | -31.2 | -40.7 | -4.7 | -50.3 | -55.1 | -14.7 | -23.1 | -15.5 |

Table 24: Phase 1 metabolism genes found to be differentially regulated. (Fold change>2 and pV<0.05).

UDP glucuronosyltransferases (Ugt) have a broad substrate specificity and mediate the glucoronidation of intermediate metabolites. Although DEX was previously shown to induce UGT transcription *in vitro* (Jemnitz et al., 2000), these results could only be confirmed for Ugt1a7 during this study. The other isoforms remained unaffected in SW-FCS culture and were reduced in expression in short term and in ML cultures.

Also of importance for xenobiotic detoxification is the transfer of sulfonate groups from 3'-phosphoadenosine 5'-phosphosulfate (PAPS) to target nucleophilic metabolites, which is mediated by sulfotransferases (Sult). These enzymes have overlapping substrate specificities with Ugts, but higher affinity and lower activity. The expression of the different isoenzymes differed from each other as well as between the different cultures. In short-term cultures and in cells cultured with FCS, all sulfotransferases were reduced whereas in FCS free cultures Sult1a1 and Sult1b1 were not affected.

## 3 RESULTS AND DISCUSSION

Glutathione is essential, not only for phase 2 metabolism, but also for intracellular redox homeostasis. Glutathione synthase (Gss) expression was induced in all types of culture, whereas the expression of several Glutathione S-transferases (Gst) was reduced. Gsts are a large group of enzymes responsible for detoxification by conjugating several electrophilic intermediates to glutathione. They are encoded by at least five gene families (alpha, mu, pi, sigma, and theta) and are an essential component of cellular antioxidant defence mechanisms. The placental Gstp1, known for its specific expression during rat hepatocarcinogenesis, is a well defined dedifferentiation marker (Vanhaecke, Elaut & Rogiers, 2001) and also used as a tumour marker (Sakai & Muramatsu, 2007). It was induced in long term cultures, especially in the presence of FCS, and minimally in SW-FCS. Gsta2, the most abundantly expressed Gst in liver, was reduced, but was more stable in SW cultured cells.

| Symbol | Accession-Nr. | Susp 1 d | Slice 1 d | ML+FCS 1 d | ML+FCS 6 d | ML+FCS 10 d | ML-FCS 1 d | ML-FCS 6 d | ML-FCS 10 d | SW+FCS 1 d | SW+FCS 6 d | SW+FCS 10 d | SW-FCS 1 d | SW-FCS 6 d | SW-FCS 10 d |
|---|---|---|---|---|---|---|---|---|---|---|---|---|---|---|---|
| Gss | NM_012962 | | 3.5 | 4.4 | 2.2 | | 2.4 | 2.5 | 2.5 | 3.8 | 2.8 | 2.5 | | 2.2 | 2.8 |
| Gsta2 | NM_017013 | -7.4 | | | -17.8 | -15.2 | -2.3 | -11.4 | -10.0 | | | | -2.6 | -4.3 | -5.5 |
| Gstm3 | NM_031154 | -9.1 | -3.2 | -8.3 | -24.0 | -21.4 | -6.5 | -16.9 | -15.8 | -7.8 | -19.1 | -18.2 | -5.9 | -7.8 | -3.8 |
| Gstp1 | XM_579338 | | 21.5 | 23.6 | 51.6 | 55.3 | 4.4 | 20.0 | 32.0 | 19.5 | 63.2 | 63.7 | | 12.6 | 11.2 |
| Sult1a1 | NM_031834 | -3.5 | -12.0 | -26.8 | -108.2 | -104.6 | | | | -19.3 | -8.2 | -12.3 | | | |
| Sult1b1 | NM_022513 | -3.1 | -2.3 | -10.3 | -29.2 | -37.0 | | | | -9.7 | -2.6 | -3.0 | | | |
| Sult1c1 | NM_031732 | -51.7 | -41.9 | -24.9 | -352.9 | -326.9 | -22.7 | -237.0 | -296.6 | -27.0 | -10.0 | -31.5 | -18.0 | -140.9 | -139.5 |
| Sult1c2 | NM_133547 | -10.3 | -3.8 | -11.2 | -17.2 | -17.4 | -9.3 | -13.6 | -11.9 | -10.3 | -12.7 | -13.4 | -5.2 | -9.3 | -12.5 |
| Ugt1a7 | NM_130407 | | | | | | 6.8 | 5.6 | 6.1 | | | | 5.7 | 6.6 | 5.5 |
| Ugt2b | NM_031533 | -3.2 | | | -5.8 | -9.3 | | | | | -2.2 | | | | |
| Ugt2b10 | XM_223299 | -5.6 | -5.9 | -6.9 | -16.9 | -8.7 | -3.1 | -3.4 | -2.9 | -5.8 | -3.0 | -3.1 | -3.0 | | |
| Ugt2b3 | NM_153314 | -3.0 | | | -4.4 | -7.2 | -2.1 | | | | -2.1 | | | | |
| Ugt2b4 | NM_001004271 | -3.1 | | | -4.8 | -4.3 | -2.0 | | | | -2.5 | | | | |
| Ugt2b4 | XM_579544 | -2.3 | | | -2.7 | -2.3 | -2.2 | | | | | | | | |
| Ugt2b5 | NM_001007264 | -3.1 | -2.4 | | -10.4 | -17.3 | -3.1 | -2.7 | | | -2.3 | -2.9 | | | |

Table 25: Genes of the phase 2 metabolism found to be differentially regulated (fold change>2 and pV<0.05).

### 3.3.6.5 Intracellular signalling and transcription factors

As mentioned earlier, ligand activated transcription factors coordinately regulate the expression of a vast number of genes involved in detoxification and many other cellular

## 3 RESULTS AND DISCUSSION

processes. They often form obligate heterodimers with the retinoid X receptor (RXR) and hence, the importance of keeping the expression levels of these genes as similar to fresh liver as possible, to preserve liver-like detoxification function, is essential. Other transcription factors are important for cellular differentiation and the regulation of genes involved in cell cycle, inflammatory processes or energy metabolism.

| Symbol | Accession-Nr. | Susp | Slice | ML+FCS | | | ML-FCS | | | SW+FCS | | | SW-FCS | | |
|---|---|---|---|---|---|---|---|---|---|---|---|---|---|---|---|
| | | 1 d | 1 d | 1 d | 6 d | 10 d | 1 d | 6 d | 10 d | 1 d | 6 d | 10 d | 1 d | 6 d | 10 d |
| Ahr | XM_579375 | -6.2 | -2.6 | -2.7 | | | -2.1 | | | -3.8 | | | -2.3 | | |
| Aif1 | NM_017196 | -2.2 | -20.0 | -36.9 | -3.7 | | -31.6 | -56.8 | -53.0 | -23.3 | -2.9 | | -31.3 | -49.1 | -45.0 |
| Arntl | NM_024362 | | | | -2.6 | -3.0 | | -2.2 | -2.1 | | -3.4 | -2.8 | | | |
| Cd53 | NM_012523 | | -4.5 | -3.7 | 2.6 | 5.7 | -4.1 | -5.2 | -4.9 | -4.0 | | 2.4 | -4.1 | -5.2 | -4.8 |
| Ctgf | NM_022266 | | 3.7 | | 30.4 | 31.3 | 30.1 | 28.4 | 26.9 | -2.3 | 33.5 | 32.0 | 21.3 | 35.4 | 33.3 |
| Egf | NM_012842 | -5.1 | -4.2 | -4.1 | -7.5 | -9.7 | -2.7 | -6.4 | -7.0 | -3.5 | -3.9 | -5.3 | -2.2 | -3.1 | -2.9 |
| Hnf4a | NM_022180 | | | | -4.3 | -3.8 | | | | -2.4 | -2.2 | | | | |
| Khdrbs1 | NM_130405 | | | 3.0 | 3.0 | | 2.1 | 2.1 | | 2.4 | 2.3 | | | | |
| Nr1h3/LXR | NM_031627 | | -2.3 | -3.3 | -5.7 | -5.4 | -2.2 | -3.2 | -3.1 | -2.7 | -3.6 | -3.2 | -3.6 | | -2.0 |
| Nr1h4/FXR | NM_021745 | | -3.1 | -4.0 | -10.6 | -13.5 | -2.5 | -4.4 | -4.6 | -3.3 | -2.0 | -2.5 | -4.7 | | -2.0 |
| Nr1i2/PXR | NM_052980 | -2.3 | -3.8 | -4.0 | -5.7 | -5.7 | | | | -2.9 | -2.7 | -2.7 | | | |
| Nr1i3/CAR | NM_022941 | | -5.2 | -5.7 | -13.1 | -13.1 | -2.5 | -6.6 | -4.8 | -4.7 | -8.2 | -8.0 | -4.6 | | |
| Nrp1 | NM_145098 | -2.1 | -5.2 | -5.5 | | | -5.7 | -5.3 | -4.3 | -5.7 | -3.9 | | -5.8 | -5.9 | -5.7 |
| Pdzk1 | NM_031712 | -2.4 | -4.7 | -4.0 | -12.4 | -15.5 | -3.5 | -4.8 | -5.7 | -2.3 | | | -3.0 | -2.7 | -2.6 |
| Rgs2 | NM_053453 | 2.2 | | | 31.8 | 34.9 | -2.6 | | 3.8 | | 15.9 | 23.2 | -2.4 | | 3.9 |
| Rgs3 | NM_019340 | | | | | 2.3 | | -3.9 | -2.7 | | 2.3 | 2.7 | | -3.9 | -3.7 |
| Rxra | NM_012805 | -2.3 | | -2.5 | -3.5 | -3.4 | | -2.6 | -2.9 | | -2.1 | -2.1 | | | |
| Tcf4 | NM_053369 | | -2.2 | | | | -2.2 | | -2.1 | -2.1 | -2.2 | | -2.1 | -2.4 | -2.3 |
| Thrb | NM_012672 | -3.2 | | -2.3 | -4.0 | -5.2 | -2.7 | -3.3 | -2.4 | | | | | | |
| Tnfsf13 | NM_001009623 | | | -3.1 | | | -3.7 | -2.3 | -2.4 | -2.4 | | | -4.0 | -3.8 | -3.6 |
| Vldlr | NM_013155 | | | 6.7 | 5.0 | 5.4 | 4.4 | | | 5.3 | 4.3 | 4.6 | 8.5 | | |

Table 26: Gene expression changes of liver enriched transcription factors (fold change>2 and pV<0.05).

Hepatocyte nuclear factor 4α (Hnf4a) plays a critical role in the maintenance of hepatocyte phenotype, lipid and bile acid metabolism (Sladek, 1994). Moreover, the expression of other transcription factors, like pregnane X receptor (PXR) and liver X receptor (LXR), and of several CYP isoforms require HNF4a activity (Tirona & Kim, 2005). In culture, FCS reduced the expression of this important TF whereas it was unchanged in serum free cultures (Table 26). Many ligand activated receptors, like RXR, PXR, CAR or Ahr, were repressed in liver slices and long-term cultures, except for SW-FCS cultures. This culture

## 3 RESULTS AND DISCUSSION

system seems to retain liver specific transcription of these important genes at physiological levels over longer times.

Epidermal growth factor (EGF) and connective tissue growth factor (Ctgf) both showed no difference in expression between the different cell cultures. Whereas EGF, important for liver regeneration and the reentry into the cell cycle after lesions, was continuously reduced in all types of culture, Ctgf was strongly induced in all but suspension cultures. Ctgf promotes cell adhesion and cell motility in nonparenchymal liver cells and therefore cell activation during liver regeneration following injury (Pi et al., 2008).

The expression of CD53, initially repressed in all cultures, was increased over time in FCS containing cultures. CD53 is a transmembrane protein mediating signal transduction events that plays a role in the regulation of cell development, growth regulation and motility by forming complexes with integrins.

### 3.3.6.6 Affected mechanisms in human hepatocytes

In contrast to rat hepatocytes, the human orthologue genes, again clustered together to functional groups, were much more stable over time (Figure 56). In most of the groups no clear differences in the dedifferentiation processes were detected over time and gene expression changes in ML and in SW cultures were comparable. Interestingly, the liver progenitor cell line HepaRG showed partly specific hepatotypic gene expression and displayed stabile expression over time. Clear differences were found in the expression of genes involved in cellular signalling, mRNA-processing, ECM-proteins, cell adhesion and metabolism.

Table 27 shows genes which displayed differences in expression in some mayor functional categories. Most important for toxicology, the deregulation of xenobiotic metabolism was less severe than in rat hepatocytes with some of the main enzymes mediating phase 1 metabolism (Cyp1a1 and 2E1) being down regulated. The glutathione system, which is encoded in distinct genomic clusters and represented here by Gstm3 and Gsp1, was less expressed in HepaRG cells, whereas Gsta was inversely regulated. Gsta´s are are the main enzymes for the detoxification of lipid peroxidation products whereas the other isoforms are mainly responsible for the detoxification of other electrophilic metabolites (Pham, Barber & Gallagher, 2004).

Some of the differences found between HepaRG cells and primary human hepatocytes can be explained by the lower expression of certain transcription factors. The activating transcription factor 3 (ATF3), CCAAT/enhancer binding protein α (CEBPA) and the

# 3 RESULTS AND DISCUSSION

glucocorticoid receptor (Nr3c1) were found to be lower expressed in HepaRG cells than in liver. This glucocorticoid receptor can act as both a transcription factor and as a regulator of other transcription factors. ATF3 is a member of the activation transcription factor/cAMP responsive element-binding (CREB) protein family and binds to certain promoter and enhancer sequences. In addition to the positive or negative regulation of transcription, CEBPA is known to inhibit cyclin dependent kinases (CDK2 and CDK4), thereby causing growth arrest in cultured cells.

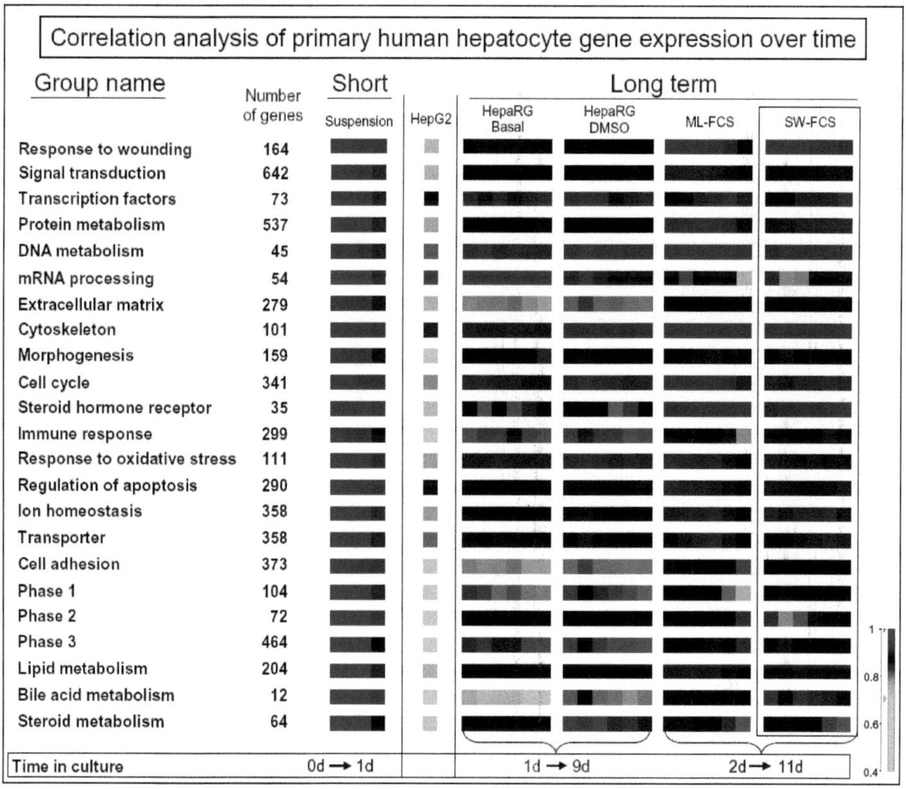

| Correlation analysis of primary human hepatocyte gene expression over time | | | | | | | | |
|---|---|---|---|---|---|---|---|---|
| Group name | Number of genes | Short | | Long term | | | | |
| | | Suspension | HepG2 | HepaRG Basal | HepaRG DMSO | ML-FCS | SW-FCS | |
| Response to wounding | 164 | | | | | | | |
| Signal transduction | 642 | | | | | | | |
| Transcription factors | 73 | | | | | | | |
| Protein metabolism | 537 | | | | | | | |
| DNA metabolism | 45 | | | | | | | |
| mRNA processing | 54 | | | | | | | |
| Extracellular matrix | 279 | | | | | | | |
| Cytoskeleton | 101 | | | | | | | |
| Morphogenesis | 159 | | | | | | | |
| Cell cycle | 341 | | | | | | | |
| Steroid hormone receptor | 35 | | | | | | | |
| Immune response | 299 | | | | | | | |
| Response to oxidative stress | 111 | | | | | | | |
| Regulation of apoptosis | 290 | | | | | | | |
| Ion homeostasis | 358 | | | | | | | |
| Transporter | 358 | | | | | | | |
| Cell adhesion | 373 | | | | | | | |
| Phase 1 | 104 | | | | | | | |
| Phase 2 | 72 | | | | | | | |
| Phase 3 | 464 | | | | | | | |
| Lipid metabolism | 204 | | | | | | | |
| Bile acid metabolism | 12 | | | | | | | |
| Steroid metabolism | 64 | | | | | | | |
| Time in culture | | 0d → 1d | | 1d → 9d | | | 2d → 11d | |

Figure 56: Group-wise correlation analysis of primary human hepatocyte gene expression. Each correlation plot represents important cellular and liver specific mechanisms for different primary rat hepatocyte culture methods. Changes in the correlation of gene expression in comparison to the reference experiments (FC) are indicated by a change of colour. The calibration bar on the right side indicates the colour scheme which was chosen for an optimal visualization.

## 3 RESULTS AND DISCUSSION

The expression levels of several genes correlating with inflammatory response and structural rearrangement, like the formiminotransferase cyclodeaminase (Ftcd), which binds vimentin intermediate filaments, thereby regulating cytoskeletal rearrangement, were found to differ from the levels in liver, implicating the onset of restructuring in primary hepatocytes which in general was different in HepaRG cells.

| Symbol | Accession-Nr. | Susp 1 d | HepaRG (Basal) 1 d | 6 d | 10 d | HepaRG (DMSO) 1 d | 6 d | 10 d | ML-FCS 1 d | 6 d | 10 d | SW-FCS 1 d | 6 d | 10 d |
|---|---|---|---|---|---|---|---|---|---|---|---|---|---|---|
| ALDH3A1 | ILMN_6390 | | 17.6 | 18.4 | 23.7 | 26.1 | 19.1 | 31.1 | | 2.6 | 2.5 | 2.8 | 3.0 | |
| APOA2 | ILMN_18670 | | -2.8 | | -2.7 | -11.3 | -8.0 | -13.2 | | | | | | |
| ATF3 | ILMN_6468 | | -4.5 | -2.8 | -4.0 | -4.4 | -3.9 | -3.5 | | 2.2 | | | | |
| CD44 | ILMN_7737 | | 2.9 | 3.5 | 3.4 | | | 2.2 | -2.1 | -2.7 | | -2.1 | -3.2 | |
| CEBPA | ILMN_27029 | | -3.6 | | -2.3 | -3.0 | -2.1 | -2.9 | -3.4 | | | | | |
| CTGF | ILMN_3374 | | 2.5 | 2.4 | 2.9 | | | | -6.0 | -2.6 | -3.7 | -8.8 | -4.3 | -3.3 |
| CYP1A2 | ILMN_19528 | -8.0 | -49.3 | -62.8 | -54.5 | -47.5 | -37.0 | -39.5 | -13.1 | -2.4 | -3.0 | -7.0 | | -3.2 |
| CYP2E1 | ILMN_27893 | | -31.1 | -11.3 | -14.8 | -9.0 | -4.7 | -12.1 | -2.4 | -20.1 | -34.5 | | -10.0 | -8.3 |
| CYP4B1 | ILMN_25411 | | 24.7 | 27.5 | 33.6 | 29.5 | 32.7 | 26.0 | | | | | | |
| EGFR | ILMN_15615 | | -3.2 | -2.6 | -2.5 | -2.4 | -2.4 | -2.0 | | | | | -2.0 | |
| FABP1 | ILMN_11988 | -3.6 | -2.3 | | -2.6 | -3.0 | | -6.5 | -24.7 | -7.6 | -9.2 | -15.2 | -3.0 | -5.1 |
| FBP1 | ILMN_16804 | -5.5 | -250.3 | -275.3 | -268.2 | -273.0 | -220.1 | -234.5 | -14.3 | -11.1 | -13.3 | -7.1 | -6.1 | -7.6 |
| FTCD | ILMN_8918 | -3.8 | -193.6 | -210.3 | -193.2 | -192.4 | -158.3 | -179.2 | -4.3 | -4.9 | -4.8 | -3.2 | -2.9 | -3.3 |
| GSTA1 | ILMN_30031 | | | | | | | -2.6 | -3.4 | -5.1 | -5.0 | -4.4 | -4.9 | -3.3 |
| GSTM3 | ILMN_2804 | | -3.0 | -3.0 | -3.1 | -3.0 | -2.7 | -2.9 | | | | | | |
| GSTP1 | ILMN_10475 | -2.8 | -11.0 | -13.2 | -13.7 | -11.2 | -10.1 | -10.1 | | -2.1 | | | | |
| HMOX1 | ILMN_25059 | 2.6 | -4.0 | -4.9 | -5.5 | -3.3 | -3.3 | -2.4 | | | | | | |
| ISL1 | ILMN_25965 | | 3.7 | 3.7 | 4.6 | 5.6 | 5.0 | 5.4 | | | | | | |
| LPL | ILMN_2233 | | 10.5 | 10.6 | 7.5 | 16.0 | 12.6 | 9.2 | | | | | | |
| MAOA | ILMN_11566 | | 2.1 | 2.1 | 2.0 | 2.5 | 2.2 | 2.2 | | | | -2.5 | | |
| MMP7 | ILMN_9188 | | 7.0 | 11.3 | 17.0 | 4.0 | 3.7 | 4.4 | | | | | | |
| NQO1 | ILMN_27575 | | | | | | | | 2.2 | 4.4 | 7.8 | 2.0 | 5.7 | 8.1 |
| NR3C1 | ILMN_21266 | | -2.7 | -3.4 | -3.2 | -2.8 | -2.4 | -2.9 | | | | | | |
| PON1 | ILMN_24208 | -7.4 | -3.3 | -3.5 | -4.5 | -5.6 | -4.4 | -6.9 | -14.7 | -8.3 | -14.2 | -11.8 | -6.3 | -8.1 |
| PPARGC1A | ILMN_16547 | -6.2 | -4.7 | -3.7 | -4.3 | -4.1 | -4.3 | -5.4 | -9.2 | -8.4 | -9.5 | -10.6 | -16.7 | -14.4 |
| S100A6 | ILMN_13161 | | -6.1 | -8.2 | -7.4 | -7.9 | -6.9 | -7.6 | 2.2 | 14.1 | 24.5 | 2.0 | 14.1 | 15.2 |
| S100A8 | ILMN_13072 | -2.5 | 4.0 | 2.4 | | 2.3 | 2.4 | 2.1 | -4.9 | -13.3 | -12.4 | -2.8 | -9.7 | -7.2 |
| SGK | ILMN_2451 | | -2.5 | -4.4 | -3.1 | -4.3 | -5.0 | -4.9 | -8.4 | -18.9 | -18.7 | -6.1 | -21.2 | -16.2 |
| SLC7A7 | ILMN_16478 | | 10.4 | 11.5 | 12.9 | 8.4 | 7.2 | 7.5 | | -2.1 | -2.0 | | | -2.2 |
| SPP1 | ILMN_9394 | | 9.7 | 8.7 | 4.6 | 2.4 | 2.2 | | -2.1 | -2.1 | -2.0 | -2.2 | -2.0 | |
| SULT2A1 | ILMN_16119 | -13.7 | -2.8 | -2.4 | -2.1 | | | | -8.9 | -9.6 | -7.2 | -14.1 | -9.8 | -7.9 |
| TIMP1 | ILMN_3162 | | 3.6 | 2.9 | 3.3 | 3.3 | 3.8 | 4.1 | | | | | | |
| TNFRSF11B | ILMN_6495 | | 22.9 | 24.0 | 9.6 | 8.5 | 7.0 | 6.5 | | | | | | |

Table 27: Subset of genes differentially expressed in human primary hepatocytes and HepaRG cells. factors (fold change>2 and pV<0.05).

# 3 RESULTS AND DISCUSSION

## 3.3.7 Confirmation of the microarray results with TaqMan PCR

Over all, more than 4000 genes were found to be differentially regulated between the different cell cultures and the liver or freshly isolated hepatocytes. The genes were selected by statistical significance (pValue<0.01) and fold change (either 1.5-fold or 2-fold). Even though the technique used (Illumina BeadChip arrays) is highly standardized, there is still a possibility to obtain false positive results.

The data obtained by microarray experiment were confirmed by two different ways. First, the comparison to previously published gene expression data, which partly covered the experiments described here (Groneberg et al. 2002; Holme, 1985; Baker et al., 2001; Boess et al., 2003; Tuschl & Müller, 2006; Beigel et al., 2008) revealed every close resemblance in the general tendencies and pathways affected. In Addition, TaqMan PCR was used to verify the results of the global gene expression measurements. Therefore, TLDA cards were designed for high, moderate and low expressed rat and human genes of toxicological importance which were found to be significantly deregulated in culture. Experiments were conducted as stated in chapter 2.2.4.3, using the same RNA as starting material which previously was used for the microarray experiments (results were generated as part of a joint work with Gregor Tuschl, PhD-student).

TaqMan PCR was conducted with samples of 15 rat cell culture conditions (FaO cells, liver slices and suspension culture after 1 d in culture, ML+/-FCS and SW+/-FCS after 1 d, 6 d and 10 d in culture) and with 43 genes of toxicological relevance resulting in an overall number of 645 genes tested in biological triplicates (Appendix 3 and Appendix 4). 530 Of these genes fulfilled the quality cut-off values of being either >2-fold deregulated in the TaqMan experiments or being >2-fold deregulated with a pValue below 0.05 in the microarray experiment. From these 530 genes, 89% (471) were accordingly detected as deregulated with both techniques. None of these 471 genes differed in terms of direction of deregulation resulting in 100% consistent results with the selected parameters for the rat experiments.

The results of human TaqMan analysis revealed slightly different results. In this case, 34 genes were tested in 13 cell culture conditions (Suspension culture after 1 d, HepaRG cells in Basal/DMSO-media, at 1 d, 2 d, and 9 d, ML-FCS and SW-FCS at 2 d, 7 d and 11 d) resulting in an overall number of 442 genes tested in biological triplicates (Appendix 5 and Appendix 6). Of these genes tested only 285 items were significantly deregulated. From these 285, only 37% (105) were commonly detected as deregulated with both techniques, but none of these items were detected to be inversely deregulated. The

# 3 RESULTS AND DISCUSSION

significantly lower rate of detection can be explained by the large human donor variation (Figure 48). The individual differences in gene expression lowered the number of genes matching the significance level cut off and therefore the overall detection rate. Nevertheless, the cut of values chosen guaranteed high quality and trustworthy results in both species. The TaqMan confirmation of some toxicologically important genes validated the results from the microarrays.

Further analysis of the entire data set might give more details of the general adaptation processes taking place after perfusion and the differences between the different culture systems. A very interesting aspect for future studies is the implementation of HepaRG as a new cell line displaying partly distinct, liver specific and stable gene expression.

## 3.3.8 Conclusions from the characterization of primary hepatocytes in culture

The application of toxicogenomic methods in combination with longer term cultured hepatocytes is a promising, but currently an error prone, approach. As gene expression is a highly dynamic and complex process, an optimization and standardization of the liver perfusion and culture conditions is crucial to maintain liver specific properties and gene expression and to generate reproducible and reliable results. Generally, the application of global gene expression serves two main goals. Firstly, it allows an exact characterization of the processes going on in the primary hepatocytes after perfusion and therefore leads to a greater understanding of these underlying processes and regulatory mechanisms controlling gene expression. Secondly, it is an essential prerequisite for each experimental model, especially for new and alternative *in vitro* models, to exactly characterize all relevant features and to estimate the capabilities and the value with respect of the expected results.

Although previous studies showed the existence of various posttranscriptional and posttranslational modifications influencing the correlation between mRNA and proteins, the relatively small dataset shown here, four CYP-isoforms measured on mRNA, protein and activity level, showed comparable results. Additionally, the results from global gene expression analysis are supported by proteomic profiling. Even though fewer mass peaks were significantly detected in comparison to the gene expression, these profiles were sufficient to support previous results. The peak patterns clearly clustered according to time in culture and separated the different culture systems suggesting that SW-FCS is the most

## 3 RESULTS AND DISCUSSION

"liver-like" long term culture system. The major disadvantage of SELDI technology is that it is not clear which proteins were present.

Changes in gene expression were detected already directly after the perfusion. These initial changes can be seen as a result of fundamental changes of cellular morphology and tissue disruption, as a result of stress during perfusion, the lack of signalling by other cell types and hormones and finally as an adaptation processes to the new *in vitro* environment. Some of these changes are inherent to the procedure of perfusion and were therefore expected. They can be minimized with the help of the serum composition. For example the lack of hormonal stimulation was balanced by the addition of Dex, a glucocorticoid analogue known to preserve metabolic activity and differentiation status in hepatocytes. Other processes are harder to avoid. The oxygen gradient between perivenous and periportal hepatocytes and Wnt signalling by endothelial cells are known for their contribution to functional liver zonation (Braeuning et al., 2006; Kienhuis et al., 2007), but are obviously missing from all culture systems.

The results of the global gene expression and from proteomic SELDI analysis clearly show the importance of an exactly defined and standardized cell culture. As the regulation of gene expression is a dynamic process, the degree of change is highly dependent on the type of culture and the time points chosen. To gain further insights into the processes taking place and to link their importance and relevance to toxicology, pathway analysis was conducted with genes found to be significantly deregulated.

Over all, more than 4000 genes were found to be differentially expressed in all of the cell cultures compared to the liver or freshly isolated hepatocytes over time. It is obvious that the multiple effects and consequences can only be partially discussed here and so the study focused on changes accumulated over time in different cultures on a global level, as well as on specific toxicologically important and functionally related sets of genes. Special emphasis was put on a key function of these cells, i.e., their metabolic competence.

Previous studies showed that most of the changes in culture are taking place during the first 24 to 48 h after plating (Beigel et al., 2008). These results were confirmed by this study. Additionally, the results of the global gene expression allowed a detailed view on the processes taking place during this time. The perfusion itself caused many changes in gene expression. Inflammatory responses and adaptation processes to the cell culture environment were characterized by the induction of many pro-inflammatory early response genes, like cytokines. In turn, this was accompanied by ECM reorganization, changes in intracellular signalling and the previously mentioned proliferative effects. Interestingly,

# 3 RESULTS AND DISCUSSION

many genes regulating blood flow and blood vessel buildup were induced, emphasizing the importance of the liver for these processes.

Previous studies suggest that phase 2 metabolism is better preserved by cells in culture than phase 1 enzymes (Kern et al., 1997; Rogiers & Vercruysse, 1998). Our data contradicted this and revealed the deviations in expression levels of these enzymes when compared to the liver. Also here the SW-FCS culture delivered the most "liver-like" gene expression over a longer time for both phase 1 and phase 2 enzymes.

The addition of Dex not only improved the morphological appearance but also significantly increased the levels of metabolic enzymes such as CYP isoforms, several phase 2 isoenzymes and cellular transporters. Dex is known to induce a variety of enzymes including phase 2 enzymes by binding to hormonal activated transcription factors (Waxman, 1999; Jemnitz et al., 2000). Figure 7 shows the main transcription factors and their complex interactions which can influence several important cellular processes. It is obvious to see that changes in transcription factors can lead to multiple modifications in cellular physiology. We showed here that the long-term culture system preserved best many transcription factors and several of the downstream processes.

The short term cultures tested (liver slices and suspension culture) both showed a rapid decline in viability and gene expression. They are used for CYP-induction, biotransformation and cell viability studies. All of these studies rely on the proteins that are still present while in the liver and therefore deliver reliable results. Because of the rapid loss of hepatotypic functionality and gene expression, gene expression analyses have to be questioned, due to their poor reliability and correlation to the *in vivo* situation. Additionally, in liver slices, an overwhelming inflammatory response was seen with extensive signalling between the cell types (especially Kupffer cells, endothelial cells and hepatocytes) leading to the generation of nitric oxide (NO), oxidative stress and therefore increasing cellular stress. In addition, liver slices are thought to represent the *in vivo* situation better by the retention of the original ECM and cellular composition, this might mask many additional changes introduced by compound treatment making this culture system only suited for special applications such as a model for non-parenchymal mediated hepatotoxicity, cell-interaction studies or for canalicular transport studies.

Primary human hepatocytes generally showed much more stabile gene expression than rat hepatocytes in ML as well as in SW culture. In contrast to rat, based on the gene expression, no clear difference between ML and SW cultures was detected. Classical dedifferentiation markers like Gstp1 were not affected in either culture and the enzymes driving metabolism were mostly stabile and closer to the liver expression than in rat. For

# 3 RESULTS AND DISCUSSION

example, the CYP isoforms 1A2 and 2E1, which were heavily reduced in rat hepatocytes at later time points were much less deregulated in human hepatocytes and showed no difference between ML and SW. The massive immune response seen in rat hepatocytes was not observed in human cells to the same extent. This might be due to the fact that the experiments started one day later after perfusion. The correlation analysis of the gene expression data suggests less oxidative stress, less perturbations in the cellular cytoskeleton and a more liver like expression of the cellular transcription factors (Figure 55 and Figure 56).

Despite the fact that primary human hepatocytes are much more difficult to obtain and much more expensive, their excellent stability makes them an ideal experimental system for toxicogenomics. Previous studies by Richert and her co-workers identified the use of cryopreserved hepatocytes as an alternative making this test system independent from surgery, time and place (Richert et al., 2006; Alexandre et al., 2002). The studies conducted were short term (24 h), therefore the possibility to prolong the time in culture with cryopreserved human hepatocytes without additional loss of specific functionality has to be proven.

When conducting studies with human hepatocytes, there are other major obstacles to be aware of. Human donors show great variability. First of all, genetic variability plays a significant role. The medical history and the moral conduct of the individuals has also a big influence, all together resulting in much larger inter-individual differences and making it harder to reach statistical cut-off values. Additionally, the genetic polymorphisms persent in phase 1, phase 2 and phase 3 enzymes in some individuals, making them exceedingly fast or slow metabolizers, influences the results of the toxicological studies. Therefore, a special emphasis has to be put on the statistical analysis of the individual human donors.

Established cell lines, both rat and human, differed significantly from all other cultures. Dramatically lower expression of many metabolically important enzymes and the lack of inducibility might result in an underestimation or even complete lack of compound toxicity. Previous studies have reported an identification rate for cytotoxicity of only 70% when compared with known toxicity in either *in vitro* assays in primary hepatocytes, in *in vivo* assays in rats, or in pre-clinical development (Westerink & Schoonen, 2007).Despite these disadvantages, hepatoma cell lines still have significant benefits as an easy-to-handle and stable test system for special applications. An exception was the human hepatoma cell line HepaRG. This relatively new established cell line has, compared to the other cell lines used, significantly elevated levels of metabolic enzymes as well as many other typical hepatocyte features (Parent et al., 2004). Previous findings from Kanebratt (Kanebratt &

## 3 RESULTS AND DISCUSSION

Andersson, 2008) were corroborated and even expanded upon these studies. They reported that the expression of CYP enzymes, transporter proteins, and transcription factors was stable in differentiated HepaRG cells over a period of 6 weeks. Most CYPs were lower but still stably expressed compared to primary hepatocytes, except for CYP3A4 and CYP7A1 (Kanebratt & Andersson, 2008). In these studies, the expression level of CYP4B1 was about 30 fold higher in HepaRG cells than in hepatocytes. This enzyme is suspected to activate certain carcinogenic compounds and thereby contribute to cellular damage. The expression of CYPs generally decreased slightly when cells were cultured in basal media without DMSO, whereas phase 2 enzymes and phase 3 transporters and other liver-specific factors were unaffected. Transporter studies showed the existence of active transporters at the contact surfaces of these cells (data not shown). Additionally, the global gene expression showed a higher correlation of these cells to primary hepatocytes than to HepG2 cells, indicating at least partially differentiated cells.

Taken together, the above described results of the morphological analyses, the functional tests, proteomic and global gene expression analysis clearly showed an advantage of the SW-FCS culture over the other cell cultures of primary rat hepatocytes. Alterations in xenobiotic metabolism and other hepatocyte-specific cellular functionalities, while still changing, were least pronounced. SW-FCS cultured cells showed the highest sensitivity to CYP inducers as well as being functionally active for over two weeks. Another important fact is the increased stability of gene expression from two days in culture up to two weeks. In some cases, even an increase in correlation to FC was observed suggesting some regenerative processes were taking place in SW-FCS.

All together, these results make SW-FCS the culture system best suited for toxicogenomic studies for the generation of high-quality quantitative data under standardised cell culture conditions.

## 3.4 Development of an *in vitro* liver toxicity prediction model based on longer term primary hepatocyte culture

### 3.4.1 Introduction to the *in vitro* prediction model

The comparison of gene expression profiles from animals exposed to compounds belonging to the same class has been reported to result in a relatively high correlation, including the comparisons between different species treated with the same compound (Amin et al., 2002; Hamadeh et al., 2002a; 2002b). The assumption that compounds causing the same toxic endpoints also generate a unique gene expression signature has led to attempts to classify compounds according to their genomic profile. Up to now, several studies e.g. by Zidek et al. (2007) and Ellinger-Ziegelbauer et al. (2008), have shown the possibility to use this approach for the successful classification of unknown compounds. However, there are still many drawbacks, which have to be resolved. All the studies reported so far were conducted *in vivo* and therefore, they do not help for early screening in drug development. The fact that huge reference databases are required to generate classification results of high quality and predictivity shows that further progress in the development of these techniques is required. Meanwhile there are commercial service providers with large databases (mainly based on *in vivo* experiments) and automated profile analysis, but they are very expensive. *In vitro* data is highly dependent of the culture system used which, as already mentioned, is not standardized yet and therefore the data generated is not totally trustworthy.

To test whether we can overcome the ethical, time and financial bottleneck of animal usage, our *in vitro* system was tested with 15 well known model compounds, as a proof of concept study. Subsequently, a blinded control study was conducted to validate the test system. Based on the results described in chapter 3.2, the SW-FCS conformation was defined as best cell system suited for further toxicogenomic studies. The aim of this study was therefore to generate a robust dataset, which could be used to generate a computational model for the classification of hepatotoxic compounds and negative controls samples *in vitro*.

### 3.4.2 Short description of the test compounds

The compounds used in this study are classic model compounds for hepatotoxicity and they were selected according to previous in-house data and published *in vivo* studies

# 3 RESULTS AND DISCUSSION

(Zidek et al., 2007). For all of the hepatotoxic compounds (Figure 57), there is already information available about their mechanism of action, or at least of their adverse effects *in vivo*. Additionally, a former drug candidate from Merck KGaA, which was stopped during development due to hepatotoxicity, was employed as a blinded control sample for the verification of the test system.

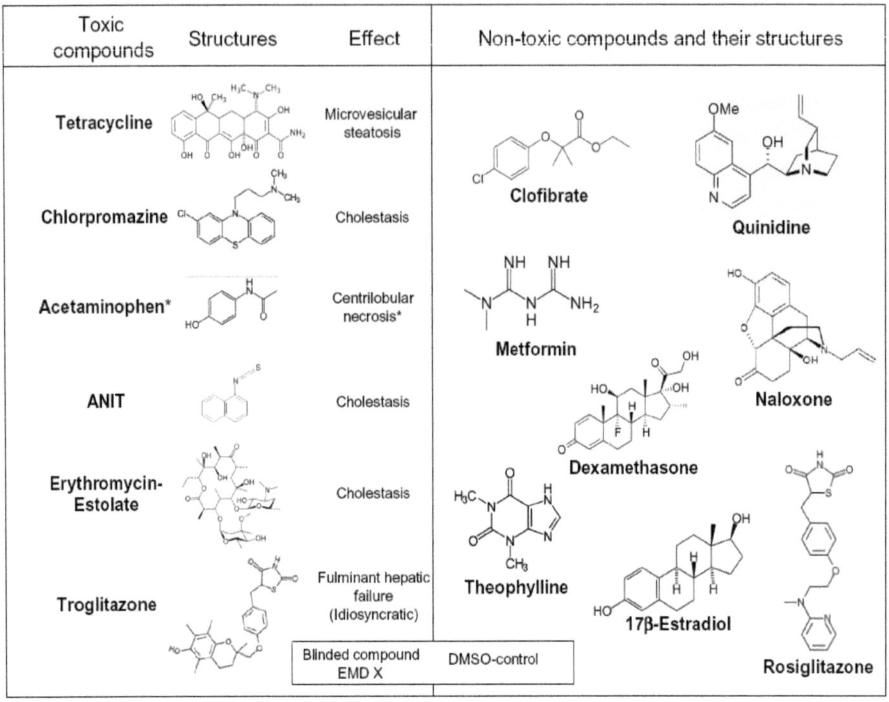

| Toxic compounds | Structures | Effect | Non-toxic compounds and their structures | | |
|---|---|---|---|---|---|
| Tetracycline | | Microvesicular steatosis | | Clofibrate | Quinidine |
| Chlorpromazine | | Cholestasis | | | |
| Acetaminophen* | | Centrilobular necrosis* | Metformin | | Naloxone |
| ANIT | | Cholestasis | | Dexamethasone | |
| Erythromycin-Estolate | | Cholestasis | Theophylline | | |
| Troglitazone | | Fulminant hepatic failure (Idiosyncratic) | | 17β-Estradiol | Rosiglitazone |
| Blinded compound EMD X | | DMSO-control | | | |

Figure 57: Molecular structures of the toxic and non-toxic compounds used in the classification model. *Acetaminophen, was not included in the model because of a lack of toxicity in the *in vitro* model (details see Figure 58)

Tetracycline is a bacteriostatic antibiotic widely used in daily practice and therefore of importance to toxicological research. Dose dependently, it causes microvesicular steatosis. The mechanism of action was discussed in detail in chapter 3.1.

Chlorpromazine (Cp) is an aliphatic phenothiazine which is used therapeutically as an anti-psycotic drug. The mechanism of action is still poorly understood, but liver injury and a

## 3 RESULTS AND DISCUSSION

periportal inflammatory reaction causes cholestasis, as well as a significant elevation of serum alanine aminotransferase (ALT).

The toxicity of *Erythromycin-Estolate* (EE), a macrolid bacteriostatic antibiotic, is clinically similar to Cp. However, the progression to chronic liver damage from this drug has not been clearly established. There is evidence that the effects of EE result from both metabolite-dependent and hypersensitivity-mediated processes (Westphal et al., 1994). EE was also reported to cause reductions of bile flow and bile acid excretion in a dose dependent manner (Gaeta et al., 1985; de Longueville et al., 2003).

In 1968, Desmet et al. reported the ability of $\alpha$-naphthyl-isothiocyanate (ANIT) to directly cause hepatobillary cholestasis in the rat. It was used as a classic model compound to study the mechanisms of intrahepatic cholestasis. Although not finally clarified, it is proposed that ANIT causes liver injury in a dose dependent way by a reduction of the hepatic antioxidant defence system mediated by SOD and catalase, which in turn could contribute to the development of hepatic lipid peroxidation (Ohta et al., 1999). Additionally, the unstable thiocarbamoyl-GSH conjugate (GS-ANIT) is exported in the bile canaliculi and, after dissociation, ANIT accumulates, thereby leading to damage of biliary endothelial cells (Jean & Roth, 1995).

The toxicity of Acetaminophen (AAP), a commonly used analgesic, is the most common cause of acute liver failure in man (Larson et al., 2005). It is catalyzed by CYP enzymes, mainly by CYP2E1 and CYP1A2, to a toxic intermediate which in turn is deactivated by building adducts with glutathione (Mutschler et al., 2008). Excessive amounts of the metabolite leads to a depletion of glutathione resulting in adduct formation and to increased susceptibility to oxidative stress. It was reported that an inhibition of metabolism led to a resistance against AAP (Zaher et al., 1998).

Troglitazone (Tro) is an anti-diabetic and anti-inflammatory drug which was withdrawn from the market in 2000 due to idiosyncratic reaction leading to drug-induced hepatitis. It belongs to the class of thiazolidinediones, the same class as Rosiglitazone (Rosi). The mechanism of action is proposed to act via activation of peroxisome proliferator-activated receptors (PPARs), mainly the $\gamma$-Type. The anti-inflammatory effects are correlated with a reduction of *nuclear factor kappa-B* (NFκB) accompanied by an increase in its inhibitor (IκB) (Aljada et al., 2001). *In vitro* studies of Tro and Rosi cytotoxicity in human

## 3 RESULTS AND DISCUSSION

hepatocytes revealed differences in the toxicity of Tro and Rosi whereby Tro appeared to be more toxic than Rosi, by all endpoints (Lloyd et al., 2002).

Another PPAR activator is one of the non-toxic compounds used in this study, Clofibrate (Clo). By activating PPARα, it causes a lowering of triglyceride-levels in the blood and activates the lipoprotein lipase (Lpl) (Mutschler et al., 2008). As with all PPAR activators, this compound may have carcinogenic potential in long-term experiments, but it causes no acute liver damage.

Metformin (Met), analogous to the thiazolidinediones Tro and Rosi, lowers glucose production in the liver and is therefore used as an oral antihyperglycemic drug in the management of type 2 diabetes. In contrast to Tro and Rosi, Met acts primarily by decreasing endogenous gluconeogenesis, whereas Tro acts by increasing the rate of insulin mediated peripheral glucose disposal (Inzucchi et al., 1998). Even so, this drug has been in clinical use for up to 40 years now and detailed molecular mechanisms remain unclear. Recent gene expression studies found several genes deregulated linked to metabolic pathways involved in gluconeogenesis and lipid metabolism (Heishi et al., 2006).

Theophylline (Theo) is a caffeine related xanthine derivative, an alkaloid which is used for the treatment of respiratory diseases. It acts by inhibition of phosphodiesterase activity and has additionally anti-inflammatory effects. It is metabolized extensively in the liver (up to 70%) and undergoes N-demethylation via cytochrome P450 1A2 (Mutschler et al., 2008). This compound is not known to cause liver damage, but nevertheless, due to its several other side effects, it is only used as a second- or even third-line clinical solution (Boswell-Smith, Cazzola & Page, 2006)

17β-Estradiol (17bEs) is an important naturally occurring steroid hormone. It acts as a female sex hormone and causes prostate enlargement in males (Mutschler et al., 2008). It was shown that in chronic studies that this compound increased the incidence of tumours in several organs (Shull et al., 1997), but no direct adverse effects on the liver are known.

The synthetic glucocorticoid Dexamethasone (DEX) has an immunosuppressive activity and also inhibits inflammatory processes. Due to these effects, it is used in clinics as an antagonist for liver damage caused by inflammation. Additionally, by binding to intracellular receptors, the transcription of multiple genes, e.g., metabolic enzymes, is modulated.

Naloxone (Nal) antagonizes opioid effects by competing for the same receptor sites. It is therefore a pure narcotic antagonist without the side effects of respiratory depression, psychotomimetical effects or pupillary constriction, it exhibits essentially no pharmacological activity (Sadée et al., 2005). It is metabolized in the liver, primarily by glucuronide conjugation and excreted in urine.

Quinidine (Q) is an antiarrhythmic agent. Additionally, it is used as an antimalarial schizonticide. It acts by inhibiting mainly the fast inward sodium transporter of neurons ($I_{Na}$). It also inhibits the CYP2D6 which can cause increased blood levels of the drug. By inhibition of transporter proteins, it can cause some peripherally acting drugs to have CNS side effects, such as respiratory depression, if the two drugs are co-administered (Sadeque et al., 2000). Quinidine is metabolized by CYP3A4 and there are several different hydroxylated metabolites, some of which have antiarrhythmic activity (Nielsen et al., 1999).

The new compound EMD X is an internal Merck Serono compound. It was accepted to be used for the verification of the classification model but detailed background information, as well as the molecular structure, are proprietary.

### 3.4.3 Experimental setup and dose finding

The culture of primary rat hepatocytes was conducted in SW-FCS conformation. After plating, cells were incubated for three days to adapt to the cell culture environment. Previous results showed that most changes in gene expression occur in the first two days after perfusion and that, in SW-FCS culture, gene expression stabilized afterwards (chapter 3.3). This time of pre-culturing was chosen to avoid a high level of false positive genes which may mask any compound specific effects.

For dose finding, two different cytotoxicity tests were conducted with membrane integrity (LDH-test) and cell viability (ATP-test) as the endpoints. For each compound, a series of multiple concentrations was run at least in biological triplicates for all time points tested to ensure statistical validity of the results. $EC_{20}$ values were calculated for both cytotoxicity tests at all time points. The $EC_{20}$ is the concentration of drug/xenobiotic required to induce

# 3 RESULTS AND DISCUSSION

a 20% loss of membrane integrity (LDH-test) or a 20% reduction in ATP content (ATP-test).

The final test concentrations for each compound were selected by combining the results from the LDH- and ATP-tests. One fifth of the $EC_{20}$ value was taken as a second concentration. This non-cytotoxic dose is still expected to have effects on gene expression.

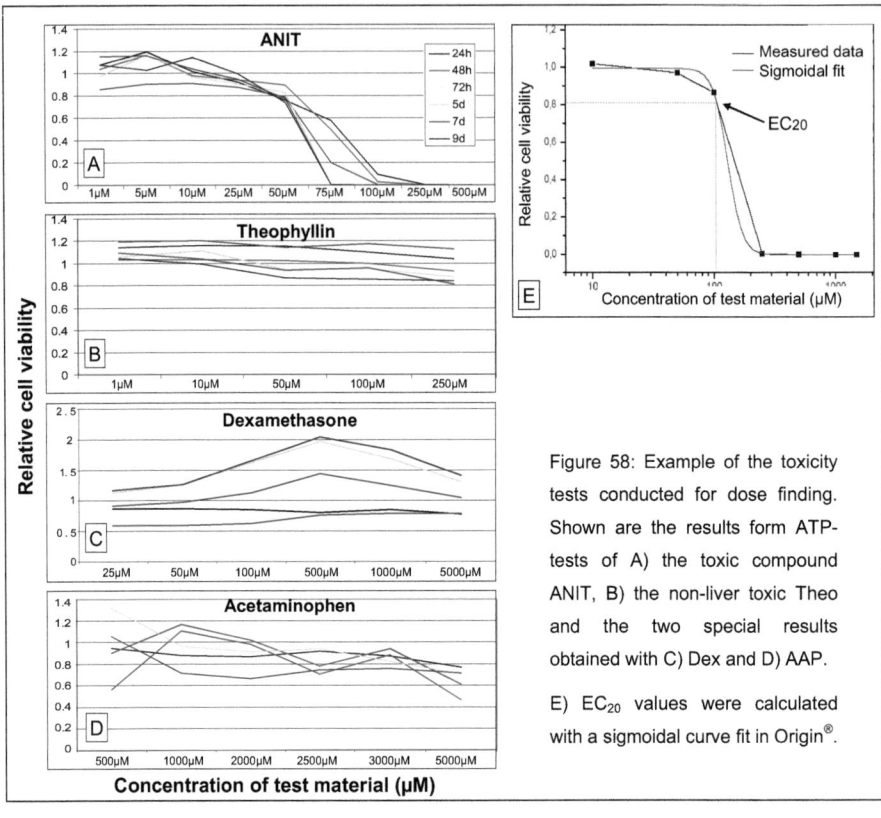

Figure 58: Example of the toxicity tests conducted for dose finding. Shown are the results form ATP-tests of A) the toxic compound ANIT, B) the non-liver toxic Theo and the two special results obtained with C) Dex and D) AAP.

E) $EC_{20}$ values were calculated with a sigmoidal curve fit in Origin®.

ANIT, as a positive compound showed a clear dose and time dependency in its cytotoxic effects, with a suggested threshold of about 50µM. For Theo, a non-liver toxic compound, no effects were detected up to the limit of solubility. In this case, the highest soluble concentration was defined as the high dose and one fifth as the low dose. Dex showed a very unusual dose response. No toxicity was detected, but instead, an increase of cellular viability at a medium concentration of 500µM was seen (Figure 58C). As discussed previously, Dex has a positive effect on liver gene expression and stabilizes cell viability

# 3 RESULTS AND DISCUSSION

and gene expression in culture. Nevertheless, at high doses, other mechanisms seem to be having a negative effect on cell viability. Additionally, morphological changes were observed at all doses (Figure 59). The number and diameter of the bile canaliculi was significantly increased. Up to the medium dose, this was accompanied by an increase of canalicular transport, demonstrated by an accumulation of a fluorescent substrate in the canaliculi. However, at high doses of Dex, even though the bile canaliculi were again increased in diameter, this transport mechanism was inhibited and biliary transport was reduced (data not shown). To allow for these findings, three doses were used for Dex.

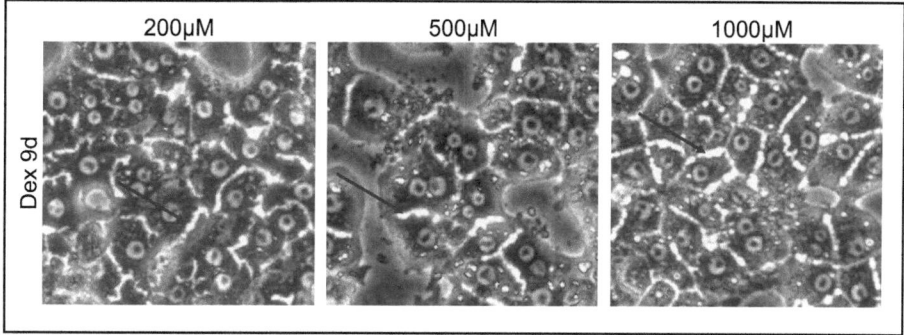

Figure 59: Primary rat hepatocytes in SW-FCS 9 d after dosing with three concentrations of Dex.

AAP, a classic liver toxic compound, did not show any toxicity in SW-FCS cultured hepatocytes. This is in contrast to previously reported studies, which clearly showed a toxic effect (Thedinga et al., 2007; Mingoia et al., 2007; Suzuki et al., 2008; Ullrich et al., 2007). A major difference between previous studies and this approach is the time in culture and the time of dosing. Whereas other studies were mainly short term with the compound treatment 4 h or 24 h, cells were treated in this study after 3 days. Looking at the mechanism of action, it becomes clear that AAP is not toxic itself but is metabolized to toxic intermediates by CYP isoforms, mainly CYP2E1. By looking at the gene expression data of rat hepatocytes in culture (Table 24), a strong reduction in CYP2E1 expression was seen. Jemnitz and his co-workers showed a clear dependency of AAP toxicity and time point of dosing with a greatly increased resistance to toxicity at later time points, in different species. Interestingly, they found no clear correlation of AAP toxicity to CYP2E1 activity ( Jemnitz et al., 2008). These results show the importance of a detailed knowledge of the test system and ideally of the mechanism of action and metabolism of the

# 3 RESULTS AND DISCUSSION

compound tested. Due to these results, AAP was removed from the dataset and was not used for the calculation of the prediction model.

As a result of the toxicity tests, the concentrations noted in Table 28 were used as the final concentrations used in the gene expression profiling experiments. For clarification, the higher concentration will be named "high" and the lower concentration will be named "low".

| Compound | Low Dose [µM] | High Dose [µM] | Compound | Low Dose [µM] | High Dose [µM] |
|---|---|---|---|---|---|
| Tet | 40 | 200 | Cp | 4 | 20 |
| Clo | 200 | 1000 | Q | 20 | 100 |
| Theo | 50 | 250 | DEX | 200/500 | 1000 |
| ANIT | 9 | 45 | Rosi | 16 | 80 |
| Nal | 12 | 60 | Tro | 14 | 70 |
| EE | 17 | 85 | Met | 300 | 1500 |
| 17bEs | 0.05 | 0.25 | EMD 335825 | 200 | 1000 |
| AAP | 1000 | 5000 | | | |

Table 28: Concentrations of the test compounds used. The high concentration resembles the approximation of the $EC_{20}$ of both cytotoxicity tests conducted (LDH- and ATP-test), the low concentration is one fifth of this value. Dex, as a special case, has a third concentration due to the fact that at this concentration a positive effect on cell viability was detected.

Cells were exposed to the test compounds continuously for 9 d with media change every second day and observed for morphological changes (Figure 60). To exclude any solvent effects which may have influenced gene expression, compounds were concordantly dissolved in DMSO as a 200x stock resulting in an end concentration of 0.5% of DMSO in the media. In the case of Met, which itself is not soluble in organic solvents, the DMSO was added directly to the media to guarantee standardized conditions. Therefore, time matched vehicle controls were treated with 0.5% DMSO.

Samples were taken at 2 h, 1 d, 3 d, 5 d, 7 d, and on day 9 after the first dosing. RNA was reverse transcribed, labelled and hybridized on Illumina RatRef-12 BeadChips. Data analysis was conducted in BeadStudio (Illumina Inc.) and Expressionist Analyst (Genedata). Data was normalized with the LOESS algorithm in order to compare multiple arrays. Fold changes and statistical analysis were calculated in regard to the time matched vehicle controls.

# 3 RESULTS AND DISCUSSION

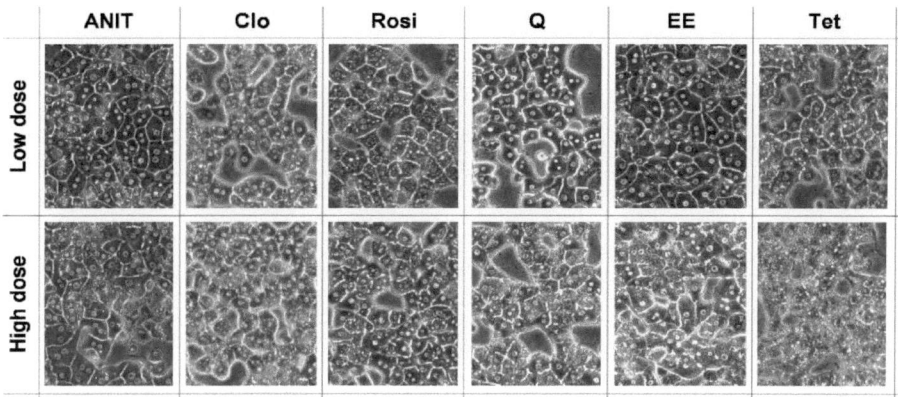

Figure 60: Cells dosed with either the high or low dose of ANIT, Clo, Rosi, Q, EE or Tet on day nine of treatment. Interestingly, not only the hepatotoxic but also non-hepatotoxic compounds caused morphological changes, including the accumulation of lipid droplets (Clo, Q). On the other hand, ANIT did not significantly alter the morphology of the hepatocytes. Most severe changes were detected in cells dosed with high concentrations of Tet. These results fit to previously published *in vivo* data (Zidek et al., 2007).

## 3.4.4 Data Analysis and establishment of an *in vitro* prediction model for hepatotoxicity

As a first overview of the data a hierarchical clustering was performed with all time points tested (2 h, 6 h, 1 d, 3 d, 5 d, and 9 d after dosing). As shown in Figure 61, no clear separation was achieved at any of these time points. On days one and five, Rosi and Clo separated from the other experiments, but on day one also the livertoxic compound Tet grouped together with them. All other experiments were organized in two large groups but clearly not based on toxicity. At later time points, cells treated with all three doses of Dex separated from the other experiments and built their own cluster. These findings were also shown by other clustering methods, such as PCA (Figure 62).

These results re-enforce the difficulty in establishing a model based on global gene expression. Also toxic compounds have specific mechanisms of action with specific gene expression changes, and these differences can be hidden by the large number of unaffected genes. To establish a model capable of discriminating between the two defined groups, other techniques are needed.

# 3 RESULTS AND DISCUSSION

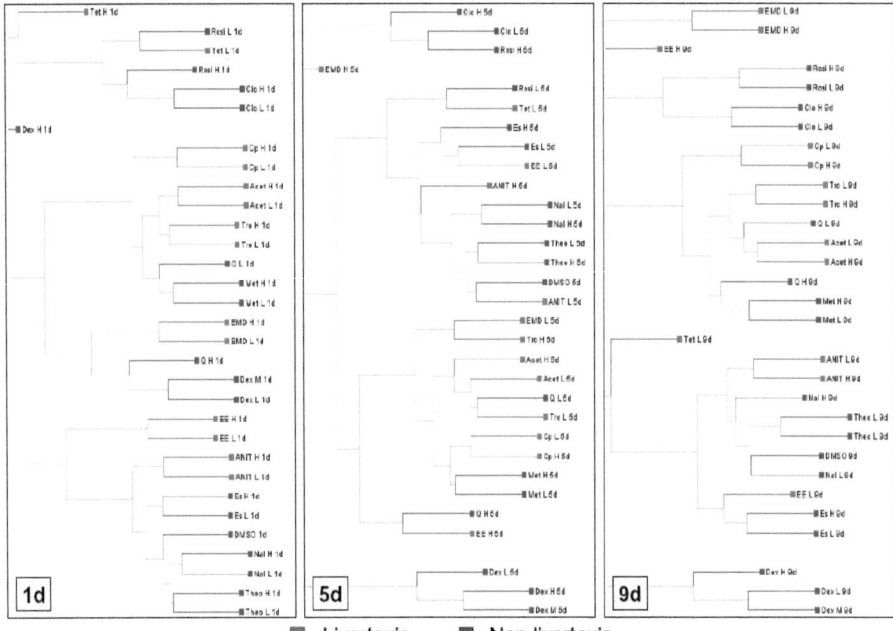

Figure 61: Hierarchical clustering from global gene expression data from compound treated primary rat hepatocytes. Shown are the results from cells dosed for 1 d, 5 d and 9 d with the previously described model compounds. No obvious separation of toxic and non-toxic compounds was achieved at any time point.

The normalized data was grouped by compound, time point, and dose. Finally two groups, toxic and non-toxic, were defined according to the previously defined toxicity (see Figure 57). First, the possibility to create a functional classification model was tested. Therefore, trainings sets were created for all time points and for the high and low doses separately as well as for both together. The classification was conducted with four different classification algorithms to account for any potential "peculiarities" in the dataset. The support vector machine algorithm (SVM), the sparse linear discriminant analysis, the fisher

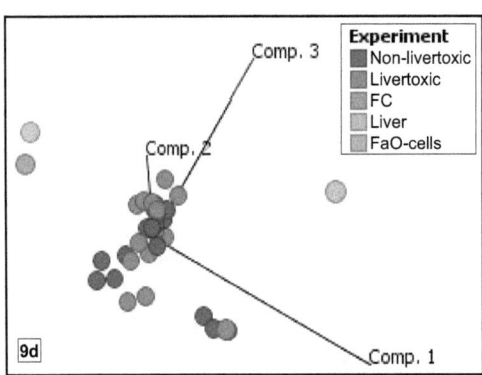

Figure 62: PCA with global gene expression data from cells treated for 9 d with previously described model compounds.

# 3 RESULTS AND DISCUSSION

linear discriminant analysis and the K-nearest neighbour analysis, all of which are supervised learning methods, were used. They were applied on the same dataset that was used for the training, but in this case, the leave-one-out cross-validation method was applied. This means that the training set was applied 1,000 times on the whole dataset, but in every run, 15% of the dataset were removed and the remaining data was classified. This classification method was checked for its accuracy afterwards and misclassification

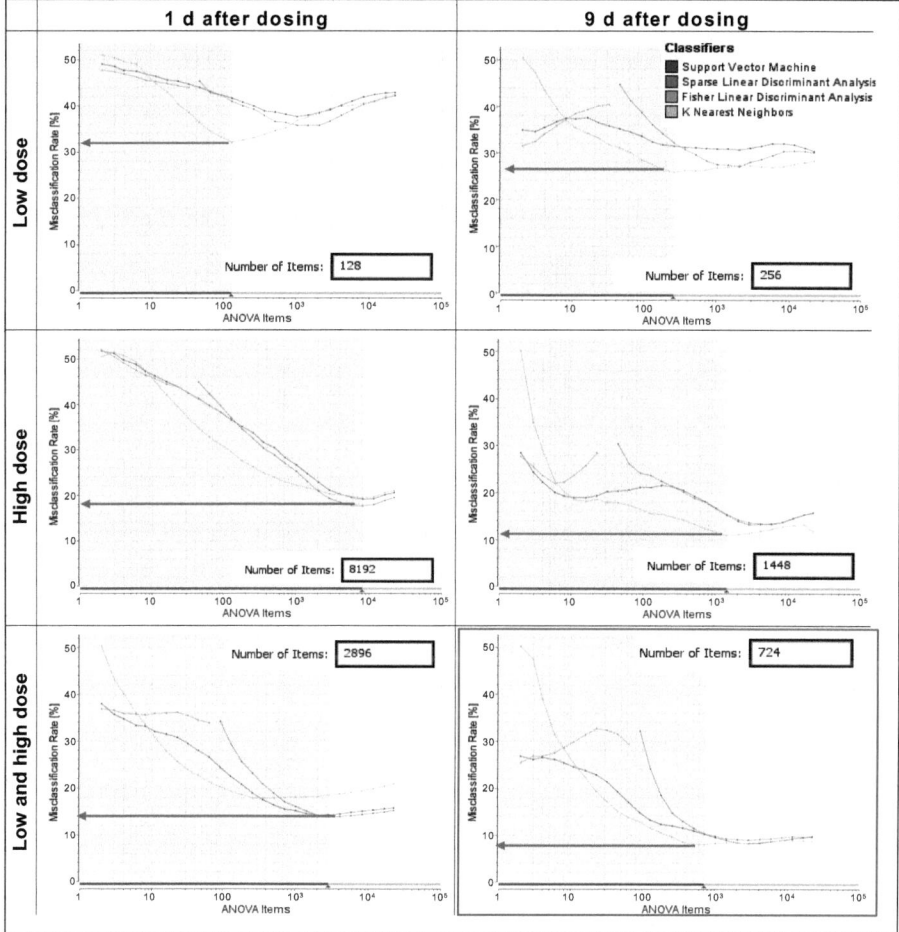

Figure 63: Construction of the classification models and gene rankings. Four different algorithms were applied to discriminate between two previously defined groups (toxic and non-toxic). For each algorithm, the misclassification rate and the number of genes needed for best results were calculated.

# 3 RESULTS AND DISCUSSION

rates for each of these algorithms were calculated. This number defines the percentage by which the samples were allocated to the wrong group. At the same time, genes were ranked according to their importance for this discrimination and the number of genes needed for best results were calculated. Results are shown in Figure 63. In most cases, the classification algorithm of K nearest neighbour resulted in the best predictions. Generally, the misclassification rates were lower for the samples treated for 9 d than for samples treated for shorter times. By analysing only the low dose samples, a misclassification rate of approximately 32% was detected one day after dosing. This result was only slightly, but not significantly, improved at later time points.

Taking only the high dose groups into the model resulted in a misclassification rate of 19% after one day of dosing and 11% after 9 d. Best results were obtained with samples dosed for 9 d in culture taking both doses together into the model. In this case, the misclassification rate was reduced to 7.5%. To reach this rate, only 724 genes were needed and were sufficient. Figure 64 shows examples of the results of the cross validations, 1 d and 9 d after dosing. It is clear to see the reduction of misclassified samples for the later time point. Whereas in the early samples the computer estimated both false positive and false negative samples, at later time points there were no falsely positive predicted samples. Only three samples were misclassified, all of which were low dose samples. One biological replicate of each, Tro, Tet and ANIT was wrongly predicted to be non-toxic. However, the whole group was still classified as toxic. All three

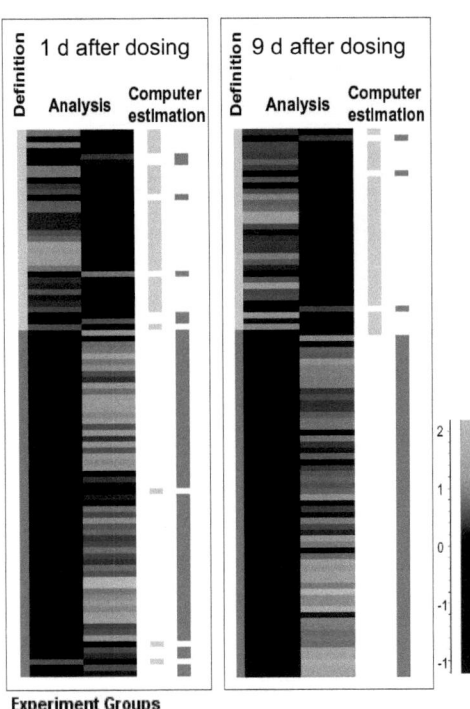

Figure 64: Visualization of the "leave one out" cross validation showing the defined groups (left side) as basis for the calculation. The computer estimation for the whole dataset is shown on the right side of the figures. Shown are the results (both doses) on day 1 and 9 after dosing.

# 3 RESULTS AND DISCUSSION

groups had a classifier output of below 0.5, which means that they were relatively close to the imaginary midline between both groups and do not significantly differ. All together, this shows the need for replicate experiments to increase robustness of the model by tolerating single experiments to be misclassified but retaining the overall correct result.

The main objective of this study was to determine whether it would be possible to distinguish between hepatotoxic and non-hepatotoxic compounds with the help of an *in vitro* system and global gene expression analysis. The clustering analysis of the global gene expression data alone did not allow such discrimination. By using the support vector machine algorithm together with a cross-validation, it was possible to obtain a subset of genes that allowed the discrimination, with a false discovery rate of only 7.5%. These results clearly show the advantage of longer term dosing for the establishment of gene expression changes, which clearly contribute to the discrimination of the two groups. Short term experiments only show the acute effects of a compound, like inflammatory or immune responses. This is not sufficient in *in vitro* experiments, because of the lack of certain cell types and therefore specific mechanisms may be missing. Dosing for longer times has the advantage of increasing compound specific gene expression changes and therefore enables the discrimination algorithms to find basic differences between toxic and non-toxic compounds in the dataset.

At the same time, the combination of two different dosing schemes also contributed to a better model. This could be simply due to the fact that more data was available for the algorithm, making the comparison more valid. Additionally, by combining high and low doses, further information hidden in the global gene expression data set may be accessible to the algorithm. It is noticeable that the low dose treated samples alone were poorly distinguishable by the algorithms but improved the result of the whole dataset. This shows that this effect is not just additive but that there is really additional information introduced into the calculation by the low dose samples. For future applications these results imply that large datasets and, if possible, two (or more) doses are required for these kind of calculations.

As detailed above, the aim of such prediction models is the classification of new data from novel compounds. This would not be possible by simple clustering methods but by ranking genes according to their contribution to the discrimination of the predefined groups and generation classifiers, this goal was achieved.

For the verification of this prediction model, the potential hepatotoxicity of EMD X was predicted. Dosing and data acquisition for this compound was conducted exactly as described for the model compounds. Additionally, the same classifier was applied to the

# 3 RESULTS AND DISCUSSION

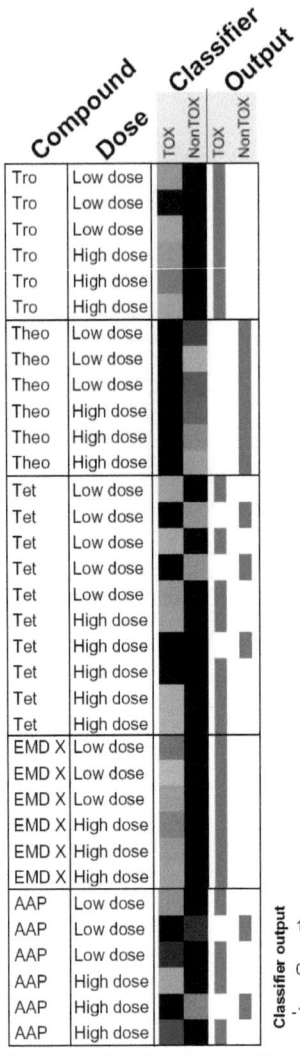

Figure 65: Result of the classification of data gained from primary rat hepatocytes treated for 9 d with Tro, Theo, Tet, EMD X and AAP. Shown are the concordances to the classifier, where light means high and dark means low concordance, and the final estimation of the algorithm.

whole dataset, including the data from AAP and the model compounds used for the calculation of this model as a retrospective verification of the previously analyzed data.

With altogether 120 experiments, the calculated misclassification rate of 7.5% would allow nine experiments to be wrongly classified (partly shown in Figure 65). Overall, only eight experiments were misclassified. In most cases, all experiments were classified correctly, independent of the dose. For Tet, two out of five low dosed and one of the high dosed experiments were misclassified. Even so, because of the five biological replicates, the majority of these experiments were still correctly classified resulting in an overall correct classification for Tet. The new compound EMD X, was classified as hepatotoxic. All experiments were clearly allocated to this group resulting in a robust classification. This result corroborated perfectly with previously obtained results from other in house studies (data not shown).

Another interesting result was obtained by the classification of AAP. Even so no toxicity was detected in the cytotoxicity tests (LDH and ATP test), the compound was still classified as hepatotoxic in both high and low dose treatment groups based on the global gene expression. A closer look on the single experiments revealed that in both doses, one experiment was classified as non toxic and two as toxic. The classifier output in most cases was unequivocal suggesting borderline classification. This means that the classification of this compound is less robust than for EMD X. Nevertheless, the classification showed an effect which could not be detected by cytotoxicity tests, but is well known *in vivo*.

# 3 RESULTS AND DISCUSSION

## 3.4.5　Analysis of the top ranked genes of the prediction model

During the process of calculating the prediction model, the genes were ranked by importance for the discrimination process. This ranking was achieved by ANOVA, a variance analysis method. The results showed 724 genes to be essential for the best classification of the experiments at 9 d (Appendix 13). These genes were analyzed for their molecular function and their involvement in toxicologically important cellular processes.

The dataset, although quite large, is certainly not sufficient to discriminate between different types of hepatotoxicity. There are multiple pathways leading to toxicity, with complex and intersecting mechanisms. The aim of this work was to evaluate the possibility to detect and predict general hepatotoxicity.

It is important to mention that the algorithm used for gene ranking is not selecting the genes according to their fold change, their statistical significance or their biological functions but according to their contribution to the classification. Nevertheless, it might be helpful to have a closer look at the genes that differentiated between hepatotoxic and non-hepatotoxic compounds.

Figure 66 shows the result of a k-means clustering, which grouped the genes according to their gene expression profile in all samples. It can be seen that none of the clusters were discriminative on their own. But taken together, the information contained in these profiles is the basis for the discrimination model generated.

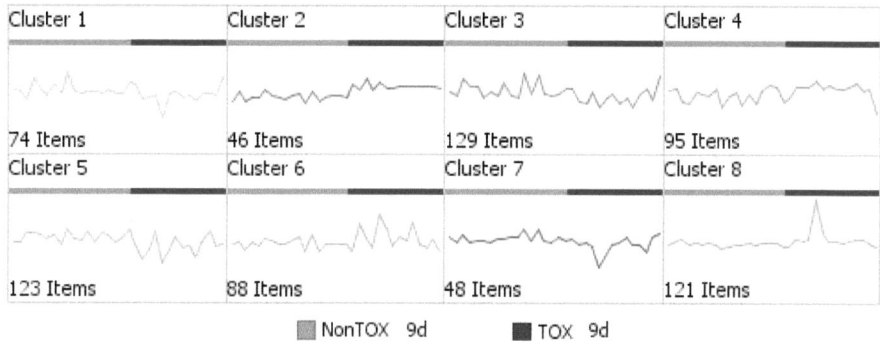

Figure 66: Results of a k-means clustering with all samples used for classifying and the 724 top ranked genes at day 9 of treatment. Genes were grouped according to their gene expression profile.

The PCA in Figure 67 was calculated with the 724 top ranked genes. In comparison to the PCA shown in Figure 62, which was calculated with the whole dataset, both groups have

## 3 RESULTS AND DISCUSSION

now separated at least to a certain degree, although still no complete separation was seen. Thus, these genes clearly have inherent information that enables the separation of these groups, but at the same time, they are not sufficient for a 100% separation, explaining the false classification rate of 7.5%.

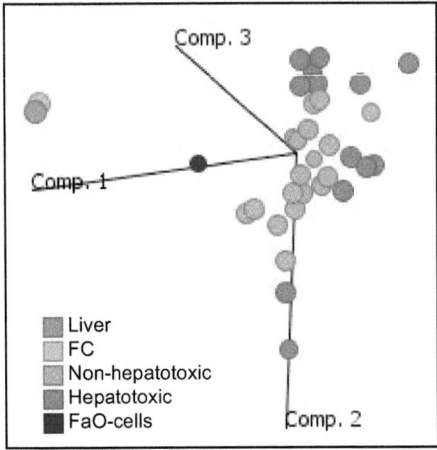

Figure 67: PCA with the 724 top ranked genes from the model previously described.

The top "hit" when a Fisher's Exact Test analysis was performed was proteasome complex and protein degradation. In total, 17 protein subunits of the proteasome were important for discrimination. The proteasome is a multiprotein complex which has an important function in protein degradation in an ATP/ubiquitin-dependent process, in a non-lysosomal related fashion. A modified proteasome, the immuno-proteasome, is responsible for the processing of class I MHC peptides and is therefore involved in immunogenic responses. Another function of the proteasome is the directionality of the cell cycle by degrading the polyubiquitinated cyclins. Changes in cell cycle are often the result of cell damage or the recovery process following, for example, a necrotic event. The impairment of the cell cycle is also documented by cyclin-dependent kinases (Cdk7) or s-phase related proteins, which were also part of this gene selection.

Several genes, Myc, Egf, the MAP kinase activated protein kinase2 (Mapkapk2), Tgfβ2 and the inhibitor of kappaB kinase (Ikbkb), play important roles in intracellular signalling and thereby influence cellular fate, growth, cell cycle or metabolism. Other signals may drive the cell in the direction of apoptosis or survival as a reaction to oxidative stress or cell damage.

# 3 RESULTS AND DISCUSSION

The involvement of energy metabolism in liver toxicity was highlighted by lactate dehydrogenase B (Ldhb), triosephosphate isomerase (Tim) and Enolase. Also directly linked to ATP production are genes such as ATP synthase C1 and d subunits, cytochrome c reductases NADH dehydrogenases. Other genes function as part of cellular adhesion complexes, for example the junctional adhesion molecule 3 (Jam3) and claudin 10, which are part of the tight junction complex and integrin-mediated cell adhesion. Both proteins are important for canalicular functionality.

Xenobiotic metabolism genes were also contained in the selection. CYPs 1A1 and 2E1 have important functions in the detoxification of a large number of compounds and therefore it is not surprising to find them included. Microsomal Gst 2 is an important phase 2 enzyme for drug detoxification and is involved in the production of leukotrienes and prostaglandin E, which are important mediators of inflammation.

Taken together it is clear that many of the discriminative genes ranked are linked to mechanisms known to be related to toxicity or cellular damage. Again, it is important to note that the compounds used for this model work via a variety of mechanisms, which is shown by many genes affecting multiple important pathways.

## 3.5 Insights into the mechanisms of action for selected compounds

From the beginning, the aim of this study was the establishment of a model that can predict general hepatotoxicity in an *in vitro* system. Nevertheless, the amount of data collected during our study allows to perform additional mechanistic analyses. The comparison of the data generated from an *in vitro* toxicogenomics study with Tet showed high correlation to the results of an *in vivo* study with the same compound (chapter 3.1.1.4). Of course, not all the compounds can be conferred here in this detail, but some interesting new findings are discussed. Details of the mechanism of action of EMD X, which clearly showed toxicity in cell culture and was classified as toxic by the predictive model is be discussed in this chapter. Additionally, AAP is discussed, because the result from the predictive model (supported by *in vivo* data) differs from the results gained with standard *in vitro* cell viability testing. To show that genomic profiling can have conflicting results, too, some effects of Dex will be discussed in the context of cell morphology.

# 3 RESULTS AND DISCUSSION

## 3.5.1 EMD X

The proprietary Merck compound EMD X, was used for validation of the model because of the availability of extensive in-house data. In fact, while being blinded for the model testing, it is known to cause hypertrophy of hepatocytes and, in high doses, bile duct inflammation, hyperplasia and liver cell necrosis. At least some of these hepatotoxic effects seem to be present *in vitro* as well, leading to a clear classification of EMD X as hepatotoxic.

Looking at the induced genes and mechanisms, it is obvious that this compound affected fatty acid and energy metabolism. The top ranked mechanisms there included the activation of fatty acid synthase activity, regulation of lipid metabolism via LXR, NF-Y and SREBP. Also fatty acid oxidation and PPAR$\alpha$ dependent genes, like Acox1, Cpt1$\alpha$ and $\beta$, Cte1 and CYP4A, were induced (Figure 68). Acyl-CoA thioesterases (Cte), which generates carboxylic acid and free Coenzyme A, were induced, whereas the generation of acetyl-CoA by acyl-CoA synthetases (ACSL) was reduced simultaneously. A metabolic activation was found to result as a response to an external stimulus, probably to EMD X treatment. Although the PPAR$\alpha$ activation is not directly proven, these results show a high correlation to the results of the *in vivo* in-house data and exhibit clear characteristics of PPAR-dependent gene expression changes.

CYP4A11 catalyzes the omega-hydroxylation of various fatty acids and was consistently induced, as was carnitine palmitoyltransferase (Cpt1a), the enzyme that catalyses the transfer of long chain fatty acids to carnitine for translocation across the mitochondrial inner membrane. These changes imply an increased need for energy of the cells after compound treatment. Whether this is a direct effect of EMD X treatment or a secondary effect due to the recovery after cellular damage can not be concluded from this data and needs to be further studied.

The strong induction of several Gst enzymes indicates a reaction to oxidative stress within the cells. This might be caused by an increased metabolism resulting in increased amounts of ROS generated or by inflammatory processes. In support of the latter is the activation of AKT kinase (mediating survival to oxidative stress) at early time points and the finding that apoptosis related mechanisms being activated including the transcriptional up-regulation of caspases.

# 3 RESULTS AND DISCUSSION

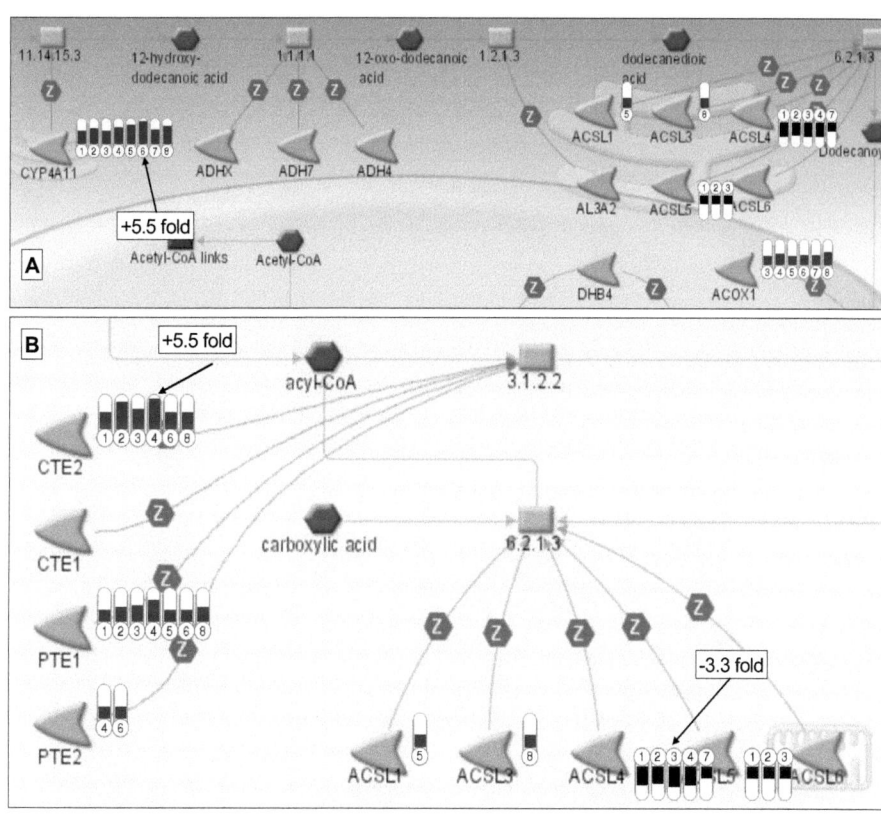

1. EMD 1d Low
2. EMD 1d High
3. EMD 3d Low
4. EMD 3d High
5. EMD 5d Low
6. EMD 5d High
7. EMD 9d Low
8. EMD 9d High

Figure 68: Details of the omega-oxidation pathway of fatty acids (A) and the CoA biosynthesis pathway (B). Both pathways were found to be induced by EMD X treatment (modified from Metacore, GeneGO).

Several genes involved in cellular adhesion, fibronectin, actin and other genes, were found to be reduced, implying cytoskeletal remodelling and a reduction of cellular anchoring, which may have been caused by the increase in cell volume, shown by histopathological investigations. Additionally, E-cadherin, which is used as a prognostic marker for hepatocellular cancer (Iso et al., 2005) was reduced at all time points and all doses.

Noticeable was the strong reduction of the complement pathway at all time points at both doses (Figure 69). This pathway, consisting of more than 30 proteins mainly synthesized in the liver (more than 90%), is part of the innate immune system and works by proteosomal activation after stimulation. The complement cascade leads to massive amplification of the response and to activation of the cell-killing membrane attack complex,

# 3 RESULTS AND DISCUSSION

thereby functioning as a pathogenic defense mechanism (Mayer, 1984). Other functions include the attracting of immune cells, increasing the permeability of vascular walls and the initiation of inflammation. Earlier studies showed that transcription is induced during acute phase response following liver injury (Prada, Zahedi & Davis, 1998; Stapp et al., 2005).

The expression of complement factors is thought to be transcriptionally controlled by several liver specific transcription factors (TFs) (such as HNF´s and C/EBP´s) (Pontoglio et al., 2001; Garnier, Circolo & Colten, 1996). Interestingly, these factors were only slightly affected. The effect that EMD X has on these TFs, and the resulting strong inhibition of the complement pathway, is important and still needs to be confirmed.

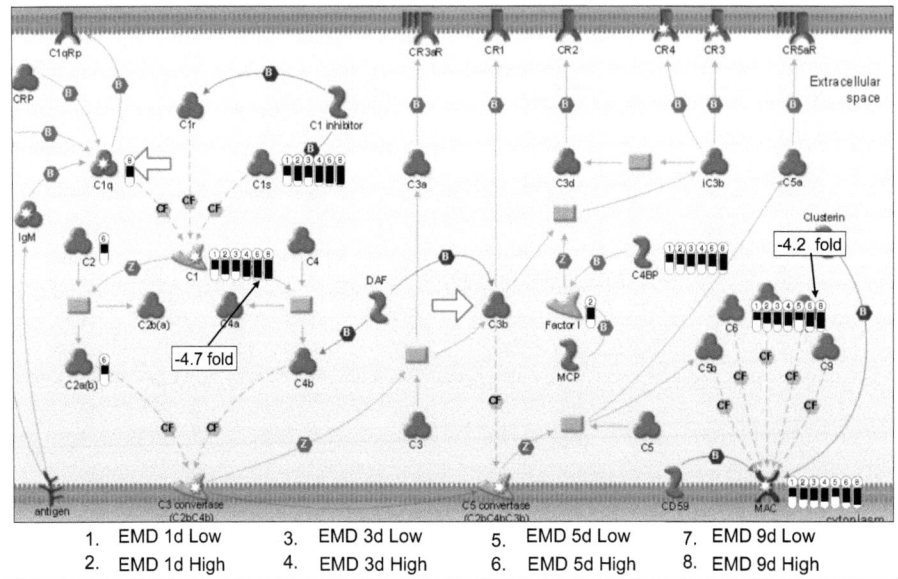

| 1. | EMD 1d Low | 3. | EMD 3d Low | 5. | EMD 5d Low | 7. | EMD 9d Low |
| 2. | EMD 1d High | 4. | EMD 3d High | 6. | EMD 5d High | 8. | EMD 9d High |

Figure 69: Genes of the classical complement pathway were found to be heavily reduced after EMD X treatment, independent of time and dose (modified from Metacore, GeneGO).

These results are in good concordance with in house *in vivo* data, where in rats treated with EMD X a reduction of C1s and C6 was detected. However, C4bp, reduced *in vitro*, was nearly unaffected *in vivo*. A loss of complement activity results in diminished liver regeneration, accompanied by transient or fatal liver failure after partial hepatectomy (Strey et al., 2003). It may therefore be concluded that an impaired recovery after cellular

## 3 RESULTS AND DISCUSSION

damage may contribute to the hepatocyte necrosis seen in the histopathology after treatment.

### 3.5.2 AAP

AAP is one of the best studied compounds in respect to liver toxicity, because of two reasons. It was previously shown that primary hepatocytes loose their sensitivity to AAP and become resistant over time in culture (Jemnitz et al., 2008). These results were confirmed by our negative cytotoxicity tests. If dosed 4 h or 1 d after plating, cells clearly showed reduced viability and increased LDH release (data not shown). Treatment 3 d after plating had no effect on ATP content or membrane integrity. Nevertheless, AAP was classified as hepatotoxic by our prediction model. The mechanistic gene expression analysis revealed clear adverse effects, but also showed a reduction of these effects over time.

AAP causes centrilobular hepatic necroses, via the CYP-generated reactive electrophilic metabolite N-acetyl-p-benzoquinone (NAPQI) (Tonge et al., 1998). The main players are the CYP-isoforms 1A2, 2E1 and 3A4. Normally, NAPQI is detoxified by an addition-reaction to GSH. This causes a depletion of GSH at higher doses and leads to covalently bound protein adducts, which finally cause the toxic effect (James, Mayeux & Hinson, 2003; Mitchell et al., 1973).

Overall, the deregulations observed were more intense at the beginning of treatment, with return to the baseline expression than at later time points of culture. CYP 1A2 and 2E1 were found to be significantly down regulated over time in cultures suggesting this as the reason for the increasing immunity of cells in culture. However, the same isoforms were found to be induced by AAP, making it possible that small amounts of the toxic metabolite may have been produced. Other isoforms, such as CYP 3A4 or 2C19, were heavily down regulated by AAP (Figure 70).

# 3 RESULTS AND DISCUSSION

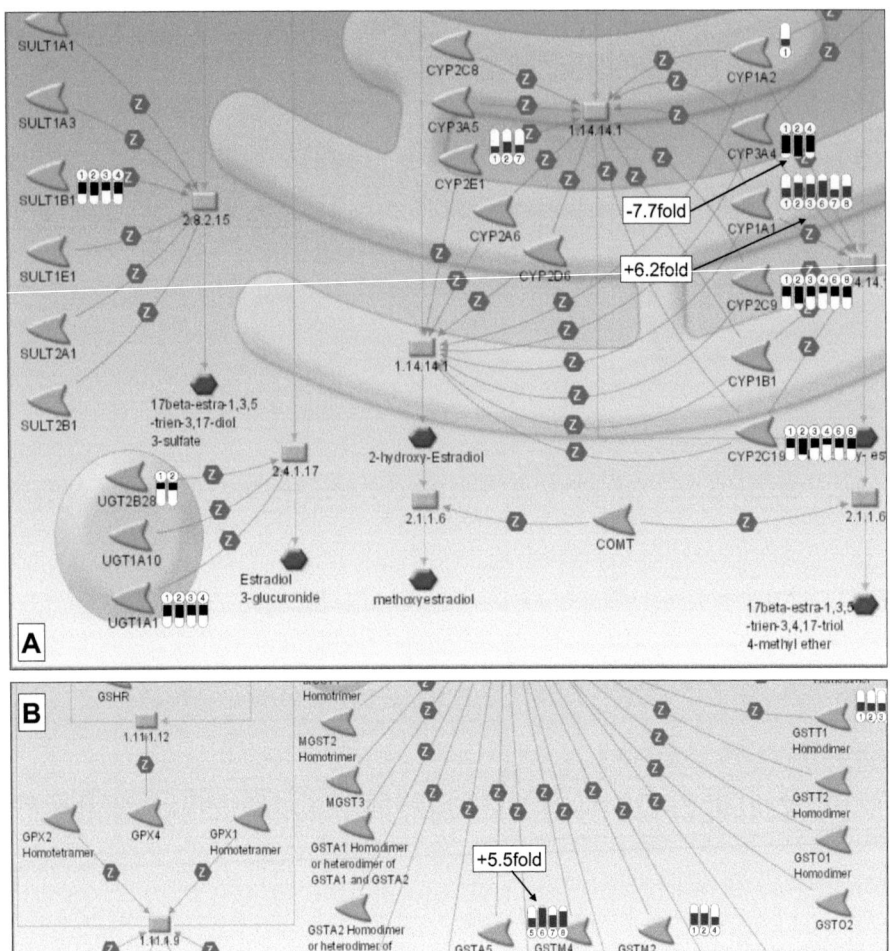

| 1. AAP 1d Low Dose | 3. AAP 3d Low Dose | 5. AAP 5d Low Dose | 7. AAP 9d Low Dose |
| 2. AAP 1d High Dose | 4. AAP 3d High Dose | 6. AAP 5d High Dose | 8. AAP 9d High Dose |

Figure 70: Genes of the phase 1 and phase 2 metabolism deregulated by AAP treatment in culture. Rising bars indicate induction, decreasing bars the repression of gene expression (modified from Metacore, GeneGO).

Generally, a reduction of phase 1 xenobiotic metabolism was observed whereas phase 2 metabolism showed an inconsistent picture. Sult1B1 and UGT isoforms were reduced, and

## 3 RESULTS AND DISCUSSION

several Gst isoforms were induced. UGTs were previously shown to be less expressed during liver regeneration after AAP treatment (Tian et al., 2005). Together, these results can be interpreted as a cellular mechanism for the protection of the cell against oxidative stress and the increased need for antioxidants, like GSH, to overcome the toxicity caused by AAP treatment. Deregulations in the AKT kinase pathway (Figure 71A) were time dependent. At early time points, HSP90, a molecular chaperone involved in ATP-dependent folding of proteins and in sequestering damaged proteins, was strongly reduced. Deregulations of genes downstream of AKT kinase imply a toxic mechanism early after dosing. MDM2 is a protein which affects the cell cycle, apoptosis and carcinogenesis by inactivating p53 and by interacting with other proteins (Bose & Ghosh, 2007). While this antagonist is repressed, p53 as well as caspase 9 and NFκB were induced, driving the cells towards apoptosis.

Figure 71B and C show the reduction of other important cellular mechanisms. CDK7 is, as a complex with cyclin H and MAT1, an essential component of the transcription factor TFIIH, which is involved in transcriptional initiation and DNA repair. All three genes were reduced initially by AAP treatment. Additionally, the initialisation of translation was reduced. Together with the building of protein adducts by NAPQI, this reduction of correctly folded proteins may contribute to the toxicity of AAP.

All these effects may be the consequence of cellular stress caused by AAP and may be the reason that our model classified AAP into the category hepatotoxic. This result suggests the possibility to detect underlying toxic mechanisms that cannot be detected with other, established *in vitro* methods. The fact that most effects detected were only transiently visible and no effects could be detected by cell viability tests may be an initial step to further studies, which are needed to uncover the mechanism of the increasing lack of response of primary hepatocytes in culture.

# 3 RESULTS AND DISCUSSION

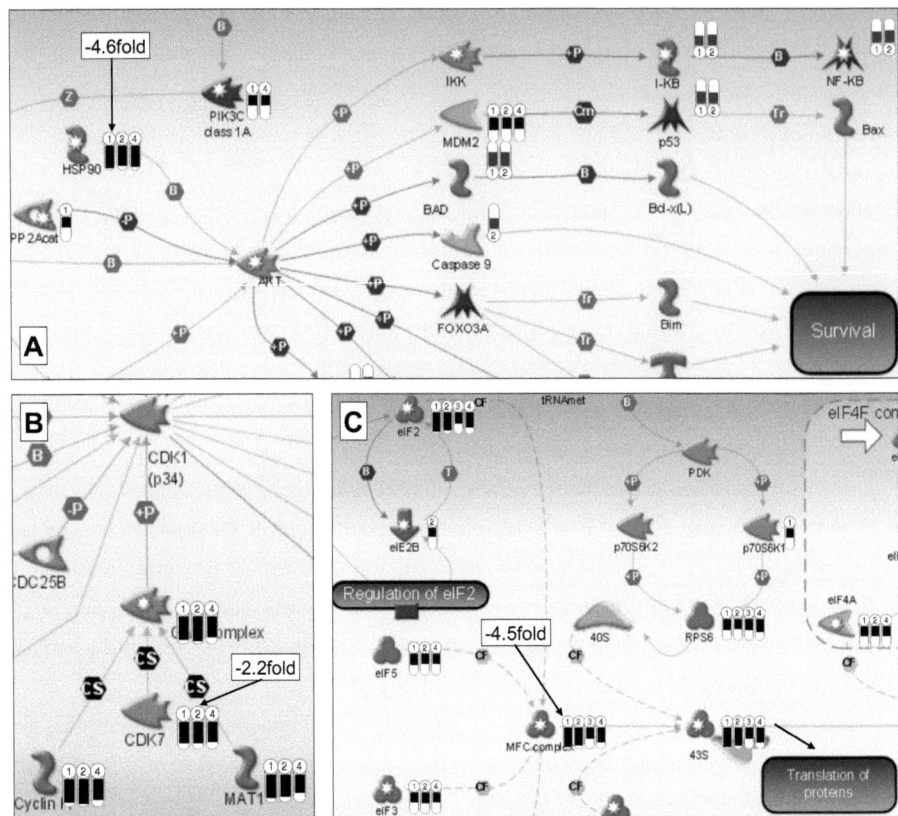

1. AAP 1d Low Dose   3. AAP 3d Low Dose   5. AAP 5d Low Dose   7. AAP 9d Low Dose
2. AAP 1d High Dose  4. AAP 3d High Dose  6. AAP 5d High Dose  8. AAP 9d High Dose

Figure 71: Deregulations caused by AAP treatment. A) AKT-kinase pathway, B) section of the cell cycle, C) translation initiation. Rising bars indicate induction, decreasing bars the repression of gene expression (modified from Metacore, GeneGO).

## 3.5.3 Dex

As previously noted, Dex had a positive effect on cell viability and biliary transport, but only at the medium dose (500µM) group. It is known from previous studies that Dex inhibits hepatocellular proliferation at high doses by inhibiting tumor necrosis factor (TNF) and IL-6 (Nagy et al. 2003). The analysis of the gene expression data revealed an induction of nucleotide metabolism and transcription by RNA polymerase II, only at the medium dose. In contrast to this, there seems to be less oxidative stress, indicated by an induction of oxidative stress related genes only in low and high dosed cells, but not in the medium

## 3 RESULTS AND DISCUSSION

dose. In contrast to this, pyruvate metabolism and insulin dependent signaling were reduced. The insulin pathway is critical for the regulation of intracellular glucose levels. The activated nucleotide production and the increased mRNA production are both energy consuming processes. At the same time, the energy producing pathways were reduced. These changes in gene expression are direct effect of Dex as a glucocorticoid and basal to the morphological and functional changes observed still needs to be analyzed. A real understanding of the underlying mechanisms taking place at the different concentrations could not be elucidated with this data.

The different compounds showed relatively large overlaps in gene expression changes. At the same time, all had some unique gene expression profiles (as discussed here). In cases were the same mechanism of action is involved, (e.g. Tro and Clo as PPAR$\alpha$ activators), known target genes like CYP4A and Cte were induced, but also clear differences were detected. For other compounds, unknown target genes and pathways were uncovered, which may give the beginning for future mechanistic investigations.

In contrast to previously conducted *in vivo* studies, no universal gene regulations were detected confined to in one of the both predefined compound-groups (Zidek et al., 2007). None of the genes were deregulated in one direction by all hepatotoxic compounds. Instead, sets of genes involved in the same cellular mechanism were detected, together building a network of regulatory processes and cellular reactions after compound treatment. Sometimes it is not easy to discriminate direct effects from secondary effects. For example, the induction of cell cycle related genes could be indicative for a mitogenic effect of a compound, or the initiation of the cell cycle could be a reaction to generated cellular damage. It is known that regenerative processes occur after liver necrosis and include proliferation (Viebahn & Yeoh, 2008).

Often energy metabolism was affected, including changes in fatty acid oxidation, glycogenolysis and acetyl-CoA synthesis. This was also true for compounds which are non hepatotoxic. In general, all cellular reactions need or deliver energy equivalents, so it is not surprising to find changes in gene expression as a reaction to the cellular need. As a normal reaction, the cells are capable of handling these changes and to produce enough energy to sustain their metabolism. If energy consumption is too high or the production falls below the minimum needed for proper function, additional mechanisms are activated causing cell damage or driving the cell into necrosis or apoptosis (Nieminen, 2003).

# 4 CONCLUDING REMARKS AND FUTURE PERSPECTIVES

In this work, new in vitro and molecular techniques were applied to establish a new, early test system for toxicological research. A wide range of alternative approaches are currently being developed to gain mechanistic information, to speed up the process of early screening in drug development, to improve the toxicological testing procedure itself and, of course, to reduce the number of animals used for toxicity testing. At the same time, new technical developments and options are being adopted into toxicology laboratories and tested for their suitability and robustness. One promising approach is the analysis of gene expression changes by microarrays (Amin et al., 2002). The combination of both of these basic approaches, in vitro experiments and modern technology, will help to answer some of the key questions faced by toxicology.

Primarily, the applicability of two commercially available gene expression platforms was examined by a thorough comparative study of data gained from in vitro as well as in vivo experiments. Our results demonstrated that the high quality and correlation of generated data on a technical level lead to a high concordance in terms of the biological interpretations, making both platforms applicable for use in toxicological studies. This result was supported by the high correlation with TaqMan gene expression data. Recently, the FDA initiated a microarray "control" study (MAQC), which clearly showed the intra- and interlaboratory comparability of microarray results as well as the consistent results obtained from different microarray platforms (Guo et al., 2006; Shi et al., 2006).

The comparison of several in vitro culture systems, each with their own advantages and disadvantages in terms of throughput, viability and metabolic activity (Table 2), on both morphological and functional levels, as well as the global gene expression level permitted insights into basal mechanisms which take place during cell culture. The combination of both global gene expression and primary hepatocytes has been performed before in smaller studies covering only limited, more specific questions, when compared to the data presented here in this thesis (Baker et al., 2001; Boess et al., 2003; Braeuning et al., 2006). This PhD work was an important step towards the understanding of how varying culture conditions affect hepatocellular differentiation and function. At the same time, this comparison and subsequent optimizations lead to the establishment of a standardized and robust long-term hepatocyte culture system with clearly characterized morphological, functional and gene expression functions.

# 4 CONCLUDING REMARKS AND FUTURE PERSPECTIVES

All of this data was necessary to allow for good data interpretation based on the background level of gene expression during culturing and to define the horizon of expectation to ensure the reliability of this test system.

The main problem of all primary hepatocyte cultures is the reduction of metabolic activity over time in culture. While this is true for short term cultures like suspension cultures, liver slices and ML cultures, our data showed a deceleration of this process by culturing the hepatocytes in the SW conformation without FCS. Not only the basal gene expression of several CYPs was found to be higher in SW- cultures, but also the treatment with well known inducers resulted in an improved inducibility of the four CYPs tested. These findings are supported by published data on both the functional level as well as in terms of gene expression (Elaut et al., 2006a; LeCluyse et al., 2000; Richert et al., 2002; Rogiers & Vercruysse, 1998; Coecke et al., 2005).

These results provided us with confidence to go forward with this in vitro culture system for a toxicogenomics study using several well known hepatotoxicants to show compound dependent gene expression changes and to compare different mechanisms of action. This data was not only used for mechanistic analyses but also to successfully develop a computer based discrimination model for hepatotoxicity. Up to now, studies employing such predictive models are based on in vivo data and are mainly focused on acute toxicity (Hamadeh et al., 2002b; Zidek et al., 2007; Ellinger-Ziegelbauer et al., 2008; Ruepp et al., 2005). This model is the first study combining in vitro toxicology and toxicogenomics to test the possibility of using primary hepatocytes dosed for 9 d to depict sub-chronic toxicity.

Surprisingly, even though a relatively small database was used, the classification of the compounds used was successfull, with a misclassification rate of only 7.5% after 9 days. Knowing the fact that multiple gene expression changes are caused by the perfusion itself and the adaption to the culture conditions, this is a high-quality result and reflects the robustness of this in vitro system to predict the in vivo outcome.

The resulting discrimination model was challenged with two blinded compounds to prove its ability do detect hepatotoxicity based on global gene expression. EMD X is a former Merck compound which was stopped in development and is known to be hepatotoxic. Using our model it was clearly predicted to be hepatotoxic. AAP has been reported to lose toxic potency in primary hepatocytes over time in culture (Jemnitz et al., 2008), which was also seen in our dose finding experiments. Nevertheless, it was predicted to be a hepatotoxin based on gene expression changes indicating that, although not visibly damaging the cells, AAP still caused changes at the gene level which would lead to

## 4 CONCLUDING REMARKS AND FUTURE PERSPECTIVES

hepatotoxicity. Further studies are needed to better understand the mechanistic processes taking place in culture and the insensitivity of primary hepatocytes to AAP toxicity.

In the last few decades, a new paradigm has emerged based on the assumption that knowing the mechanism of action of a toxic compound would enable the development of predictive models which would help new, safer compounds to be brought quicker onto the market. The search for adaptive changes in gene expression has resulted in many genes being proposed as predictive biomarkers, although only a few of them have been shown to be really decisive. Currently, new techniques in bioinformatic analysis has lead to the identification of gene signatures and networks which seem to contain more information and therefore to be more reliable than single gene biomarkers (Khor et al., 2006).

The ultimate goal of these in vitro toxicogenomic studies is the establishment of a predictive screening model which is easy to use and which delivers reliable, high quality results. The results presented here are very promising, but this study is just the starting point for a more thorough classification process. As mentioned before, the size of the database used for classification is crucial for the validity of the system. This is highlighted by the fact that the best results were obtained with the whole dataset (low and high dose together). Is it really beneficial to combine two dosing schemes, or is the improvement due to the increasing size of the dataset? The high dose was chosen due to the reduction of cell viability, but changes in gene expression resulting from low dose treatment were seen as well. These low-dose effects may also contain important information for the prediction model.

Another important point to consider is the dosing-scheme itself. Always controversially discussed (Monro, 1990; Campbell & Ings, 1988) and of central importance to the outcome of any in vitro experiment, there are currently no specific guidelines available. To avoid false positive or negative results, a list of general criteria would be helpful to exclude unsuitable samples due to incorrect dosing or differences in the culturing conditions. In toxicology testing, doses greatly in excess of pharmacologically active doses are used to induce adverse effects, therefore there might be effects obtained also for (in vivo) non toxic compounds, leading to false results. On the other hand, if a threshold value is not achieved, even toxic compounds may be classified as non toxic. A potential solution would be the application of a minimum number of deregulated genes according to t-test statistic and/or fold-change. A minimum set of deregulated genes might be adequate for discrimination. Whereas for non toxic compounds the genes affected should either be involved in non-damaging processes or random, toxic compounds should generate gene profiles clearly connected to adverse cellular fate and viability. The conduction of these

## 4 CONCLUDING REMARKS AND FUTURE PERSPECTIVES

tests with multiple doses, which is enabled by in vitro experiments, is also a possibility to increase data quality.

The compound selection allowed a proof of concept for the constructed prediction model, although it was too small to cover all of the various potential mechanisms of hepatotoxicity. The gene set of 724 genes was capable of discriminating the compounds used to build the model, as well as to correctly classify newly added compounds with a misclassification rate of 7.5%. These results need to be further validated and refined, by including more compounds with specific modes of action or to focus a certain compound classes. This will increase the robustness of the predictive system and facilitate improved data interpretation.

Finally, the insecurity of extrapolating the results in between species, especially to men, may be overcome by the possibility to conduct these experiments with human hepatocytes. Also human hepatocytes can be successfully cultured in either ML- or SW-conformation, there is still the need to optimize the culture conditions. Because of the difficulties and the costs of getting high quality human hepatocytes in a sufficient amount, there might also be other options like the new HepaRG cell line which may be considered. Yet, the data obtained during this work is promising but not sufficient to attest the qualification of either possibility.

To conclude, screening tests alone do not allow for a final estimation of the hazard and risk of a compound, but molecular toxicology can contribute by improving the mechanistic understanding, refining the predictivity of toxicological outcomes and to significantly reduce animal usage in toxicology and, more generally, in drug discovery. We have now a robust, semi-validated long-term cell culture system that can be used in drug discovery for predicting hepatotoxicity as well as helping the toxicologist to understand a compounds mechanism of action. Therefore, the development of this predictive in vitro test system can be seen as a contribution to the efforts to implement the principles of 3R into the daily toxicological work.

# 5 REFERENCES

Aardema, M. J. & MacGregor, J. T. (2002). Toxicology and genetic toxicology in the new era of "toxicogenomics": impact of "-omics" technologies. *Mutat Res, 499*(1), 13-25.

Akerboom, T. P., Narayanaswami, V., Kunst, M. & Sies, H. (1991). ATP-dependent S-(2,4-dinitrophenyl)glutathione transport in canalicular plasma membrane vesicles from rat liver. *J Biol Chem, 266*(20), 13147-52.

Alexandre, E., Viollon-Abadie, C., David, P., Gandillet, A., Coassolo, P., Heyd, B., Heyd, B., Mantion, G., Wolf, P., Bachellier, P., Jaeck, D. & Richert, L. (2002). Cryopreservation of adult human hepatocytes obtained from resected liver biopsies. *Cryobiology, 44*(2), 103-13.

Aljada, A., Garg, R., Ghanim, H., Mohanty, P., Hamouda, W., Assian, E. & Dandona, P. (2001). Nuclear factor-kappaB suppressive and inhibitor-kappaB stimulatory effects of troglitazone in obese patients with type 2 diabetes: evidence of an antiinflammatory action? *J Clin Endocrinol Metab, 86*(7), 3250-6.

Ames, B. N., Lee, F. D. & Durston, W. E. (1973). An improved bacterial test system for the detection and classification of mutagens and carcinogens. *Proc Natl Acad Sci U S A., 70*(3), 782-6.

Amin, R. P., Hamadeh, H. K., Bushel, P. R., Bennett, L., Afshari, C. A. & Paules, R. S. (2002). Genomic interrogation of mechanism(s) underlying cellular responses to toxicants. *Toxicology, 181-182*, 555-63.

Anderson, N. L. & Anderson, N. G. (2002). The human plasma proteome: history, character, and diagnostic prospects. *Mol Cell Proteomics, 1*(11), 845-67.

Andrade, R. J., Camargo, R., Lucena, M. I. & González-Grande, R. (2004). Causality assessment in drug-induced hepatotoxicity. *Expert Opin Drug Drug Saf, 3*(4), 329-44.

Bader, A., Frühauf, N., Zech, K., Haverich, A. & Borlak, J. T. (1998). Development of a small-scale bioreactor for drug metabolism studies maintaining hepatospecific functions. *Xenobiotica, 28*(9), 815-25.

Bailly-Maitre, B., de Sousa, G., Zucchini, N., Gugenheim, J., Boulukos, K. E. & Rahmani, R. (2002). Spontaneous apoptosis in primary cultures of human and rat hepatocytes: molecular mechanisms and regulation by dexamethasone. *Cell Death Differ, 9*(9), 945-55.

Baker, T. K., Carfagna, M. A., Gao, H., Dow, E. R., Li, Q., Searfoss, G. H. & Ryan, T. P. (2001). Temporal gene expression analysis of monolayer cultured rat hepatocytes. *Chem Res Toxicol, 14*(9), 1218-31.

# 6 REFERENCES

Ballet, F. (1997). Hepatotoxicity in drug development: detection, significance and solutions. *J Hepatol, 26 Suppl 2*, 26-36.

Bandara, L. R. & Kennedy, S. (2002). Toxicoproteomics - a new preclinical tool. *Drug Discov Today, 7*(7), 411-8.

Bayad, J., Sabolovic, N., Bagrel, D., Magdalou, J. & Siest, G. (1991). Influence of the isolation method on the stability of differentiated phenotype in cultured rat hepatocytes. *J Pharmacol Methods, 25*(1), 85-94.

Bedossa, P. & Paradis, V. (2003). Liver extracellular matrix in health and disease. *J Pathol, 200*(4), 504-15.

Begue, J. M., Guguen-Guillouzo, C., Pasdeloup, N. & Guillouzo A. (1994). Prolonged maintenance of active cytochrome P-450 in adult rat hepatocytes co-cultured with another liver cell type. *Hepatology, 4*(5), 839-42.

Beigel, J., Fella, K., Kramer, P., Kroeger, M. & Hewitt, P. (2008). Genomics and proteomics analysis of cultured primary rat hepatocytes. *Toxicol in vitro, 22*(1), 171-81.

Benoit, G., Cooney, A., Giguere, V., Ingraham, H., Lazar, M., Muscat, G., Perlmann, T., Renaud, J. P., Schwabe, J., Sladek, F., Tsai, M. J. & Laudet, V. (2006). International Union of Pharmacology. LXVI. Orphan nuclear receptors. *Pharmacol Rev, 58*(4), 798-836.

Berridge, M. V., Herst, P. M. & Tan, A. S. (2005). Tetrazolium dyes as tools in cell biology: new insights into their cellular reduction. *Biotechnol Annu Rev, 11*, 127-52.

Berthiaume, F., Moghe, P. V., Toner, M. & Yarmush, M. L. (1996). Effect of extracellular matrix topology on cell structure, function, and physiological responsiveness: hepatocytes cultured in a sandwich configuration. *FASEB J, 10*(13), 1471-84.

Besaratinia, A. & Pfeifer, G. P. (2005). DNA adduction and mutagenic properties of acrylamide. *Mutat Res, 580*(1-2), 31-40.

Blouin, A., Bolender, R. P. & Weibel, E. R. (1977). Distribution of organelles and membranes between hepatocytes and nonhepatocytes in the rat liver parenchyma. A stereological study. *J Cell Biol, 72*(2), 441-55.

Boelsterli, U. A. (2003). Disease-related determinants of susceptibility to drug-induced idiosyncratic hepatotoxicity. *Curr Opin Drug Discov Devel, 6*(1), 81-91.

Boess, F., Kamber, M., Romer, S., Gasser, R., Muller, D., Albertini, S. & Suter, L.. (2003). Gene expression in two hepatic cell lines, cultured primary hepatocytes, and liver slices compared to the in vivo liver gene expression in rats: possible implications for toxicogenomics use of in vitro systems. *Toxicol Sci, 73*(2), 386-402.

Bose, I. & Ghosh, B. (2007). The p53-MDM2 network: from oscillations to apoptosis. *J of BioSci, 32*(5), 991-7.

# 6 REFERENCES

Boswell-Smith, V., Cazzola, M. & Page, C. P. (2006). Are phosphodiesterase 4 inhibitors just more theophylline? *J Allergy Clin Immunol*, 117(6), 1237-43.

Braeuning, A., Ittrich, C., Köhle, C., Hailfinger, S., Bonin, M., Buchmann, A. & Schwarz, M. (2006). Differential gene expression in periportal and perivenous mouse hepatocytes. *FEBS J*, 273(22), 5051-61.

Brandon, E. F. A., Raap, C. D., Meijerman, I., Beijnen, J. H. & Schellens, J. H. M. (2003). An update on in vitro test methods in human hepatic drug biotransformation research: pros and cons. *Toxicol Appl Pharmacol*, 189(3), 233-46.

Brock, C., Schaefer, M., Reusch, H. P., Czupalla, C., Michalke, M., Spicher, K., Schultz, G. & Nürnberg, B. (2003). Roles of G beta gamma in membrane recruitment and activation of p110 gamma/p101 phosphoinositide 3-kinase gamma. *J Cell Biol*, 160(1), 89-99.

Brown, P. O. & Botstein, D. (1999). Exploring the new world of the genome with DNA microarrays. *Nat Genet*, 21(1 Suppl), 33-7.

Bulera, S. J., Eddy, S. M., Ferguson, E., Jatkoe, T. A., Reindel, J. F., Bleavins, M. R. & De La Iglesia, F. A. (2001). RNA expression in the early characterization of hepatotoxicants in Wistar rats by high-density DNA microarrays. *Hepatology*, 33(5), 1239-58.

Burchiel, S. W., Knall, C. M., Davis, J. W., Paules, R. S., Boggs, S. E. & Afshari, C. A. (2001). Analysis of genetic and epigenetic mechanisms of toxicity: potential roles of toxicogenomics and proteomics in toxicology. *Toxicol Sci*, 59(2), 193-5.

Burke, M. D., Thompson, S., Elcombe, C. R., Halpert, J., Haaparanta, T. & Mayer, R. T. (1985). Ethoxy-, pentoxy- and benzyloxyphenoxazones and homologues: a series of substrates to distinguish between different induced cytochromes P-450. *Biochem Pharmacol*, 34(18), 3337-45.

Burke-Gaffney, A., Callister, M. E. J. & Nakamura, H. (2005). Thioredoxin: friend or foe in human disease? *Trends Pharmacol Sci*, 26(8), 398-404.

Butte, A. (2002). The use and analysis of microarray data. *Nat Rev Drug Discov*, 1(12), 951-60.

Callander, R. D., Mackay, J. M., Clay, P., Elcombe, C. R. & Elliott, B. M. (1995). Evaluation of phenobarbital/beta-naphthoflavone as an alternative S9-induction regime to Aroclor 1254 in the rat for use in in vitro genotoxicity assays. *Mutagenesis*, 10(6), 517-22.

Campbell, D. B. & Ings, R. M. (1988). New approaches to the use of pharmacokinetics in toxicology and drug development. *Hum Toxicol*, 7(5), 469-79.

Cesaratto, L., Vascotto, C., Calligaris, S. & Tell, G. (2004). The importance of redox state in liver damage. *Ann Hepatol*, 3(3), 86-92.

# 6 REFERENCES

Chapman, G. S., Jones, A. L., Meyer, U. A. & Montgomery Bissell, D. (1973). Parenchymal cells from adult rat liver in nonproliverating monolayer culture: II. Ultrastructural studies. *J Cell Biol, 59*(3), 735-47.

Chen, G., Gharib, T. G., Huang, C., Taylor, J. M. G., Misek, D. E., Kardia, S. L., Giordano, T. J., Iannettoni, M. D., Orringer, M. B., Hanash, S. M. & Beer, D. G. (2002). Discordant protein and mRNA expression in lung adenocarcinomas. *Mol Cell Proteomics, 1*(4), 304-13.

Chen, J. J., Hsueh, H., Delongchamp, R. R., Lin, C. & Tsai, C. (2007). Reproducibility of microarray data: a further analysis of microarray quality control (MAQC) data. *BMC Bioinformatics, 8*, 412.

Chin, K. & Kong, A. N. T. (2002). Application of DNA microarrays in pharmacogenomics and toxicogenomics. *Pharm Res, 19*(12), 1773-8.

Ching, K. Z., Tenney, K. A., Chen, J. & Morgan, E. T. (1996). Suppression of constitutive cytochrome P450 gene expression by epidermal growth factor receptor ligands in cultured rat hepatocytes. *Drug Metab Dispos, 24*(5), 542-6.

Clayton, D. F., Weiss, M. & Darnell, J. E. (1985). Liver-specific RNA metabolism in hepatoma cells: variations in transcription rates and mRNA levels. *Mol Cell Biol, 5*(10), 2633-41.

Coecke, S., Blaauboer, B. J., Elaut, G., Freeman, S., Freidig, A., Gensmantel, N., Hoet, P., Kapoulas, V. M., Ladstetter, B., Langley, G. Leahy, D., Mannens, G., Meneguz, A., Monshouwer, M., Nemery, B., Pelkonen, O., Pfaller, W., Prieto, P., Proctor, N., Rogiers, V., Rostami-Hodjegan, A., Sabbioni, E., Steiling, W. & van de Sandt, J. J. (2005). Toxicokinetics and metabolism. *Altern Lab Anim, 33 Suppl 1*, 147-75.

Coyle, B., Freathy, C., Gant, T. W., Roberts, R. A. & Cain, K. (2003). Characterization of the transforming growth factor-beta 1-induced apoptotic transcriptome in FaO hepatoma cells. *J Biol Chem, 278*(8), 5920-8.

Cross, D. M. & Bayliss, M. K. (2000). A commentary on the use of hepatocytes in drug metabolism studies during drug discovery and development. *Drug Metab Rev, 32*(2), 219-40.

Czaja, M. J. (2002). Induction and regulation of hepatocyte apoptosis by oxidative stress. *Antioxid Redox Signal, 4*(5), 759-67.

Davila, J. C. & Morris, D. L. (1999). Analysis of cytochrome P450 and phase 2 conjugating enzyme expression in adult male rat hepatocytes. *In Vitro Cell Dev Biol Anim, 35*(3), 120-30.

# 6 REFERENCES

De Smet, K., Beken, S., Vanhaecke, T., Pauwels, M., Vercruysse, A. & Rogiers, V. (1998). Isolation of rat hepatocytes. *Methods Mol Biol, 107*, 295-301.

Desmet, V. J., Krstulović, B. & Damme, B. V. (1968). Histochemical study of rat liver in alpha-naphthyl isothiocyanate (ANIT) induced cholestasis. *Methods Mol Biol, 52*(2), 401–421.

Dhainaut, J. F., Marin, N., Mignon, A. & Vinsonneau, C. (2001). Hepatic response to sepsis: interaction between coagulation and inflammatory processes. *Crit Care Med, 29*(7 Suppl), S42-7.

Dickins, M. (2004). Induction of cytochromes P450. *Curr Top Med Chem, 4*(16), 1745-66.

Dix, D. J., Gallagher, K., Benson, W. H., Groskinsky, B. L., McClintock, J. T., , Dearfield, K. L. & Farland, W. H. (2006). A framework for the use of genomics data at the EPA. *Nat Biotechnol, 24*(9), 1108-11.

Donato, M. T., Castell, J. V. & Gómez-Lechón, M. J. (1994). Cytochrome P450 activities in pure and co-cultured rat hepatocytes. Effects of model inducers. *In Vitro Cell Dev Biol Anim, 30A*(12), 825-32.

Dunn, J. C., Tompkins, R. G. & Yarmush, M. L. (1991). Long-term in vitro function of adult hepatocytes in a collagen sandwich configuration. *Biotechnol Prog, 7*(3), 237-45.

Dunn, J. C., Yarmush, M. L., Koebe, H. G. & Tompkins, R. G. (1989). Hepatocyte function and extracellular matrix geometry: long-term culture in a sandwich configuration. *FASEB J, 3*(2), 174-7.

Ekins, S., Murray, G. I., Burke, M. D., Williams, J. A., Marchant, N. C. & Hawksworth, G. M. (1995). Quantitative differences in phase 1 and II metabolism between rat precision-cut liver slices and isolated hepatocytes. *Drug Metab Dispos, 23*(11), 1274-9.

Elaut, G., Henkens, T., Papeleu, P., Snykers, S., Vinken, M., Vanhaecke, T. & Rogiers, V. (2006). Molecular mechanisms underlying the dedifferentiation process of isolated hepatocytes and their cultures. *Curr Drug Metab, 7*(6), 629-60.

Elaut, G., Papeleu, P., Vinken, M., Henkens, T., Snykers, S., Vanhaecke, T. & Rogiers, V. (2006). Hepatocytes in suspension. *Methods Mol Biol, 320*, 255-63.

El-Bahay, C., Gerber, E., Horbach, M., Tran-Thi, Q. H., Röhrdanz, E. & Kahl, R. (1999). Influence of tumor necrosis factor-alpha and silibin on the cytotoxic action of alpha-amanitin in rat hepatocyte culture. *Toxicol Appl Pharmacol, 158*(3), 253-60.

Elias, E. & Mills, C. O. (2007). Coordinated defence and the liver. *Clin Med, 7*(2), 180-4.

Ellinger-Ziegelbauer, H., Gmuender, H., Bandenburg, A. & Ahr, H. J. (2008). Prediction of a carcinogenic potential of rat hepatocarcinogens using toxicogenomics analysis of short-term in vivo studies. *Mutat Res, 637*(1-2), 23-39.

# 6 REFERENCES

Ellinger-Ziegelbauer, H., Stuart, B., Wahle, B., Bomann, W. & Ahr, H. (2004). Characteristic expression profiles induced by genotoxic carcinogens in rat liver. *Toxicol Sci, 77*(1), 19-34.

Enat, R., Jefferson, D. M., Ruiz-Opazo, N., Gatmaitan, Z., Leinwand, L. A. & Reid, L. M. (1984). Hepatocyte proliferation in vitro: its dependence on the use of serum-free hormonally defined medium and substrata of extracellular matrix. *Proc Natl Acad Sci U S A, 81*(5), 1411-5.

Enomoto, K., Nishikawa, Y., Omori, Y., Tokairin, T., Yoshida, M., Ohi, N., Nishimura, T., Yamamoto, Y. & Li, Q. (2004). Cell biology and pathology of liver sinusoidal endothelial cells. *Med Electron Microsc, 37*(4), 208-15.

Etienne, P. L., Baffet, G., Desvergne, B., Boisnard-Rissel, M., Glaise, D. & Guguen-Guillouzo, C. (1988). Transient expression of c-fos and constant expression of c-myc in freshly isolated and cultured normal adult rat hepatocytes. *Oncogene Res, 3*(3), 255-62.

Evans, W. E. & Relling, M. V. (1999). Pharmacogenomics: translating functional genomics into rational therapeutics. *Science, 286*(5439), 487-91.

Farkas, D. & Tannenbaum, S. R. (2005a). In vitro methods to study chemically-induced hepatotoxicity: a literature review. *Curr Drug Metab, 6*(2), 111-25.

Farkas, D. & Tannenbaum, S. R. (2005b). Characterization of chemically induced hepatotoxicity in collagen sandwiches of rat hepatocytes. *Toxicol Sci, 85*(2), 927-34.

Fella, K., Glückmann, M., Hellmann, J., Karas, M., Kramer, P. & Kröger, M. (2005). Use of two-dimensional gel electrophoresis in predictive toxicology: identification of potential early protein biomarkers in chemically induced hepatocarcinogenesis. *Proteomics, 5*(7), 1914-27.

Fielden, M. R. & Zacharewski, T. R. (2001). Challenges and limitations of gene expression profiling in mechanistic and predictive toxicology. *Toxicol Sci, 60*(1), 6-10.

Förster, T. (1948). Zwischenmolekulare Energiewanderung und Fluoreszenz. *Annalen der Physik, 437*(1-2), 55-75.

Fréneaux, E., Labbe, G., Letteron, P., The Le Dinh, Degott, C., Genève, J., Larrey, D. & Pessayre, D. (1988). Inhibition of the mitochondrial oxidation of fatty acids by tetracycline in mice and in man: possible role in microvesicular steatosis induced by this antibiotic. *Hepatology, 8*(5), 1056-62.

Friedman, S. L. (1997). Molecular mechanisms of hepatic fibrosis and principles of therapy. *J Gastroenterol, 32*(3), 424-30.

Gabler, W. L. & Creamer, H. R. (1991). Suppression of human neutrophil functions by tetracyclines. *J Periodontal Res, 26*(1), 52-8.

# 6 REFERENCES

Gaeta, G. B., Utili, R., Adinolfi, L. E., Abernathy, C. O. & Giusti, G. (1985). Characterization of the effects of erythromycin estolate and erythromycin base on the excretory function of the isolated rat liver. *Toxicol Appl Pharmacol, 80*(2), 185-92.

Gallai, M., Kovalszky, I., Knittel, T., Neubauer, K., Armbrust, T. & Ramadori, G. (1996). Expression of extracellular matrix proteoglycans perlecan and decorin in carbon-tetrachloride-injured rat liver and in isolated liver cells. *Methods Mol Biol, 148*(5), 1463-71.

Garnier, G., Circolo, A. & Colten, H. R. (1996). Constitutive expression of murine complement factor B gene is regulated by the interaction of its upstream promoter with hepatocyte nuclear factor 4. *J Biol Chem, 271*(47), 30205-11.

Gatzidou, E. T., Zira, A. N. & Theocharis, S. E. (2007). Toxicogenomics: a pivotal piece in the puzzle of toxicological research. *J Appl Toxicol, 27*(4), 302-9.

Gautam, A., Ng, O. C. & Boyer, J. L. (1987). Isolated rat hepatocyte couplets in short-term culture: structural characteristics and plasma membrane reorganization. *Hepatology, 7*(2), 216-23.

Gebhardt R, Hengstler JG, Müller D, Glöckner R, Buenning P, Laube B, Schmelzer E, Ullrich M, Utesch D, Hewitt N, Ringel M, Hilz BR, Bader A, Langsch A, Koose T, Burger HJ, Maas J & Oesch F. (2003). New hepatocyte in vitro systems for drug metabolism: metabolic capacity and recommendations for application in basic research and drug development, standard operation procedures. *Drug Metab Rev, 35*(2-3), 145-213.

Giancotti, F. G. & Ruoslahti, E. (1999). Integrin signaling. *Science, 285*(5430), 1028-32.

Giancotti, F. G. & Tarone, G. (2003). Positional control of cell fate through joint integrin/receptor protein kinase signaling. *Annu Rev Cell Dev Biol, 19*, 173-206.

Gómez-Lechón, M. J., Donato, T., Ponsoda, X. & Castell, J. V. (2003). Human hepatic cell cultures: in vitro and in vivo drug metabolism. *Altern Lab Anim, 31*(3), 257-65.

Gómez-Lechón, M. J., Ponsoda, X., Bort, R. & Castell, J. V. (2004). The use of cultured hepatocytes to investigate the metabolism of drugs and mechanisms of drug hepatotoxicity. *Altern Lab Anim, 29*(3), 225-31.

González, H. E., Eugenín, E. A., Garcés, G., Solís, N., Pizarro, M., Accatino, L. & Sáez, J. C. (2002). Regulation of hepatic connexins in cholestasis: possible involvement of Kupffer cells and inflammatory mediators. *Am J Physiol Gastrointest Liver, 282*(6), G991-G1001.

Goodman, L. S., Limbird, L. E., Milinoff, P. B., Ruddon, R. W. & Gilman, A. G. (1996). *Goodman and Gilman's: The Pharmacological Basis of Therapeutics* (9th ed., p. 1905). Mcgraw-Hill, Columbus.

# 6 REFERENCES

Gordon, E. M., Douglas, M. C., Jablonski, P., Owen, J. A., Sali, A. & Watts, J. M. (1972). Gastroduodenal hormones and bile-secretion studies in the isolated perfused pig liver. *Surgery*, 72(5), 708-21.

Gracie, J. A., Robertson, S. E. & McInnes, I. B. (2003). Interleukin-18. *J Leukoc Biol*, 73(2), 213-24.

Graf, J. & Boyer, J. L. (1990). The use of isolated rat hepatocyte couplets in hepatobiliary physiology. *J Hepatol*, 10(3), 387-94.

Gripon, P., Rumin, S., Urban, S., Le Seyec, J., Glaise, D., Cannie, I., Guyomard, C., Lucas, J., Trepo, C. & Guguen-Guillouzo, C. (2002). Infection of a human hepatoma cell line by hepatitis B virus. *Proc Natl Acad Sci U S A*, 99(24), 15655-60.

Groneberg, D. A., Grosse-Siestrup, C. & Fischer, A. (2002). In vitro models to study hepatotoxicity. *Toxicol Pathol*, 30(3), 394-9.

Guengerich, F. P. (2003). Cytochromes P450, drugs, and diseases. *Mol. Interv*, 3(4), 194-204.

Guigoz, Y., Werffeli, P., Favre, D., Juillerat, M., Wellinger, R. & Honegger, P. (1987). Aggregate cultures of foetal rat liver cells: development and maintenance of liver gene expression. *Biol Cell*, 60(3), 163-71.

Gunderson, K. L., Kruglyak, S., Graige, M. S., Garcia, F., Kermani, B. G., Zhao, C., Che, D., Dickinson, T., Wickham, E., Bierle, J., Doucet, D., Milewski, M., Yang, R., Siegmund, C., Haas, J., Zhou, L., Oliphant, A., Fan, J. B., Barnard, S. & Chee, M. S. (2004). Decoding randomly ordered DNA arrays. *Genome Res*, 14(5), 870-7.

Guo, L., Lobenhofer, E. K., Wang, C., Shippy, R., Harris, S. C., Zhang, L., Mei, N., Chen, T., Herman, D., Goodsaid, F. M., Hurban, P., Phillips, K. L., Xu, J., Deng, X., Sun, Y. A., Tong, W., Dragan, Y. P. & Shi, L. (2006). Rat toxicogenomic study reveals analytical consistency across microarray platforms. *Nat Biotechnol*, 24(9), 1162-9.

Gygi, S. P., Rochon, Y., Franza, B. R. & Aebersold, R. (1999). Correlation between protein and mRNA abundance in yeast. *Mol Cell Biol*, 19(3), 1720-30.

Hakkola, J., Hu, Y. & Ingelman-Sundberg, M. (2003). Mechanisms of down-regulation of CYP2E1 expression by inflammatory cytokines in rat hepatoma cells. *J Pharmacol Exp Ther*, 304(3), 1048-54.

Hamadeh, H.K., Bushel, P.R., Jayadev, S., DiSorbo, O., Bennett, L., Li, L., Tennant, R., Stoll, R., Barrett, J.C., Paules, R.S., Blanchard, K. & Afshari, C.A. (2002). Prediction of compound signature using high density gene expression profiling. *Toxicol Sci*, 67(2), 232-40.

# 6 REFERENCES

Hamadeh, H.K., Bushel, P.R., Jayadev, S., Martin, K., DiSorbo, O., Sieber, S., Bennett, L., Tennant, R., Stoll, R., Barrett, J.C., Blanchard, K., Paules, R.S. & Afshari, C.A. (2002). Gene expression analysis reveals chemical-specific profiles. *Toxicol Sci*, 67(2), 219-31.

Hamilton, G. A., Jolley, S. L., Gilbert, D., Coon, D. J., Barros, S. & LeCluyse, E. L. (2001). Regulation of cell morphology and cytochrome P450 expression in human hepatocytes by extracellular matrix and cell-cell interactions. *Cell Tissue Res*, 306(1), 85-99.

Hamilton, G. A., Westmorel, C. & George, A. E. (2001). Effects of medium composition on the morphology and function of rat hepatocytes cultured as spheroids and monolayers. *In Vitro Cell Dev Biol Anim*, 37(10), 656-67.

Häussinger, D., Reinehr, R. & Schliess, F. (2006). The hepatocyte integrin system and cell volume sensing. *Acta physiologica (Oxford, England)*, 187(1-2), 249-55.

Hayashi, R., Wada, H., Ito, K. & Adcock, I. M. (2004). Effects of glucocorticoids on gene transcription. *Eur J Clin Pharmacol*, 500(1-3), 51-62.

Heinrich, P. C., Behrmann, I., Haan, S., Hermanns, H. M., Müller-Newen, G. & Schaper, F. (2003). Principles of interleukin (IL)-6-type cytokine signalling and its regulation. *Biochem J*, 374(Pt 1), 1-20.

Heishi, M., Ichihara, J., Teramoto, R., Itakura, Y., Hayashi, K., Ishikawa, H., Gomi, H., Sakai, J., Kanaoka, M., Taiji, M. & Kimura, T. (2006). Global gene expression analysis in liver of obese diabetic db/db mice treated with metformin. *Diabetologia*, 49(7), 1647-55.

Hengstler, J. G., Utesch, D., Steinberg, P., Platt, K. L., Diener, B., Ringel, M., Swales, N., Fischer, T., Biefang, K., Gerl, M., Böttger, T. & Oesch, F. (2000). Cryopreserved primary hepatocytes as a constantly available in vitro model for the evaluation of human and animal drug metabolism and enzyme induction. *Drug Metab Rev*, 32(1), 81-118.

Heredi-Szabo, K., Kis, E., Molnar, E., Gyorfi, A. & Krajcsi, P. (2008). Characterization of 5(6)-Carboxy-2,'7'-Dichlorofluorescein Transport by MRP2 and Utilization of this Substrate as a Fluorescent Surrogate for LTC4. *J Biomol Screen*, 13(4), 295-301.

Hewitt, N. J. & Hewitt, P. (2004). Phase 1 and II enzyme characterization of two sources of HepG2 cell lines. *Xenobiotica*, 34(3), 243-56.

Hiroi, J., Kimura, K., Aikawa, M., Tojo, A., Suzuki, Y., Nagamatsu, T., Omata, M., Yazaki, Y. & Nagai, R. (1996). Expression of a nonmuscle myosin heavy chain in glomerular cells differentiates various types of glomerular disease in rats. *Kidney Int*, 49(5), 1231-41.

Holme, J. A. (1985). Xenobiotic metabolism and toxicity in primary monolayer cultures of hepatocytes. *NIPH Ann*, 8(2), 49-63.

Howard, R. B., Christensen, A. K., Gibbs, F. A. & Pesch, L. A. (1967). The enzymatic preparation of isolated intact parenchymal cells from rat liver. *J Cell Biol*, 35(3), 675-84.

# 6 REFERENCES

Hutchens, T. W. & Yip, T. (1993). New desorption strategies for the mass spectrometric analysis of macromolecules. *Rapid Commun Mass Spectrom*, 7(7), 576-580.

Illenberger, D., Walliser, C., Nurnberg, B., Diaz Lorente, M. & Gierschik, P. (2003). Specificity and structural requirements of phospholipase C-beta stimulation by Rho GTPases versus G protein beta gamma dimers. *J Biol Chem*, 278(5), 3006-14.

Imai, T., Jiang, M., Kastner, P., Chambon, P. & Metzger, D. (2001). Selective ablation of retinoid X receptor alpha in hepatocytes impairs their lifespan and regenerative capacity. *Proc Natl Acad Sci U S A*, 98(8), 4581-6.

Ingelman-Sundberg, M., Ronis, M. J., Lindros, K. O., Eliasson, E. & Zhukov, A. (1994). Ethanol-inducible cytochrome P4502E1: regulation, enzymology and molecular biology. *Alcohol, Supplement*, 2, 131-9.

Inzucchi, S. E., Maggs, D. G., Spollett, G. R., Page, S. L., Rife, F. S., Walton, V. & Shulman, G. I. (1998). Efficacy and metabolic effects of metformin and troglitazone in type II diabetes mellitus. *N Engl J Medl*, 338(13), 867-72.

Irigaray, P., Newby, J. A., Clapp, R., Hardell, L., Howard, V., Montagnier, L., Epstein S. & Belpomme D. (2007). Lifestyle-related factors and environmental agents causing cancer: an overview. *Biomedicine & pharmacoTher*, 61(10), 640-58.

Irizarry, R. A., Hobbs, B., Collin, F., Beazer-Barclay, Y. D., Antonellis, K. J., Scherf, U. & Speed T. P. (2003). Exploration, normalization, and summaries of high density oligonucleotide array probe level data. *Biostatistics*, 4(2), 249-64.

Iso, Y., Sawada, T., Okada, T. & Kubota, K. (2005). Loss of E-cadherin mRNA and gain of osteopontin mRNA are useful markers for detecting early recurrence of HCV-related hepatocellular carcinoma. *Eur J Surg Oncol*, 92(4), 304-11.

Jaeschke, H., Gores, G. J., Cederbaum, A. I., Hinson, J. A., Pessayre, D. & Lemasters, J. J. (2002). Mechanisms of hepatotoxicity. *Toxicol Sci*, 65(2), 166-76.

James, L. P., Mayeux, P. R. & Hinson, J. A. (2003). Acetaminophen-induced hepatotoxicity. *Drug Metab Dispos*, 31(12), 1499-506.

Jean, P. A. & Roth, R. A. (1995). Naphthylisothiocyanate disposition in bile and its relationship to liver glutathione and toxicity. *Biochem Pharmacol*, 50(9), 1469-74.

Jemnitz, K., Veres, Z., Monostory, K. & Vereczkey, L. (2000). Glucuronidation of thyroxine in primary monolayer cultures of rat hepatocytes: in vitro induction of UDP-glucuronosyltranferases by methylcholanthrene, clofibrate, and dexamethasone alone and in combination. *Drug Metab Dispos*, 28(1), 34-7.

# 6 REFERENCES

Jemnitz, K., Veres, Z., Monostory, K., Kóbori, L. & Vereczkey, L. (2008). Interspecies differences in acetaminophen sensitivity of human, rat, and mouse primary hepatocytes. *Toxicol In Vitro, 22*(4), 961-7.

Kanebratt, K. P. & Andersson, T. B. (2008). Evaluation of HepaRG cells as an in vitro model for human drug metabolism studies. *Drug Metab Dispos, 36*(7), 1444-52.

Kaplowitz, N. (2001). Drug-induced liver disorders: implications for drug development and regulation. *Drug Drug Saf, 24*(7), 483-90.

Kern, A., Bader, A., Pichlmayr, R. & Sewing, K. F. (1997). Drug metabolism in hepatocyte sandwich cultures of rats and humans. *Biochem Pharmacol, 54*(7), 761-72.

Kersten, S., Mandard, S., Escher, P., Gonzalez, F. J., Tafuri, S., Desvergne, B. & Wahli, W. (2001). The peroxisome proliferator-activated receptor alpha regulates amino acid metabolism. *FASEB J, 15*(11), 1971-8.

Kessova, I. & Cederbaum, A. I. (2003). CYP2E1: biochemistry, toxicology, regulation and function in ethanol-induced liver injury. *Curr Mol Med, 3*(6), 509-18.

Kevresan, S., Kuhajda, K., Kandrac, J., Fawcett, J. P. & Mikov, M. (2007). Biosynthesis of bile acids in mammalian liver. *Eur J Drug Metab Pharmacokinet, 31*(3), 145-56.

Khor, T. O., Ibrahim, S. & Kong, A. T. (2006). Toxicogenomics in drug discovery and drug development: potential applications and future challenges. *Pharm Res, 23*(8), 1659-64.

Kienhuis, A. S., Wortelboer, H. M., Maas, W. J., van Herwijnen, M., Kleinjans, J. C. S., van Delft, J. H. M. & Stierum, R. H. (2007). A sandwich-cultured rat hepatocyte system with increased metabolic competence evaluated by gene expression profiling. *Toxicol In Vitro, 21*(5), 892-901.

Kipp, H. & Arias, I. M. (2002). Trafficking of canalicular ABC transporters in hepatocytes. *Annu Rev Physiol, 64*, 595-608.

Klebanov, L. & Yakovlev, A. (2007). How high is the level of technical noise in microarray data? *Biol Direct, 2*, 9.

Kliewer, S. A., Lehmann, J. M., Milburn, M. V. & Willson, T. M. (1999). The PPARs and PXRs: nuclear xenobiotic receptors that define novel hormone signaling pathways. *Recent Prog Horm Res, 54*, 345-67; discussion 367-8.

Kmieć, Z. (2001). Cooperation of liver cells in health and disease. *Adv Anat Embryol Cell Biol, 161*, III-XIII, 1-151.

Knasmüller, S., Mersch-Sundermann, V., Kevekordes, S., Darroudi, F., Huber, W. W., Hoelzl, C., Bichler, J. & Majer, B. J. (2004). Use of human-derived liver cell lines for the detection of environmental and dietary genotoxicants; current state of knowledge. *Toxicology, 198*(1-3), 315-28.

# 6 REFERENCES

Kohonen, T., (1997). *Self-organizing maps*. Springer-Verlag New York, Inc., Secaucus, NJ.

König, B. & Eder, K. (2006). Differential action of 13-HPODE on PPARalpha downstream genes in rat Fao and human HepG2 hepatoma cell lines. *J Nutr Biochem*, 17(6), 410-8.

Kostrubsky, V. E., Strom, S. C., Hanson, J., Urda, E., Rose, K., Burliegh, J., Zocharsk,i P., Cai, H., Sinclair, J. F. & Sahi, J. (2003). Evaluation of hepatotoxic potential of drugs by inhibition of bile-acid transport in cultured primary human hepatocytes and intact rats. *Toxicol Sci*, 76(1), 220-8.

Kroeger, M. (2006). How omics technologies can contribute to the '3R' principles by introducing new strategies in animal testing. *Trends Biotechnol*, 24(8), 343-6.

Krumdieck, C. L., dos Santos, J. E. & Ho, K. J. (1980). A new instrument for the rapid preparation of tissue slices. *Anal Biochem*, 104(1), 118-23.

Kuo, W. P., Liu, F., Trimarchi, J., Punzo, C., Lombardi, M., Sarang, J., Whipple, M. E., Maysuria, M., Serikawa, K., Lee, S. Y., McCrann, D., Kang, J., Shearstone, J. R., Burke, J., Park, D. J., Wang, X., Rector, T. L., Ricciardi-Castagnoli, P., Perrin, S., Choi, S., Bumgarner, R., Kim, J. H., Short, G. F. 3rd, Freeman, M. W., Seed, B., Jensen, R., Church, G. M., Hovig, E., Cepko, C. L., Park, P., Ohno-Machado, L. & Jenssen, T. K.. (2006). A sequence-oriented comparison of gene expression measurements across different hybridization-based technologies. *Nat Biotechnol*, 24(7), 832-40.

Kurokawa, S., Ishibashi, H., Hayashida, K., Tsuchiya, Y., Hirata, Y., Sakaki, Y., Okubo, H. & Niho, Y. (1987). Kupffer cell stimulation of alpha 2-macroglobulin synthesis in rat hepatocytes and the role of glucocorticoid. *Cell Struct Funct*, 12(1), 35-42.

Kutty, R. K., Daniel, R. F., Ryan, D. E., Levin, W. & Maines, M. D. (1988). Rat liver cytochrome P-450b, P-420b, and P-420c are degraded to biliverdin by heme oxygenase. *Arch Biochem Biophys*, 260(2), 638-44.

LaBrecque, D. (1994). Liver regeneration: a picture emerges from the puzzle. *The American J Gastroenterol*, 89(8 Suppl), S86-96.

Laishes, B. A. & Williams, G. M. (1976). Conditions affecting primary cell cultures of functional adult rat hepatocytes. 1. The effect of insulin. *In Vitro*, 12(7), 521-32.

Landry, J., Bernier, D., Ouellet, C., Goyette, R. & Marceau, N. (1985). Spheroidal aggregate culture of rat liver cells: histotypic reorganization, biomatrix deposition, and maintenance of functional activities. *J Cell Biol*, 101(3), 914-23.

Larson, A. M., Polson, J., Fontana, R. J., Davern, T. J., Lalani, E., Hynan, L. S., Reisch, J. S., Schiødt, F. V., Ostapowicz, G., Shakil, A. O., Lee, W. M.; Acute Liver Failure Study

# 6 REFERENCES

Group., (2005). Acetaminophen-induced acute liver failure: results of a United States multicenter, prospective study. *Hepatology.* 2005 Dec;42(6):1364-72.

Latruffe, N., Passilly, P., Jannin, B., Motojima, K., Cherkaoui Malki, M., Schohn, H., Clemencet, M. C., Boscoboinik, D. & Dauça, M. (2000). Relationship between signal transduction and PPAR alpha-regulated genes of lipid metabolism in rat hepatic-derived Fao cells. *Cell Biochem Biophys, 32 (Spring),* 213-20.

Lawyer, F. C., Stoffel, S., Saiki, R. K., Chang, S. Y., Landre, P. A., Abramson, R. D. & Gelfand, D. H. (1993). High-level expression, purification, and enzymatic characterization of full-length Thermus aquaticus DNA polymerase and a truncated form deficient in 5' to 3' exonuclease activity. *PCR Methods Appl, 2*(4), 275-87.

LeCluyse, E. L., Ahlgren-Beckendorf, J. A., Carroll, K., Parkinson, A. & Johnson, J. (2000). Regulation of glutathione S-transferase enzymes in primary cultures of rat hepatocytes maintained under various matrix configurations. *Toxicol in vitro, 14*(2), 101-15.

LeCluyse, E. L., Audus, K. L. & Hochman, J. H. (1994). Formation of extensive canalicular networks by rat hepatocytes cultured in collagen-sandwich configuration. *Am J Physiol, 266*(6 Pt 1), C1764-74.

LeCluyse, E. L., Fix, J. A., Audus, K. L. & Hochman, J. H. (2000). Regeneration and maintenance of bile canalicular networks in collagen-sandwiched hepatocytes. *Toxicol in vitro, 14*(2), 117-32.

LeCluyse, E., Madan, A., Hamilton, G., Carroll, K., DeHaan, R. & Parkinson, A. (2000). Expression and regulation of cytochrome P450 enzymes in primary cultures of human hepatocytes. *J Biochem Mol Toxicol, 14*(4), 177-88.

LeCluyse, E. L., Alexandre, E., Hamilton, G. A., Viollon-Abadie, C., Coon, D. J., Jolley, S. & Richert, L. (2005). Isolation and culture of primary human hepatocytes. *Methods Mol Biol, 290,* 207-29.

LeCluyse, E., Bullock, P., Madan, A., Carroll, K. & Parkinson, A. (1999). Influence of extracellular matrix overlay and medium formulation on the induction of cytochrome P-450 2B enzymes in primary cultures of rat hepatocytes. *Drug Metab Dispos, 27*(8), 909-15.

Lee, W. M. (2003). Drug-induced hepatotoxicity. *N Engl J Medl, 349*(5), 474-85.

Lerche-Langr, C. & Toutain, H. J. (2000). Precision-cut liver slices: characteristics and use for in vitro pharmaco-toxicology. *Toxicology, 153*(1-3), 221-253.

Lesko, L. J. & Woodcock, J. (2004). Translation of pharmacogenomics and pharmacogenetics: a regulatory perspective. *Nat Rev Drug Discov, 3*(9), 763-9.

Lettieri, T. (2006). Recent applications of DNA microarray technology to toxicology and ecotoxicology. *Environ Health Perspect, 114*(1), 4-9.

# 6 REFERENCES

Lewis, J. H. (2002). Drug-induced liver disease. *Curr Opin Gastroenterol 18*(3), 307-13.

Li, J., Pankratz, M. & Johnson, J. A. (2002). Differential gene expression patterns revealed by oligonucleotide versus long cDNA arrays. *Toxicol Sci, 69*(2), 383-90.

Li, W., Liang, X., Leu, J. I., Kovalovich, K., Ciliberto, G. & Taub, R. (2001). Global changes in interleukin-6-dependent gene expression patterns in mouse livers after partial hepatectomy. *Hepatology, 33*(6), 1377-86.

Linke, K., Schanz, J., Hansmann, J., Walles, T., Brunner, H. & Mertsching, H. (2007). Engineered liver-like tissue on a capillarized matrix for applied research. *Tissue Eng, 13*(11), 2699-707.

Liu, X., Brouwer, K. L., Gan, L. S., Brouwer, K. R., Stieger, B., Meier, P. J., Audus, K. L. & LeCluyse, E. L. (1998). Partial maintenance of taurocholate uptake by adult rat hepatocytes cultured in a collagen sandwich configuration. *Pharm Res, 15*(10), 1533-9.

Liu, X., Chism, J. P., LeCluyse, E. L., Brouwer, K. R. & Brouwer, K. L. (1999). Correlation of biliary excretion in sandwich-cultured rat hepatocytes and in vivo in rats. *Drug Metab Dispos, 27*(6), 637-44.

Lloyd, S., Hayden, M. J., Sakai, Y., Fackett, A., Silber, P. M., Hewitt, N. J. & Li, A. P. (2002). Differential in vitro hepatotoxicity of troglitazone and rosiglitazone among cryopreserved human hepatocytes from 37 donors. *Chem Biol Interact, 142*(1-2), 57-71.

Lottaz, C., Yang, X., Scheid, S. & Spang, R. (2006). OrderedList--a bioconductor package for detecting similarity in ordered gene lists. *Bioinformatics, 22*(18), 2315-6.

de Longueville, F., Atienzar, F. A., Marcq, L., Dufrane, S., Evrard, S., Wouters, L., Leroux, F., Bertholet, V., Gerin, B., Whomsley, R., Arnould, T., Remacle, J. & Canning, M. (2003). Use of a low-density microarray for studying gene expression patterns induced by hepatotoxicants on primary cultures of rat hepatocytes. *Toxicol Sci, 75*(2), 378-92.

Loyer, P., Ilyin, G., Cariou, S., Glaise, D., Corlu, A. & Guguen-Guillouzo, C. (1996). Progression through G1 and S phases of adult rat hepatocytes. *Prog Cell Cycle Res, 2*, 37-47.

Lu, H., Chua, K., Zhang, P., Lim, W., Ramakrishna, S., Leong, K. W. & Mao, H. Q. (2005). Three-dimensional co-culture of rat hepatocyte spheroids and NIH/3T3 fibroblasts enhances hepatocyte functional maintenance. *Acta Biomater, 1*(4), 399-410.

Lupp, A., Danz, M. & Müller, D. (2001). Morphology and cytochrome P450 isoforms expression in precision-cut rat liver slices. *Toxicology, 161*(1-2), 53-66.

Luttringer, O., Theil, F. P., Lavé, T., Wernli-Kuratli, K., Guentert, T. W. & de Saizieu, A. (2002). Influence of isolation procedure, extracellular matrix and dexamethasone on the

# 6 REFERENCES

regulation of membrane transporters gene expression in rat hepatocytes. *Biochem Pharmacol*, *64*(11), 1637-50.

Lyu, J. & Joo, C. (2005). Wnt-7a up-regulates matrix metalloproteinase-12 expression and promotes cell proliferation in corneal epithelial cells during wound healing. *J Biol Chem*, 280(22), 21653-60.

Mah, N., Thelin, A., Lu, T., Nikolaus, S., Kühbacher, T., Gurbuz, Y., Eickhoff, H., Klöppel, G., Lehrach, H., Mellgård, B., Costello, C. M. & Schreiber, S. (2004). A comparison of oligonucleotide and cDNA-based microarray systems. *Physiol Genomics*, *16*(3), 361-70.

Makowski, P. & Pikuła, S. (1997). Participation of the multispecific organic anion transporter in hepatobiliary excretion of glutathione S-conjugates, drugs and other xenobiotics. *Pol J Pharmacol*, *49*(6), 387-94.

Marquardt, H. & Schäfer, S. G. (2004). *Lehrbuch der Toxikologie*. (2nd ed.). Wissenschaftliche Verlagsgesellschaft, Stuttgart.

Marquardt, H., Schafer, S. G., McClellan, R. & Welch, F., (1999), Toxicology, Academic Press, NY.

Matsumoto, T. & Kawakami, M. (1982). The unit-concept of hepatic parenchyma-a re-examination based on angioarchitectural studies. *Acta Pathol Jpn*, *32 Suppl 2*, 285-314.

Mattes, W. B., Pettit, S. D., Sansone, S., Bushel, P. R. & Waters, M. D. (2004). Database development in toxicogenomics: issues and efforts. *Environ Health Perspect*, *112*(4), 495-505.

Mayer, M. M. (1984). Complement. Historical perspectives and some current issues. *Complement*, *1*(1), 2-26.

McGall, G. H. & Fidanza, J. A. (2001). Photolithographic synthesis of high-density oligonucleotide arrays. *Methods Mol Biol*, *170*, 71-101.

McKee, E. E., Ferguson, M., Bentley, A. T. & Marks, T. A. (2006). Inhibition of Mammalian Mitochondrial Protein Synthesis by Oxazolidinones. *Antimicrob Agents Chemother*, *50*(6), 2042–2049.

Merrick, B. A. & Madenspacher, J. H. (2005). Complementary gene and protein expression studies and integrative approaches in toxicogenomics. *Toxicol Appl Pharmacol*, *207*(2 Suppl), 189-94.

Milani, S., Herbst, H., Schuppan, D., Hahn, E. G. & Stein, H. (1989). In situ hybridization for procollagen types I, III and IV mRNA in normal and fibrotic rat liver: evidence for predominant expression in nonparenchymal liver cells. *Hepatology*, *10*(1), 84-92.

Mingoia, R. T., Nabb, D. L., Yang, C. & Han, X. (2007). Primary culture of rat hepatocytes in 96-well plates: effects of extracellular matrix configuration on cytochrome P450 enzyme

# 6 REFERENCES

activity and inducibility, and its application in in vitro cytotoxicity screening. *Toxicol In Vitro*, 21(1), 165-73.

Miranti, C. K. (2002). Application of cell adhesion to study signaling networks. *Methods Cell Biol*, 69, 359-83.

Mitchell, J. R., Jollow, D. J., Gillette, J. R. & Brodie, B. B. (1973). Drug metabolism as a cause of drug toxicity. *Drug Metab Dispos*, 1(1), 418-23.

Mohammed, F. F., Pennington, C. J., Kassiri, Z., Rubin, J. S., Soloway, P. D., Ruther, U., Edwards, D. R. & Khokha, R. (2005). Metalloproteinase inhibitor TIMP-1 affects hepatocyte cell cycle via HGF activation in murine liver regeneration. *Hepatology*, 41(4), 857-867.

Monro, A. M. (1990). Interspecies comparisons in toxicology: the utility and futility of plasma concentrations of the test substance. *Regul Toxicol Pharmacol*, 12(2), 137-60.

Montoudis, A., Seidman, E., Boudreau, F., Beaulieu, J., Menard, D., Elchebly, M., Mailhot, G., Sane, A. T., Lambert, M., Delvin, E. & Levy, E. (2008). Intestinal fatty acid binding protein regulates mitochondrion beta-oxidation and cholesterol uptake. *J Lipid Res*, 49(5), 961-72.

Müller, D., Glöckner, R., Rost, M. & Steinmetzer, P. (1998). Monooxygenation, cytochrome P450-mRNA expression and other functions in precision-cut rat liver slices. *Exp Toxicol Pathol*, 50(4-6), 507-13.

Müller, A. S. & Pallauf, J. (2003). Effect of increasing selenite concentrations, vitamin E supplementation and different fetal calf serum content on GPx1 activity in primary cultured rabbit hepatocytes. *J Trace Elem Med Biol*, 17(3), 183-92.

Musat, A. I., Sattler, C. A., Sattler, G. L. & Pitot, H. C. (1993). Reestablishment of cell polarity of rat hepatocytes in primary culture. *Hepatology*, 18(1), 198-205.

Mutschler, E., Geisslinger, G., Kroemer, H. K., Ruth, P. & Schäfer-Korting, M. (2008). *Arzneimittelwirkungen: Mit einführenden Kapiteln in die Anatomie, Physiologie und Pathophysiologie* (9th ed.). Wissenschaftliche Verlagsgesellschaft, Stuttgart.

Nagy, P., Kiss, A., Schnur, J. & Thorgeirsson, S. S. (2003). Dexamethasone inhibits the proliferation of hepatocytes and oval cells but not bile duct cells in rat liver. *Hepatology*. 28(2):423-9.

Nielsen, T. L., Rasmussen, B. B., Flinois, J., Beaune, P. & Brosen, K. (1999). In Vitro Metabolism of Quinidine: The (3S)-3-Hydroxylation of Quinidine Is a Specific Marker Reaction for Cytochrome P-4503A4 Activity in Human Liver Microsomes. *J Pharmacol Exp Ther*, 289(1), 31-37.

# 6 REFERENCES

Nieminen, A. (2003). Apoptosis and necrosis in health and disease: role of mitochondria. *Int Rev Cytol*, *224*, 29-55.

Nikkilä, J., Törönen, P., Kaski, S., Venna, J., Castrén, E. & Wong, G. (2002). Analysis and visualization of gene expression data using self-organizing maps. *Neural Netw*, *15*(8-9), 953-66.

Nuwaysir, E. F., Bittner, M., Trent, J., Barrett, J. C. & Afshari, C. A. (1999). Microarrays and toxicology: the advent of toxicogenomics. *Mol Carcinog*, *24*(3), 153-9.

O'Brien, P. J., Chan, K. & Silber, P. M. (2004). Human and animal hepatocytes in vitro with extrapolation in vivo. *Chem Biol Interact*, *150*(1), 97-114.

Ohta, Y., Kongo, M., Sasaki, E. & Harada, N. (1999). Change in hepatic antioxidant defense system with liver injury development in rats with a single naphthylisothiocyanate intoxication. *Toxicology*, *139*(3), 265-75.

Ogata, I., Mochida, S., Tomiya, T. & Fujiwara, K. (1991). Minor contribution of hepatocytes to collagen production in normal and early fibrotic rat livers. *Hepatology*, *14*(2), 361-7.

Ogata, K., Ohno, R., Terao, K., Iwasaki, K. & Endo, Y. (2000). Some properties and the possible role of intrinsic ATPase of rat liver 80S ribosomes in peptide bond elongation. *J Biochem*, *127*(2), 221-31.

Ohira, H., Abe, K., Yokokawa, J., Takiguchi, J., Rai, T., Shishido, S. & Sato, Y. (2003). Adhesion molecules and CXC chemokines in endotoxin-induced liver injury. *Fukushima J Med Sci*, *49*(1), 1-13.

Olson, H., Betton, G., Robinson, D., Thomas, K., Monro, A., Kolaja, G., Lilly, P., Sanders, J., Sipes, G., Bracken, W., Dorato, M., Van Deun, K., Smith, P., Berger, B. & Heller, A. (2000). Concordance of the toxicity of pharmaceuticals in humans and in animals. *Regul Toxicol Pharmacol*, *32*(1), 56-67.

Olson, H., Betton, G., Stritar, J. & Robinson, D. (1998). The predictivity of the toxicity of pharmaceuticals in humans from animal data- an interim assessment. *Toxicol Lett*, *102-103*, 535-8.

Orphanides, G. (2003). Toxicogenomics: challenges and opportunities. *Toxicol Lett*, *140-141*, 145-8.

Oude Elferink, R. P., Meijer, D. K., Kuipers, F., Jansen, P. L., Groen, A. K. & Groothuis, G. M. (1995). Hepatobiliary secretion of organic compounds; molecular mechanisms of membrane transport. *Biochim Biophys Acta*, *1241*(2), 215-68.

Page, J. L., Johnson, M. C., Olsavsky, K. M., Strom, S. C., Zarbl, H. & Omiecinski, C. J. (2007). Gene Expression Profiling of Extracellular Matrix as an Effector of Human Hepatocyte Phenotype in Primary Cell Culture. *Toxicol. Sci*, *97*(2), 384-397.

# 6 REFERENCES

Paine, A. J. & Andreakos, E. (2004). Activation of signalling pathways during hepatocyte isolation: relevance to Toxicol in vitro. *Toxicol In Vitro*, *18*(2), 187-93.

Papeleu, P., Vanhaecke, T., Henkens, T., Elaut, G., Vinken, M., Snykers, S. & Rogiers, V. (2006). Isolation of rat hepatocytes. *Methods Mol Biol*, *320*, 229-37.

Parent, R. & Beretta, L. (2008). Translational control plays a prominent role in the hepatocytic differentiation of HepaRG liver progenitor cells. *Genome Biol*, *9*(1), R19.

Parent, R., Marion, M., Furio, L., Trépo, C. & Petit, M. (2004). Origin and characterization of a human bipotent liver progenitor cell line. *Gastroenterology*, *126*(4), 1147-56.

Parrish, M. L., Wei, N., Duenwald, S., Tokiwa, G. Y., Wang, Y., Holder, D., Dai, H., Zhang, X., Wright, C., Hodor, P., Cavet, G., Phillips, R. L., Sun, B. I. & Fare, T. L. (2004). A microarray platform comparison for neuroscience applications. *J Neurosci Methods*, *132*(1), 57-68.

Pascussi, J. M., Gerbal-Chaloin, S., Fabre, J. M., Maurel, P. & Vilarem, M. J. (2000). Dexamethasone enhances constitutive androstane receptor expression in human hepatocytes: consequences on cytochrome P450 gene regulation. *Mol Pharmacol*, *58*(6), 1441-50.

Pennie, W. D. (2000). Use of cDNA microarrays to probe and understand the toxicological consequences of altered gene expression. *Toxicol Lett*, *112-113*, 473-7.

Pennie, W. D., Tugwood, J. D., Oliver, G. J. & Kimber, I. (2000). The principles and practice of toxicogenomics: applications and opportunities. *Toxicol Sci*, *54*(2), 277-83.

Pfaffl, M. W. (2001). A new mathematical model for relative quantification in real-time RT-PCR. *Nucleic Acids Res*, *29*(9), e45.

Pham, R. T., Barber, D. S., & Gallagher, E. P., (2004). GSTA is a major glutathione S-transferase gene responsible for 4-hydroxynonenal conjugation in largemouth bass liver. Mar Environ Res, 58 (2-5), 485-488.

Pi, L., Ding, X., Jorgensen, M., Pan, J., Oh, S., Pintilie, D., Brown, A., Song, W. Y. & Petersen, B. E. (2008). Connective tissue growth factor with a novel fibronectin binding site promotes cell adhesion and migration during rat oval cell activation. *Hepatology*, *47*(3), 996-1004.

Pontoglio, M., Pausa, M., Doyen, A., Viollet, B., Yaniv, M. & Tedesco, F. (2001). Hepatocyte nuclear factor 1alpha controls the expression of terminal complement genes. *J Exp Med*, *194*(11), 1683-9.

Powers, M. J., Domansky, K., Kaazempur-Mofrad, M. R., Kalezi, A., Capitano, A., Upadhyaya, A., Upadhyaya, A., Kurzawski, P., Wack, K. E., Stolz, D. B., Kamm, R. &

# 6 REFERENCES

Griffith, L. G. (2002). A microfabricated array bioreactor for perfused 3 d liver culture. *Biotechnol Bioeng, 78*(3), 257-69.

Prada, A. E., Zahedi, K. & Davis, A. E. (1998). Regulation of C1 inhibitor synthesis. *Immunobiology, 199*(2), 377-88.

Püschel, G. P. & Jungermann, K. (1994). Integration of function in the hepatic acinus: intercellular communication in neural and humoral control of liver metabolism. *Prog Liver Dis, 12*, 19-46.

Pusztai, L. (2006). Chips to Bedside: Incorporation of Microarray Data into Clinical Practice. *Clin Cancer Res, 12*(24), 7209-7214.

Radisavljevic, Z. M. & González-Flecha, B. (2004). TOR kinase and ran are downstream from PI3K/Akt in $H_2O_2$-induced mitosis. *J Cell Biochem, 91*(6), 1293-1300.

Ramadori, G. & Armbrust, T. (2001). Cytokines in the liver. *Eur J Gastroenterol Hepatol, 13*(7), 777-84.

Rannug, A., Alexandrie, A. K., Persson, I. & Ingelman-Sundberg, M. (1995). Genetic polymorphism of cytochromes P450 1A1, 2 d6 and 2E1: regulation and toxicological significance. *J occup environ med, 37*(1), 25-36.

Raudys, S. (2000). How good are support vector machines? *Neural Netw, 13*(1), 17-9.

Reid, L. M., Fiorino, A. S., Sigal, S. H., Brill, S. & Holst, P. A. (1992). Extracellular matrix gradients in the space of Disse: relevance to liver biology. *Hepatology, 15*(6), 1198-203.

Rialland, L., Guyomard, C., Scotte, M., Chesné, C. & Guillouzo, A. (2000). Viability and drug metabolism capacity of alginate-entrapped hepatocytes after cryopreservation. *Cell Biol Toxicol, 16*(2), 105-16.

Richert, L., Alexandre, E., Lloyd, T., Orr, S., Viollon-Abadie, C., Patel, R., Kingston, S., Berry, D., Dennison, A., Heyd, B., Mantion, G. & Jaeck, D. (2004). Tissue collection, transport and isolation procedures required to optimize human hepatocyte isolation from waste liver surgical resections. A multilaboratory study. *Liver Int, 24*(4), 371-8.

Richert, L., Binda, D., Hamilton, G., Viollon-Abadie, C., Alexandre, E., Bigot-Lasserre, D., Bars, R., Coassolo, P. & LeCluyse, E. (2002). Evaluation of the effect of culture configuration on morphology, survival time, antioxidant status and metabolic capacities of cultured rat hepatocytes. *Toxicol in vitro, 16*(1), 89-99.

Richert, L., Liguori, M. J., Abadie, C., Heyd, B., Mantion, G., Halkic, N. & Waring, J. F. (2006). Gene expression in human hepatocytes in suspension after isolation is similar to the liver of origin, is not affected by hepatocyte cold storage and cryopreservation, but is strongly changed after hepatocyte plating. *Drug Metab Dispos, 34*(5), 870-9.

# 6 REFERENCES

Rodríguez-Antona, C., Donato, M. T., Boobis, A., Edwards, R. J., Watts, P. S., Castell, J. V. & Gómez-Lechón, M. J. (2002). Cytochrome P450 expression in human hepatocytes and hepatoma cell lines: molecular mechanisms that determine lower expression in cultured cells. *Xenobiotica, 32*(6), 505-20.

Rogiers, V. & Vercruysse, A. (1998). Hepatocyte cultures in drug metabolism and toxicological research and testing. *Methods Mol Biol, 107*, 279-94.

Roter, A. H. (2005). Large-scale integrated databases supporting drug discovery. *Curr Opin Drug Discov Devel, 8*(3), 309-15.

Ruepp, S., Boess, F., Suter, L., de Vera, M. C., Steiner, G., Steele, T., Weiser, T. & Albertini, S. (2005). Assessment of hepatotoxic liabilities by transcript profiling. *Toxicol Appl Pharmacol, 207*(2 Suppl), 161-70.

Russell, W. & Burch, R. (1959). *The Principles of Humane Experimental Technique*. Methuen, London.

Sadée, W., Wang, D. & Bilsky, E. J. (2005). Basal opioid receptor activity, neutral antagonists, and therapeutic opportunities. *Life Sci, 76*(13), 1427-1437.

Sadeque, A. J., Wandel, C., He, H., Shah, S. & Wood, A. J. (2000). Increased drug delivery to the brain by P-glycoprotein inhibition. *Clin Pharmacol Ther, 68*(3), 231-7.

Sahu, S. C. (2008). *Hepatotoxicity: From Genomics to in Vitro and in Vivo Models* (1st ed., p. 704). Wiley & Sons, West Sussex.

Sakai, M. & Muramatsu, M. (2007). Regulation of GST-P gene expression during hepatocarcinogenesis. *Methods Enzymol, 401*, 42-61.

Sampath, H. & Ntambi, J. M. (2004). Polyunsaturated fatty acid regulation of gene expression. *Nutr Rev, 62*(9), 333-9.

Schena, M. (1996). Genome analysis with gene expression microarrays. *Bioessays, 18*(5), 427-31.

Scholz, G., Pohl, I., Genschow, E., Klemm, M. & Spielmann, H. (1999). Embryotoxicity screening using embryonic stem cells in vitro: correlation to in vivo teratogenicity. *Cells Tissues Organs, 165*(3-4), 203-11.

Schoonen, W. G. E. J., Westerink, W. M. A., de Roos, J. A. D. M. & Débiton, E. (2005). Cytotoxic effects of 100 reference compounds on Hep G2 and HeLa cells and of 60 compounds on ECC-1 and CHO cells I. Mechanistic assays on ROS, glutathione depletion and calcein uptake. *Toxicol in vitro, 19*(4), 505-16.

Schuetz, E. G., Li, D., Omiecinski, C. J., Muller-Eberhard, U., Kleinman, H. K., Elswick, B. & Guzelian, P. S. (1988). Regulation of gene expression in adult rat hepatocytes cultured on a basement membrane matrix. *J Cell Physiol, 134*(3), 309-23.

# 6 REFERENCES

Schuster, D., Laggner, C. & Langer, T. (2005). Why drugs fail- a study on side effects in new chemical entities. *Curr Pharm Des, 11*(27), 3545-59.

Scoazec, J. Y. & Feldmann, G. (1994). The cell adhesion molecules of hepatic sinusoidal endothelial cells. *J Hepatol, 20*(2), 296-300.

Seglen, P. O. (1976). Preparation of isolated rat liver cells. *Methods Cell Biol, 13*, 29-83.

Sell, S. (2001).The role of progenitor cells in repair of liver injury and in liver transplantation. *Wound Repair Regen, 9*(6), 467-82.

Shi, L., Reid, L. H., Jones, W. D., Shippy, R., Warrington, J. A., Baker, S. C., Collins, P. J., de Longueville, F., Kawasaki, E. S., Lee, K. Y., Luo, Y., Sun, Y. A., Willey, J.C., Setterquist, R.A., Fischer, G. M., Tong, W., Dragan, Y. P., Dix, D. J., Frueh, F. W., Goodsaid, F. M., Herman, D., Jensen, R. V., Johnson, C. D., Lobenhofer, E. K., Puri, R. K., Schrf, U., Thierry-Mieg, J., Wang, C., Wilson, M., Wolber, P. K., Zhang, L., Amur, S., Bao, W., Barbacioru, C. C., Lucas, A. B., Bertholet, V., Boysen, C., Bromley, B., Brown, D., Brunner, A., Canales, R., Cao, X. M., Cebula, T. A., Chen, J. J., Cheng, J., Chu, T. M., Chudin, E., Corson, J., Corton, J. C., Croner, L. J., Davies, C., Davison, T. S., Delenstarr, G., Deng, X., Dorris, D., Eklund, A. C., Fan, X. H., Fang, H., Fulmer-Smentek, S., Fuscoe, J. C., Gallagher, K., Ge, W., Guo, L., Guo, X., Hager, J., Haje, P. K., Han, J., Han, T., Harbottle, H. C., Harris, S. C., Hatchwell, E., Hauser, C. A., Hester, S., Hong, H., Hurban, P., Jackson, S. A., Ji, H., Knight, C. R., Kuo, W. P., LeClerc, J. E., Levy, S., Li, Q. Z., Liu, C., Liu, Y., Lombardi, M. J., Ma, Y., Magnuson, S. R., Maqsodi, B., McDaniel, T., Mei, N., Myklebost, O., Ning, B., Novoradovskaya, N., Orr, M. S., Osborn, T. W., Papallo, A., Patterson, T. A., Perkins, R. G., Peters, E. H., Peterson, R., Philips, K. L., Pine, P. S., Pusztai, L., Qian, F., Ren, H., Rosen, M., Rosenzweig, B. A., Samaha, R. R., Schena, M., Schroth G. P., Shchegrova, S., Smith, D. D., Staedtler, F., Su, Z., Sun, H., Szallasi, Z., Tezak, Z., Thierry-Mieg, D., Thompson, K. L., Tikhonova, I., Turpaz, Y., Vallanat, B., Van, C., Walker, S. J., Wang, S. J., Wang, Y., Wolfinger, R., Wong, A., Wu, J., Xiao, C., Xie, Q., Xu, J., Yang, W., Zhang, L., Zhong, S., Zong, Y. & Slikker, W. Jr. (2006). The MicroArray Quality Control (MAQC) project shows inter- and intraplatform reproducibility of gene expression measurements. *Nat Biotechnol, 24*(9), 1151-61.

Shull, J., Spady, T., Snyder, M., Johansson, S. & Pennington, K. (1997). Ovary-intact, but not ovariectomized female ACI rats treated with 17beta-estradiol rapidly develop mammary carcinoma. *Carcinogenesis, 18*(8), 1595-1601.

Sidhu, J. S., Liu, F. & Omiecinski, C. J. (2004). Phenobarbital responsiveness as a uniquely sensitive indicator of hepatocyte differentiation status: requirement of

# 6 REFERENCES

dexamethasone and extracellular matrix in establishing the functional integrity of cultured primary rat hepatocytes. *Exp Cell Res*, 292(2), 252-64.

Sidhu, J. S. & Omiecinski, C. J. (1995). Modulation of xenobiotic-inducible cytochrome P450 gene expression by dexamethasone in primary rat hepatocytes. *Pharmacogenetics*, 5(1), 24-36.

Siegenthaler, Blum, (2006). *Klinische Pathophysiologie*. p. 860, Georg Thieme Verlag KG, Stuttgart.

Sigal, S. H., Rajvanshi, P., Gorla, G. R., Sokhi, R. P., Saxena, R., Gebhard, D. R., Reid, L. M. & Gupta, S. (1999). Partial hepatectomy-induced polyploidy attenuates hepatocyte replication and activates cell aging events. *Am J Physiol*, 276(5 Pt 1), G1260-72.

Simon, R., Radmacher, M. D., Dobbin, K. & McShane, L. M. (2003). Pitfalls in the use of DNA microarray data for diagnostic and prognostic classification. *J Natl Cancer Inst*, 95(1), 14-8.

Sivaraman, A., Leach, J. K., Townsend, S., Iida, T., Hogan, B. J., Stolz, D. B., Fry, R., Samson, L. D., Tannenbaum, S. R. & Griffith, L. G. (2005). A microscale in vitro physiological model of the liver: predictive screens for drug metabolism and enzyme induction. *Curr Drug Metab*, 6(6), 569-91.

Skett, P. & Bayliss, M. (1996). Time for a consistent approach to preparing and culturing hepatocytes? *Xenobiotica*, 26(1), 1-7.

Sladek, F. M. (1994). Orphan receptor HNF-4 and liver-specific gene expression. *Receptor*, 4(1), 64.

Slaughter, M. R., Thakkar, H. & O'Brien, P. J. (2002). Effect of diquat on the antioxidant system and cell growth in human neuroblastoma cells. *Toxicol Appl Pharmacol*, 178(2), 63-70.

Smith, R. D. (2000). Probing proteomes--seeing the whole picture? *Nat Biotechnol*, 18(10), 1041-2.

Southern, E. M. (1975). Detection of specific sequences among DNA fragments separated by gel electrophoresis. *J Mol Biol*, 98(3), 503-17.

Stafford, P. & Brun, M. (2007). Three methods for optimization of cross-laboratory and cross-platform microarray expression data. *Nucleic Acids Res*, 35(10), e72.

Stapp, J. M., Sjoelund, V., Lassiter, H. A., Feldhoff, R. C. & Feldhoff, P. W. (2005). Recombinant rat IL-1beta and IL-6 synergistically enhance C3 mRNA levels and complement component C3 secretion by H-35 rat hepatoma cells. *Cytokine*, 30(2), 78-85.

# 6 REFERENCES

Strey, C. W., Markiewski, M., Mastellos, D., Tudoran, R., Spruce, L. A., Greenbaum, L. E. & Lambris, J. D. (2003). The proinflammatory mediators C3a and C5a are essential for liver regeneration. *J Exp Med*, *198*(6), 913-23.

Stubberfield, C. R. & Page, M. J. (1999). Applying proteomics to drug discovery. *Expert Opin Investig Drugs*, *8*(1), 65-70.

Stupack, D. G. (2007). The biology of integrins. *Oncology (Williston Park)*, *21*(9 Suppl 3), 6-12.

Suter, L., Babiss, L. E. & Wheeldon, E. B. (2004). Toxicogenomics in predictive toxicology in drug development. *Chem Biol*, *11*(2), 161-71.

Suzuki, H., Inoue, T., Matsushita, T., Kobayashi, K., Horii, I., Hirabayashi, Y. & Inoue, T. (2008). In vitro gene expression analysis of hepatotoxic drugs in rat primary hepatocytes. *J Appl Toxicol*, *28*(2), 227-36.

Talamini, M. A., Kappus, B. & Hubbard, A. (1997). Repolarization of hepatocytes in culture. *Hepatology*, *25*(1), 167-72.

Terry, T. L. & Gallin, W. J. (1994). Effects of fetal calf serum and disruption of cadherin function on the formation of bile canaliculi between hepatocytes. *Exp Cell Res*, *214*(2), 642-53.

Thedinga, E., Ullrich, A., Drechsler, S., Niendorf, R., Kob, A., Runge, D., Keuer, A., Freund, I., Lehmann, M. & Ehret, R. (2007). In vitro system for the prediction of hepatotoxic effects in primary hepatocytes. *ALTEX*, *24*(1), 22-34.

Tian, H., Ou, J., Strom, S. C. & Venkataramanan, R. (2005). Activity and expression of various isoforms of uridine diphosphate glucuronosyltransferase are differentially regulated during hepatic regeneration in rats. *Pharm Res*, *22*(12), 2007-15.

Tirona, R. G. & Kim, R. B. (2005). Nuclear receptors and drug disposition gene regulation. *J Pharm Sci*, *94*(6), 1169-1186.

Tonge, R. P., Kelly, E. J., Bruschi, S. A., Kalhorn, T., Eaton, D. L., Nebert, D. W. & Nelson, S. D. (1998). Role of CYP1A2 in the hepatotoxicity of acetaminophen: investigations using Cyp1a2 null mice. *Toxicol Appl Pharmacol*, *153*(1), 102-8.

Tsutsui, H., Adachi, K., Seki, E. & Nakanishi, K. (2003). Cytokine-induced inflammatory liver injuries. *Curr Mol Med*, *3*(6), 545-59.

Turncliff, R. Z., Meier, P. J. & Brouwer, K. L. R. (2004). Effect of dexamethasone treatment on the expression and function of transport proteins in sandwich-cultured rat hepatocytes. *Drug Metab Dispos*, *32*(8), 834-9.

# 6 REFERENCES

Turncliff, R. Z., Tian, X. & Brouwer, K. L. R. (2006). Effect of culture conditions on the expression and function of Bsep, Mrp2, and Mdr1a/b in sandwich-cultured rat hepatocytes. *Biochem Pharmacol*, *71*(10), 1520-9.

Tuschl, G. & Müller, S. O. (2006). Effects of cell culture conditions on primary rat hepatocytes-cell morphology and differential gene expression. *Toxicology*, *218*(2-3), 205-15.

Ulrich, R. G., Bacon, J. A., Cramer, C. T., Peng, G. W., Petrella, D. K., Stryd, R. P. & Sun, E. L. (1995). Cultured hepatocytes as investigational models for hepatic toxicity: practical applications in drug discovery and development. *Toxicol Lett*, *82-83*, 107-15.

Ulrich, R. G. (2003). The toxicogenomics of nuclear receptor agonists. *Curr Opin Chem Biol* 7, 505-10.

Ullrich, A., Berg, C., Hengstler, J. G. & Runge, D. (2007). Use of a standardised and validated long-term human hepatocyte culture system for repetitive analyses of drugs: repeated administrations of acetaminophen reduces albumin and urea secretion. *ALTEX*, *24*(1), 35-40.

Vanhaecke, T., Elaut, G. & Rogiers, V. (2001). Effect of oxygen concentration on the expression of glutathione S-transferase activity in periportal and perivenous rat hepatocyte cultures. *Toxicol in vitro*, *15*(4-5), 387-92.

Veenstra, T. D. & Conrads, T. P. (2003). Serum protein fingerprinting. *Curr Opin Mol Ther*, *5*(6), 584-93.

Viebahn, C. S. & Yeoh, G. C. T. (2008). What fires prometheus? The link between inflammation and regeneration following chronic liver injury. *Int J Biochem Cell Biol*, *40*(5), 855-73.

Vinken, M., Elaut, G., Henkens, T., Papeleu, P., Snykers, S., Vanhaecke, T. & Rogiers, V. (2006). Rat hepatocyte cultures: collagen gel sandwich and immobilization cultures. *Methods Mol Biol*, *320*, 247-54.

Wakabayashi, Y., Kipp, H. & Arias, I. M. (2006). Transporters on demand: intracellular reservoirs and cycling of bile canalicular ABC transporters. *J Biol Chem, 281*(38), 27669-73.

Warburg, O. (1923). Versuche an überlebendem Karzinomgewebe. *Biochem Z*, (142), 317-333.

Waring, J. F., Jolly, R. A., Ciurlionis, R., Lum, P. Y., Praestgaard, J. T., Morfitt, D. C., Buratto, B., Roberts, C., Schadt, E. & Ulrich, R. G. (2001). Clustering of hepatotoxins based on mechanism of toxicity using gene expression profiles. *Toxicol Appl Pharmacol, 175*(1), 28-42.

# 6 REFERENCES

Waxman, D. J. (1999). P450 gene induction by structurally diverse xenochemicals: central role of nuclear receptors CAR, PXR, and PPAR. *Arch Biochem Biophys*, *369*(1), 11-23.

Westerink, W. M. A. & Schoonen, W. G. E. J. (2007). Cytochrome P450 enzyme levels in HepG2 cells and cryopreserved primary human hepatocytes and their induction in HepG2 cells. *Toxicol In Vitro*, *21*(8), 1581-91.

Westphal, J. F., Vetter, D. & Brogard, J. M. (1994). Hepatic side-effects of antibiotics. *J Antimicrob Chemother*, *33*(3), 387-401.

Wetmore, B. A. & Merrick, B. A. (2004) Toxicoproteomics: proteomics applied to toxicology and pathology. *Toxicol Pathol*, *32*(6), 619-42.

Wettschureck, N. & Offermanns, S. (2005). Mammalian G proteins and their cell type specific functions. *Physiol Rev*, *85*(4), 1159-204.

Widmann, J. J., Cotran, R. S. & Fahimi, H. D. (1972). Mononuclear phagocytes (Kupffer cells) and endothelial cells. Identification of two functional cell types in rat liver sinusoids by endogenous peroxidase activity. *J Cell Biol*, *52*(1), 159-70.

Wilkening, S., Stahl, F. & Bader, A. (2003). Comparison of primary human hepatocytes and hepatoma cell line Hepg2 with regard to their biotransformation properties. *Drug Metab Dispos*, *31*(8), 1035-42.

Wilkinson, R. C. & Dickson, A. J. (2001). Expression of CCAAT/enhancer binding protein family genes in monolayer and sandwich culture of hepatocytes: induction of stress-inducible GADD153. *Biochem Biophys Res Commun*, *289*(5), 942-9.

Williams, G. M., Bermudez, E. & Scaramuzzino, D. (1977). Rat hepatocyte primary cell cultures III. Improved dissociation and attachment techniques and the enhancement of survival by culture medium. *In vitro*, *13*(12), 809-17.

Winwood, P. J. & Arthur, M. J. (1993). Kupffer cells: their activation and role in animal models of liver injury and human liver disease. *Semin Liver Dis*, *13*(1), 50-9.

Wisse, E. (1977a). Ultrastructure and function of Kupffer cells and other sinusoidal cells in the liver. *Med Chir Dig*, *6*(7), 409-18.

Wisse, E. (1977b). On the endothelial cells of rat liver sinusoids. *Bibliotheca anatomica*, (16 Pt 2), 373-6.

Wolfrum, C., Borrmann, C. M., Borchers, T. & Spener, F. (2001). Fatty acids and hypolipidemic drugs regulate peroxisome proliferator-activated receptors alpha - and gamma-mediated gene expression via liver fatty acid binding protein: a signaling path to the nucleus. *Proc Natl Acad Sci U S A*, *98*(5), 2323-8.

Wolfrum, C. & Spener, F. (2000). Fatty acids as regulators of lipid metabolism. *Eur J Lipid Sci Technol*, *102*(12), 746-62.

# 6 REFERENCES

Woolfson, A. M. (1983). Amino acids--their role as an energy source. *Proc Nutr Soc, 42*(3), 489-95.

Wrighton, S. A. & Stevens, J. C. (1992). The human hepatic cytochromes P450 involved in drug metabolism. *Crit Rev Toxicol, 22*(1), 1-21.

Wunder, C. & Potter, R. F. (2003). The heme oxygenase system: its role in liver inflammation. *Curr Drug Targets Cardiovasc Haematol Disord, 3*(3), 199-208.

Wysowski, D. K. & Swartz, L. (2005). Adverse Drug Event Surveillance and Drug Withdrawals in the United States, 1969-2002: The Importance of Reporting Suspected Reactions. *Arch Intern Med, 165*(12), 1363-69.

Xu, C., Li, C. Y. & Kong, A. T. (2005). Induction of phase 1, II and III drug metabolism/transport by xenobiotics. *Arch Pharm Res, 28*(3), 249-68.

Xu, J. J., Diaz, D. & O'Brien, P. J. (2004). Applications of cytotoxicity assays and pre-lethal mechanistic assays for assessment of human hepatotoxicity potential. *Chem Biol Interact, 150*(1), 115-28.

Yamada, S., Otto, P. S., Kennedy, D. L. & Whayne, T. F. (1980). The effects of dexamethasone on metabolic activity of hepatocytes in primary monolayer culture. *In Vitro, 16*(7), 559-70.

Yamazaki, M., Suzuki, H. & Sugiyama, Y. (1996). Recent advances in carrier-mediated hepatic uptake and biliary excretion of xenobiotics. *Pharm Res, 13*(4), 497-513.

Yan, Z. & Caldwell, G. W. (2001). Metabolism profiling, and cytochrome P450 inhibition & induction in drug discovery. *Curr Top Med Chem, 1*(5), 403-25.

Yeung, K. Y. & Ruzzo, W. L. (2001). Principal component analysis for clustering gene expression data. *Bioinformatics, 17*(9), 763-74.

Yin, H., Kim, M., Kim, J., Kong, G., Lee, M., Kang, K., Yoon, B. I., Kim, H. L. & Lee, B. H. (2006). Hepatic Gene Expression Profiling and Lipid Homeostasis in Mice Exposed to Steatogenic Drug, Tetracycline. *Toxicol Sci, 94*, 206-16.

You, L. (2004). Steroid hormone biotransformation and xenobiotic induction of hepatic steroid metabolizing enzymes. *Chem Biol Interact, 147*(3), 233-46.

Zaher, H., Buters, J. T., Ward, J. M., Bruno, M. K., Lucas, A. M., Stern, S. T., Cohen, S. D. & Gonzalez, F. J. (1998). Protection against acetaminophen toxicity in CYP1A2 and CYP2E1 double-null mice. *Toxicol Appl Pharmacol, 152*(1), 193-9.

Zidek, N., Hellmann, J., Kramer, P. & Hewitt, P. G. (2007). Acute hepatotoxicity: a predictive model based on focused illumina microarrays. *Toxicol Sci, 99*(1), 289-302.

Zvibel, I., Smets, F. & Soriano, H. (2002). Anoikis: roadblock to cell transplantation? *Cell Transplant, 11*(7), 621-30.

# APPENDIX

# APPENDIX

Appendix 1: Results of the one sided tests comparing gene lists ranked by p Value.

Settings

| | |
|---|---|
| List comparison | |
| Assessing similarity of | top ranks |
| Length of lists | 7263 |
| Quantile of invariant genes | 0.5 |
| Number of random samples | 1000 |

**Affymetrix_In vivo, high dose_24h  vs.  Illumina_In vivo, high dose_24h**

| | Genes | Scores | p.values | Rev.Scores | Rev.p.values |
|---|---|---|---|---|---|
| 0.115 | 100 | 3.396578 | 0.021 | 0.00E+00 | 0.942 |
| 0.077 | 150 | 12.872106 | 0 | 0.00E+00 | 0.999 |
| 0.058 | 200 | 29.560405 | 0 | 2.55E-04 | 1 |
| 0.038 | 300 | 87.649945 | 0 | 2.17E-02 | 1 |
| 0.029 | 400 | 183.980918 | 0 | 1.72E-01 | 1 |
| 0.023 | 500 | 324.038894 | 0 | 6.33E-01 | 1 |
| 0.015 | 750 | 891.757136 | 0 | 4.39E+00 | 1 |
| 0.012 | 1000 | 1806.952651 | 0 | 1.45E+01 | 1 |
| 0.008 | 1500 | 4819.958101 | 0 | 7.07E+01 | 1 |
| 0.006 | 2000 | 9604.577392 | 0 | 2.09E+02 | 1 |
| 0.005 | 2500 | 16356.67251 | 0 | 4.71E+02 | 1 |

**Affymetrix_In vivo, high dose_6 h  vs.  Illumina_In vivo, high dose_6 h**

| | Genes | Scores | p.values | Rev.Scores | Rev.p.values |
|---|---|---|---|---|---|
| 0.115 | 100 | 4.496039 | 0.012 | 0.00E+00 | 0.95 |
| 0.077 | 150 | 16.355067 | 0 | 0.00E+00 | 0.998 |
| 0.058 | 200 | 36.734735 | 0 | 0.00E+00 | 1 |
| 0.038 | 300 | 105.510524 | 0 | 5.53E-04 | 1 |
| 0.029 | 400 | 215.222581 | 0 | 1.41E-02 | 1 |
| 0.023 | 500 | 369.287354 | 0 | 9.00E-02 | 1 |
| 0.015 | 750 | 966.487184 | 0 | 1.39E+00 | 1 |
| 0.012 | 1000 | 1895.079548 | 0 | 7.04E+00 | 1 |
| 0.008 | 1500 | 4853.82513 | 0 | 5.12E+01 | 1 |
| 0.006 | 2000 | 9419.988236 | 0 | 1.76E+02 | 1 |
| 0.005 | 2500 | 15740.11764 | 0 | 4.28E+02 | 1 |

# APPENDIX

**Affymetrix_In vivo, high dose_72 h  vs.  Illumina_In vivo, high dose_72 h**

|  | Genes | Scores | p.values | Rev.Scores | Rev.p.values |
|---|---|---|---|---|---|
| 0.115 | 100 | 0.0820066 | 0.394 | 0.00E+00 | 0.936 |
| 0.077 | 150 | 0.9049201 | 0.351 | 0.00E+00 | 0.998 |
| 0.058 | 200 | 3.5427757 | 0.288 | 1.45E-03 | 0.999 |
| 0.038 | 300 | 17.8166802 | 0.16 | 9.41E-02 | 1 |
| 0.029 | 400 | 48.203631 | 0.058 | 7.56E-01 | 1 |
| 0.023 | 500 | 97.9639087 | 0.02 | 2.88E+00 | 1 |
| 0.015 | 750 | 319.699483 | 0 | 2.12E+01 | 1 |
| 0.012 | 1000 | 697.2417988 | 0 | 6.92E+01 | 1 |
| 0.008 | 1500 | 1994.939427 | 0 | 3.06E+02 | 1 |
| 0.006 | 2000 | 4137.290714 | 0 | 8.25E+02 | 1 |
| 0.005 | 2500 | 7258.68298 | 0 | 1.75E+03 | 1 |

**Affymetrix_In vivo, low dose_24h  vs.  Illumina_In vivo, low dose_24h**

|  | Genes | Scores | p.values | Rev.Scores | Rev.p.values |
|---|---|---|---|---|---|
| 0.115 | 100 | 1.991168 | 0.057 | 2.09E-04 | 0.888 |
| 0.077 | 150 | 6.969976 | 0.041 | 1.57E-02 | 0.902 |
| 0.058 | 200 | 15.638143 | 0.018 | 1.37E-01 | 0.91 |
| 0.038 | 300 | 45.759576 | 0 | 1.43E+00 | 0.919 |
| 0.029 | 400 | 95.184211 | 0 | 5.27E+00 | 0.946 |
| 0.023 | 500 | 166.214749 | 0 | 1.24E+01 | 0.976 |
| 0.015 | 750 | 451.538273 | 0 | 4.61E+01 | 0.999 |
| 0.012 | 1000 | 913.753175 | 0 | 1.06E+02 | 1 |
| 0.008 | 1500 | 2469.962063 | 0 | 3.34E+02 | 1 |
| 0.006 | 2000 | 5014.659594 | 0 | 7.77E+02 | 1 |
| 0.005 | 2500 | 8703.099602 | 0 | 1.52E+03 | 1 |

**Affymetrix_In vivo, low dose_6 h  vs.  Illumina_In vivo, low dose_6 h**

|  | Genes | Scores | p.values | Rev.Scores | Rev.p.values |
|---|---|---|---|---|---|
| 0.115 | 100 | 7.283426 | 0.006 | 0 | 0.955 |
| 0.077 | 150 | 19.243393 | 0 | 0 | 1 |
| 0.058 | 200 | 36.969171 | 0 | 0.00001 | 1 |
| 0.038 | 300 | 92.427889 | 0 | 0.01222236 | 1 |
| 0.029 | 400 | 180.357296 | 0 | 0.12293679 | 1 |
| 0.023 | 500 | 306.936003 | 0 | 0.55805418 | 1 |
| 0.015 | 750 | 822.530248 | 0 | 5.62455642 | 1 |
| 0.012 | 1000 | 1662.852982 | 0 | 22.7816052 | 1 |
| 0.008 | 1500 | 4442.275855 | 0 | 126.114992 | 1 |
| 0.006 | 2000 | 8804.673908 | 0 | 371.034203 | 1 |
| 0.005 | 2500 | 14842.6007 | 0 | 814.456991 | 1 |

# APPENDIX

**Affymetrix_In vivo, low dose_72 h  vs.  Illumina_In vivo, low dose_72 h**

|       | Genes | Scores      | p.values | Rev.Scores | Rev.p.values |
|-------|-------|-------------|----------|------------|--------------|
| 0.115 | 100   | 0.6533219   | 0.148    | 1.02E-04   | 0.931        |
| 0.077 | 150   | 2.9582573   | 0.134    | 9.83E-03   | 0.945        |
| 0.058 | 200   | 6.9889852   | 0.122    | 8.04E-02   | 0.963        |
| 0.038 | 300   | 19.9385361  | 0.11     | 7.65E-01   | 0.977        |
| 0.029 | 400   | 40.3567281  | 0.106    | 2.73E+00   | 0.993        |
| 0.023 | 500   | 70.3485953  | 0.118    | 6.51E+00   | 1            |
| 0.015 | 750   | 201.443388  | 0.15     | 2.79E+01   | 1            |
| 0.012 | 1000  | 436.0229586 | 0.188    | 7.63E+01   | 1            |
| 0.008 | 1500  | 1310.829829 | 0.305    | 3.15E+02   | 1            |
| 0.006 | 2000  | 2856.292467 | 0.548    | 8.42E+02   | 1            |
| 0.005 | 2500  | 5208.756318 | 0.818    | 1.77E+03   | 1            |

**Affymetrix_Tet_in vitro, 200µM_24h  vs.  Illumina_Tet_in vitro, 200µM_24h**

|       | Genes | Scores      | p.values | Rev.Scores | Rev.p.values |
|-------|-------|-------------|----------|------------|--------------|
| 0.115 | 100   | 5.486148    | 0.009    | 0.00E+00   | 0.935        |
| 0.077 | 150   | 19.204741   | 0        | 0.00E+00   | 0.999        |
| 0.058 | 200   | 42.889678   | 0        | 2.55E-04   | 1            |
| 0.038 | 300   | 125.232997  | 0        | 2.22E-02   | 1            |
| 0.029 | 400   | 260.821096  | 0        | 1.85E-01   | 1            |
| 0.023 | 500   | 454.645129  | 0        | 7.13E-01   | 1            |
| 0.015 | 750   | 1213.559971 | 0        | 5.37E+00   | 1            |
| 0.012 | 1000  | 2392.390421 | 0        | 1.81E+01   | 1            |
| 0.008 | 1500  | 6122.928476 | 0        | 8.29E+01   | 1            |
| 0.006 | 2000  | 11833.59296 | 0        | 2.21E+02   | 1            |
| 0.005 | 2500  | 19662.67078 | 0        | 4.58E+02   | 1            |

**Affymetrix_Tet_in vitro, 200µM_6 h  vs.  Illumina_Tet_in vitro, 200µM_6 h**

|       | Genes | Scores      | p.values | Rev.Scores | Rev.p.values |
|-------|-------|-------------|----------|------------|--------------|
| 0.115 | 100   | 1.48309     | 0.069    | 0.00E+00   | 0.928        |
| 0.077 | 150   | 7.153101    | 0.032    | 1.47E-03   | 0.981        |
| 0.058 | 200   | 18.694907   | 0.006    | 2.48E-02   | 0.985        |
| 0.038 | 300   | 62.205048   | 0        | 4.50E-01   | 0.988        |
| 0.029 | 400   | 135.584691  | 0        | 2.20E+00   | 0.998        |
| 0.023 | 500   | 241.308089  | 0        | 6.24E+00   | 0.999        |
| 0.015 | 750   | 659.85671   | 0        | 3.12E+01   | 1            |
| 0.012 | 1000  | 1318.54695  | 0        | 8.42E+01   | 1            |
| 0.008 | 1500  | 3440.196261 | 0        | 3.09E+02   | 1            |
| 0.006 | 2000  | 6749.990373 | 0        | 7.60E+02   | 1            |
| 0.005 | 2500  | 11362.82429 | 0        | 1.54E+03   | 1            |

# APPENDIX

**Affymetrix_Tet_in vitro, 200µM_72 h    vs.    Illumina_Tet_in vitro, 200µM_72 h**

|       | Genes | Scores   | p.values | Rev.Scores | Rev.p.values |
|-------|-------|----------|----------|------------|--------------|
| 0.115 | 100   | 0.00E+00 | 0.953    | 3.29E-04   | 0.899        |
| 0.077 | 150   | 1.32E-03 | 0.994    | 1.71E-02   | 0.922        |
| 0.058 | 200   | 2.81E-02 | 0.994    | 1.24E-01   | 0.944        |
| 0.038 | 300   | 6.53E-01 | 0.992    | 1.07E+00   | 0.974        |
| 0.029 | 400   | 3.87E+00 | 0.99     | 3.64E+00   | 0.991        |
| 0.023 | 500   | 1.28E+01 | 0.986    | 8.33E+00   | 0.999        |
| 0.015 | 750   | 8.52E+01 | 0.948    | 3.16E+01   | 1            |
| 0.012 | 1000  | 2.76E+02 | 0.856    | 7.53E+01   | 1            |
| 0.008 | 1500  | 1.21E+03 | 0.491    | 2.49E+02   | 1            |
| 0.006 | 2000  | 3.17E+03 | 0.179    | 5.90E+02   | 1            |
| 0.005 | 2500  | 6.42E+03 | 0.054    | 1.16E+03   | 1            |

**Affymetrix_Tet_in vitro, 40µM_24h    vs.    Illumina_Tet_in vitro, 40µM_24h**

|       | Genes | Scores     | p.values | Rev.Scores | Rev.p.values |
|-------|-------|------------|----------|------------|--------------|
| 0.115 | 100   | 2.385667   | 0.054    | 4.10E-02   | 0.504        |
| 0.077 | 150   | 7.646565   | 0.027    | 3.67E-01   | 0.525        |
| 0.058 | 200   | 16.499255  | 0.008    | 1.20E+00   | 0.572        |
| 0.038 | 300   | 47.125522  | 0        | 4.46E+00   | 0.706        |
| 0.029 | 400   | 97.431035  | 0        | 9.62E+00   | 0.851        |
| 0.023 | 500   | 169.010198 | 0        | 1.66E+01   | 0.942        |
| 0.015 | 750   | 449.565631 | 0        | 4.36E+01   | 0.999        |
| 0.012 | 1000  | 897.035527 | 0        | 9.09E+01   | 1            |
| 0.008 | 1500  | 2417.73594 | 0        | 2.92E+02   | 1            |
| 0.006 | 2000  | 4950.564876| 0        | 7.23E+02   | 1            |
| 0.005 | 2500  | 8652.718524| 0        | 1.49E+03   | 1            |

**Affymetrix_Tet_in vitro, 40µM_6 h    vs.    Illumina_Tet_in vitro, 40µM_6 h**

|       | Genes | Scores      | p.values | Rev.Scores | Rev.p.values |
|-------|-------|-------------|----------|------------|--------------|
| 0.115 | 100   | 1.54447     | 0.07     | 1.64E-02   | 0.588        |
| 0.077 | 150   | 5.855951    | 0.052    | 2.09E-01   | 0.628        |
| 0.058 | 200   | 12.736524   | 0.035    | 8.40E-01   | 0.665        |
| 0.038 | 300   | 32.172252   | 0.02     | 4.06E+00   | 0.74         |
| 0.029 | 400   | 57.293263   | 0.031    | 1.04E+01   | 0.822        |
| 0.023 | 500   | 87.786004   | 0.049    | 2.05E+01   | 0.893        |
| 0.015 | 750   | 196.205276  | 0.163    | 6.66E+01   | 0.982        |
| 0.012 | 1000  | 375.311426  | 0.415    | 1.53E+02   | 1            |
| 0.008 | 1500  | 1069.383307 | 0.771    | 5.04E+02   | 1            |
| 0.006 | 2000  | 2385.423526 | 0.939    | 1.18E+03   | 1            |
| 0.005 | 2500  | 4494.577654 | 0.997    | 2.31E+03   | 1            |

# APPENDIX

**Affymetrix_Tet_in vitro, 40µM_72 h    vs.   Illumina_Tet_in vitro, 40µM_72 h**

|  | Genes | Scores | p.values | Rev.Scores | Rev.p.values |
|---|---|---|---|---|---|
| 0.115 | 100 | 0.2532672 | 0.257 | 3.25E-02 | 0.527 |
| 0.077 | 150 | 1.4725369 | 0.249 | 3.15E-01 | 0.563 |
| 0.058 | 200 | 4.2493281 | 0.236 | 1.06E+00 | 0.609 |
| 0.038 | 300 | 16.3431309 | 0.184 | 4.06E+00 | 0.745 |
| 0.029 | 400 | 40.0437893 | 0.134 | 8.79E+00 | 0.866 |
| 0.023 | 500 | 78.6345881 | 0.089 | 1.52E+01 | 0.956 |
| 0.015 | 750 | 258.6040214 | 0.032 | 4.22E+01 | 1 |
| 0.012 | 1000 | 584.9951258 | 0.01 | 9.56E+01 | 1 |
| 0.008 | 1500 | 1780.971792 | 0.002 | 3.34E+02 | 1 |
| 0.006 | 2000 | 3846.553298 | 0.003 | 8.34E+02 | 1 |
| 0.005 | 2500 | 6931.927263 | 0.007 | 1.70E+03 | 1 |

Appendix 2: Results of the two sided tests comparing gene lists ranked by score.

Settings

List comparison

Assessing similarity of    : top and bottom ranks

Length of lists           : 7263

Quantile of invariant genes : 0.5

Number of random samples   : 1000

**Affymetrix_In vivo, high dose_24h  vs.  Illumina_In vivo, high dose_24h**

|  | Genes | Scores | p.values | Rev.Scores | Rev.p.values |
|---|---|---|---|---|---|
| 0.115 | 100 | 49.55621 | 0 | 0.00E+00 | 0.997 |
| 0.077 | 150 | 111.19045 | 0 | 0.00E+00 | 1 |
| 0.058 | 200 | 197.40218 | 0 | 0.00E+00 | 1 |
| 0.038 | 300 | 450.91057 | 0 | 1.65E-04 | 1 |
| 0.029 | 400 | 823.02235 | 0 | 8.51E-03 | 1 |
| 0.023 | 500 | 1322.53258 | 0 | 5.84E-02 | 1 |
| 0.015 | 750 | 3165.93227 | 0 | 8.55E-01 | 1 |
| 0.012 | 1000 | 5908.00598 | 0 | 3.74E+00 | 1 |
| 0.008 | 1500 | 14271.93084 | 0 | 2.11E+01 | 1 |
| 0.006 | 2000 | 26729.61978 | 0 | 6.50E+01 | 1 |
| 0.005 | 2500 | 43541.83669 | 0 | 1.59E+02 | 1 |

# APPENDIX

**Affymetrix_In vivo, high dose_6 h vs. Illumina_In vivo, high dose_6 h**

|        | Genes | Scores      | p.values | Rev.Scores | Rev.p.values |
|--------|-------|-------------|----------|------------|--------------|
| 0.115  | 100   | 54.99712    | 0        | 0.00E+00   | 0.996        |
| 0.077  | 150   | 129.93003   | 0        | 0.00E+00   | 1            |
| 0.058  | 200   | 236.95433   | 0        | 0.00E+00   | 1            |
| 0.038  | 300   | 547.40588   | 0        | 3.00E-03   | 1            |
| 0.029  | 400   | 989.25309   | 0        | 4.92E-02   | 1            |
| 0.023  | 500   | 1566.37151  | 0        | 2.62E-01   | 1            |
| 0.015  | 750   | 3621.70696  | 0        | 2.78E+00   | 1            |
| 0.012  | 1000  | 6586.25333  | 0        | 1.03E+01   | 1            |
| 0.008  | 1500  | 15395.64479 | 0        | 4.79E+01   | 1            |
| 0.006  | 2000  | 28266.90455 | 0        | 1.29E+02   | 1            |
| 0.005  | 2500  | 45425.74841 | 0        | 2.82E+02   | 1            |

**Affymetrix_In vivo, high dose_72 h vs. Illumina_In vivo, high dose_72 h**

|        | Genes | Scores      | p.values | Rev.Scores | Rev.p.values |
|--------|-------|-------------|----------|------------|--------------|
| 0.115  | 100   | 29.60283    | 0        | 0.00E+00   | 0.997        |
| 0.077  | 150   | 66.67136    | 0        | 5.59E-03   | 1            |
| 0.058  | 200   | 116.08303   | 0        | 7.25E-02   | 1            |
| 0.038  | 300   | 251.04498   | 0        | 1.14E+00   | 1            |
| 0.029  | 400   | 436.85835   | 0        | 5.47E+00   | 1            |
| 0.023  | 500   | 677.59694   | 0        | 1.59E+01   | 1            |
| 0.015  | 750   | 1542.033    | 0        | 8.53E+01   | 1            |
| 0.012  | 1000  | 2816.62934  | 0        | 2.41E+02   | 1            |
| 0.008  | 1500  | 6748.06413  | 0        | 8.96E+02   | 1            |
| 0.006  | 2000  | 12749.18053 | 0        | 2.13E+03   | 1            |
| 0.005  | 2500  | 21071.31965 | 0        | 4.07E+03   | 1            |

**Affymetrix_In vivo, low dose_24h vs. Illumina_In vivo, low dose_24h**

|        | Genes | Scores      | p.values | Rev.Scores | Rev.p.values |
|--------|-------|-------------|----------|------------|--------------|
| 0.115  | 100   | 38.01436    | 0        | 0.00E+00   | 0.997        |
| 0.077  | 150   | 82.74386    | 0        | 0.00E+00   | 1            |
| 0.058  | 200   | 145.71855   | 0        | 1.52E-03   | 1            |
| 0.038  | 300   | 328.20886   | 0        | 6.04E-02   | 1            |
| 0.029  | 400   | 588.14631   | 0        | 4.20E-01   | 1            |
| 0.023  | 500   | 928.80845   | 0        | 1.48E+00   | 1            |
| 0.015  | 750   | 2162.53377  | 0        | 9.97E+00   | 1            |
| 0.012  | 1000  | 3998.17757  | 0        | 3.17E+01   | 1            |
| 0.008  | 1500  | 9708.97803  | 0        | 1.43E+02   | 1            |
| 0.006  | 2000  | 18443.33018 | 0        | 4.10E+02   | 1            |
| 0.005  | 2500  | 30493.33326 | 0        | 9.33E+02   | 1            |

# APPENDIX

## Affymetrix_In vivo, low dose_6 h vs. Illumina_In vivo, low dose_6 h

|       | Genes | Scores    | p.values | Rev.Scores | Rev.p.values |
|-------|-------|-----------|----------|------------|--------------|
| 0.115 | 100   | 35.45322  | 0        | 0.00E+00   | 0.997        |
| 0.077 | 150   | 79.64536  | 0        | 0.00E+00   | 1            |
| 0.058 | 200   | 147.2389  | 0        | 0.00E+00   | 1            |
| 0.038 | 300   | 363.52957 | 0        | 2.47E-03   | 1            |
| 0.029 | 400   | 696.20846 | 0        | 4.67E-02   | 1            |
| 0.023 | 500   | 1150.19933| 0        | 2.74E-01   | 1            |
| 0.015 | 750   | 2835.18092| 0        | 3.57E+00   | 1            |
| 0.012 | 1000  | 5332.80084| 0        | 1.56E+01   | 1            |
| 0.008 | 1500  | 12882.55084| 0       | 9.08E+01   | 1            |
| 0.006 | 2000  | 24036.39917| 0       | 2.73E+02   | 1            |
| 0.005 | 2500  | 39035.32004| 0       | 6.14E+02   | 1            |

## Affymetrix_In vivo, low dose_72 h vs. Illumina_In vivo, low dose_72 h

|       | Genes | Scores     | p.values | Rev.Scores | Rev.p.values |
|-------|-------|------------|----------|------------|--------------|
| 0.115 | 100   | 2.976163   | 0.055    | 0.00E+00   | 0.998        |
| 0.077 | 150   | 13.061734  | 0.007    | 2.96E-03   | 1            |
| 0.058 | 200   | 32.230139  | 0.001    | 4.58E-02   | 1            |
| 0.038 | 300   | 99.511169  | 0        | 7.66E-01   | 1            |
| 0.029 | 400   | 205.774151 | 0        | 3.63E+00   | 1            |
| 0.023 | 500   | 351.213881 | 0        | 1.02E+01   | 1            |
| 0.015 | 750   | 891.186768 | 0        | 5.26E+01   | 1            |
| 0.012 | 1000  | 1705.079388| 0        | 1.49E+02   | 1            |
| 0.008 | 1500  | 4329.08781 | 0        | 6.02E+02   | 1            |
| 0.006 | 2000  | 8608.793868| 0        | 1.58E+03   | 1            |
| 0.005 | 2500  | 14905.12842| 0        | 3.31E+03   | 1            |

## Affymetrix_Tet_in vitro, 200µM_24h vs. Illumina_Tet_in vitro, 200µM_24h

|       | Genes | Scores     | p.values | Rev.Scores | Rev.p.values |
|-------|-------|------------|----------|------------|--------------|
| 0.115 | 100   | 22.58013   | 0        | 0.00E+00   | 0.996        |
| 0.077 | 150   | 60.57986   | 0        | 0.00E+00   | 1            |
| 0.058 | 200   | 120.59625  | 0        | 0.00E+00   | 1            |
| 0.038 | 300   | 314.46124  | 0        | 0.00E+00   | 1            |
| 0.029 | 400   | 616.46887  | 0        | 5.43E-04   | 1            |
| 0.023 | 500   | 1034.53955 | 0        | 1.10E-02   | 1            |
| 0.015 | 750   | 2619.72023 | 0        | 3.59E-01   | 1            |
| 0.012 | 1000  | 5028.59504 | 0        | 2.33E+00   | 1            |
| 0.008 | 1500  | 12577.73879| 0        | 1.99E+01   | 1            |
| 0.006 | 2000  | 24149.41609| 0        | 7.53E+01   | 1            |
| 0.005 | 2500  | 40096.48161| 0        | 2.03E+02   | 1            |

# APPENDIX

**Affymetrix_Tet_in vitro, 200µM_6 h vs. Illumina_Tet_in vitro, 200µM_6 h**

|        | Genes | Scores     | p.values | Rev.Scores | Rev.p.values |
|--------|-------|------------|----------|------------|--------------|
| 0.115  | 100   | 14.55154   | 0        | 0.4838354  | 0.315        |
| 0.077  | 150   | 35.10029   | 0        | 2.4942963  | 0.306        |
| 0.058  | 200   | 66.10476   | 0        | 6.397284   | 0.308        |
| 0.038  | 300   | 160.92214  | 0        | 19.4572677 | 0.387        |
| 0.029  | 400   | 302.45276  | 0        | 38.4889048 | 0.579        |
| 0.023  | 500   | 495.35045  | 0        | 62.8119617 | 0.798        |
| 0.015  | 750   | 1237.08209 | 0        | 146.950646 | 0.996        |
| 0.012  | 1000  | 2412.99373 | 0        | 269.555034 | 1            |
| 0.008  | 1500  | 6337.90474 | 0        | 670.206743 | 1            |
| 0.006  | 2000  | 12724.42496| 0        | 1363.97036 | 1            |
| 0.005  | 2500  | 21927.40605| 0        | 2470.59178 | 1            |

**Affymetrix_Tet_in vitro, 200µM_72 h vs. Illumina_Tet_in vitro, 200µM_72 h**

|        | Genes | Scores      | p.values | Rev.Scores | Rev.p.values |
|--------|-------|-------------|----------|------------|--------------|
| 0.115  | 100   | 16.85476    | 0        | 0.00E+00   | 0.998        |
| 0.077  | 150   | 46.75645    | 0        | 0.00E+00   | 1            |
| 0.058  | 200   | 95.6189     | 0        | 0.00E+00   | 1            |
| 0.038  | 300   | 253.80153   | 0        | 1.70E-03   | 1            |
| 0.029  | 400   | 498.04828   | 0        | 2.77E-02   | 1            |
| 0.023  | 500   | 835.2868    | 0        | 1.45E-01   | 1            |
| 0.015  | 750   | 2126.6926   | 0        | 1.47E+00   | 1            |
| 0.012  | 1000  | 4127.58671  | 0        | 5.50E+00   | 1            |
| 0.008  | 1500  | 10549.77083 | 0        | 3.23E+01   | 1            |
| 0.006  | 2000  | 20588.51822 | 0        | 1.22E+02   | 1            |
| 0.005  | 2500  | 34607.73555 | 0        | 3.43E+02   | 1            |

**Affymetrix_Tet_in vitro, 40µM_24h vs. Illumina_Tet_in vitro, 40µM_24h**

|        | Genes | Scores      | p.values | Rev.Scores | Rev.p.values |
|--------|-------|-------------|----------|------------|--------------|
| 0.115  | 100   | 1.016569    | 0.219    | 0.103141   | 0.617        |
| 0.077  | 150   | 5.186208    | 0.149    | 0.6876056  | 0.698        |
| 0.058  | 200   | 13.919643   | 0.085    | 1.983603   | 0.781        |
| 0.038  | 300   | 49.101183   | 0.021    | 7.0161555  | 0.924        |
| 0.029  | 400   | 114.181156  | 0.002    | 15.9344595 | 0.976        |
| 0.023  | 500   | 216.395932  | 0        | 29.8661677 | 0.997        |
| 0.015  | 750   | 677.855438  | 0        | 95.230228  | 1            |
| 0.012  | 1000  | 1506.573843 | 0        | 218.768469 | 1            |
| 0.008  | 1500  | 4573.798813 | 0        | 699.055785 | 1            |
| 0.006  | 2000  | 9930.830092 | 0        | 1584.58575 | 1            |
| 0.005  | 2500  | 17961.08234 | 0        | 3004.01755 | 1            |

# APPENDIX

**Affymetrix_Tet_in vitro, 40µM_6 h  vs.  Illumina_Tet_in vitro, 40µM_6 h**

|       | Genes | Scores      | p.values | Rev.Scores  | Rev.p.values |
|-------|-------|-------------|----------|-------------|--------------|
| 0.115 | 100   | 0.2559717   | 0.461    | 1.523661    | 0.148        |
| 0.077 | 150   | 1.6982916   | 0.443    | 5.871424    | 0.117        |
| 0.058 | 200   | 5.2381833   | 0.423    | 13.314133   | 0.089        |
| 0.038 | 300   | 21.1078175  | 0.385    | 36.409515   | 0.082        |
| 0.029 | 400   | 51.7865426  | 0.361    | 69.01333    | 0.118        |
| 0.023 | 500   | 100.3429219 | 0.357    | 111.300757  | 0.229        |
| 0.015 | 750   | 322.5465651 | 0.389    | 272.773391  | 0.659        |
| 0.012 | 1000  | 738.0425118 | 0.437    | 546.638554  | 0.934        |
| 0.008 | 1500  | 2368.086474 | 0.591    | 1589.41331  | 1            |
| 0.006 | 2000  | 5336.811315 | 0.838    | 3531.41974  | 1            |
| 0.005 | 2500  | 9905.492391 | 0.978    | 6631.43868  | 1            |

**Affymetrix_Tet_in vitro, 40µM_72 h  vs.  Illumina_Tet_in vitro, 40µM_72 h**

|       | Genes | Scores    | p.values | Rev.Scores | Rev.p.values |
|-------|-------|-----------|----------|------------|--------------|
| 0.115 | 100   | 8.16E-01  | 0.246    | 0.1634394  | 0.523        |
| 0.077 | 150   | 5.11E+00  | 0.132    | 0.9225119  | 0.584        |
| 0.058 | 200   | 1.56E+01  | 0.048    | 2.4006937  | 0.683        |
| 0.038 | 300   | 6.13E+01  | 0.004    | 7.3470961  | 0.881        |
| 0.029 | 400   | 1.47E+02  | 0        | 15.1555819 | 0.977        |
| 0.023 | 500   | 2.77E+02  | 0        | 26.5637358 | 0.997        |
| 0.015 | 750   | 8.23E+02  | 0        | 76.8447866 | 1            |
| 0.012 | 1000  | 1.73E+03  | 0        | 172.214448 | 1            |
| 0.008 | 1500  | 4.78E+03  | 0        | 588.618738 | 1            |
| 0.006 | 2000  | 9.79E+03  | 0        | 1472.45966 | 1            |
| 0.005 | 2500  | 1.71E+04  | 0        | 3013.93168 | 1            |

# APPENDIX

Appendix 3: Number of genes deregulated between different typers of primary rat hepatocyte culture. Shown are the results of an ANOVA concerning the effect of culture condition and the effect of time. Light grey means up regulated genes and the darker grey means down regulated genes.

| Culture condition | Nr. of genes deregulated between culture conditions | Nr. of genes deregulated over time of culture |
|---|---|---|
| Liver/FC | 336 | |
| | 693 | |
| Liver/FaO | 2178 | |
| | 1405 | |
| Liver Slices | 123 | 922 |
| | 178 | 610 |
| FC Susp. | 253 | 924 |
| | 267 | 1124 |
| FC/ML + FCS | 1320 | 463 |
| | 992 | 383 |
| FC/ML - FCS | 864 | 260 |
| | 722 | 204 |
| FC/SW + FCS | 910 | 235 |
| | 826 | 98 |
| FC/SW - FCS | 1199 | 105 |
| | 919 | 168 |

# APPENDIX

Appendix 4: Number of genes deregulated between time points of rat hepatocyte cultures were calculated with T-test statistics (<pV 0.01; >1.5fold). Light grey means up regulated genes and the darker grey means down regulated genes.

| Short term cultures | Nr. of genes deregulated | ML cultures | Nr. of genes deregulated | SW cultures | Nr. of genes deregulated |
|---|---|---|---|---|---|
| Liver/FC | 742 / 868 | FC/ML +FCS 1 d | 2099 / 1681 | FC/SW +FCS 1 d | 1650 / 1462 |
| Liver/FaO | 2828 / 2023 | ML +FCS 1 d/2 d | 143 / 137 | SW +FCS 1 d/2 d | 191 / 78 |
| Liver Slices | 452 / 622 | ML +FCS 1 d/4 d | 346 / 264 | SW +FCS 1 d/4 d | 396 / 260 |
| Slices 0 h/2 h | 248 / 54 | ML +FCS 1 d/6 d | 990 / 836 | SW +FCS 1 d/6 d | 512 / 328 |
| Slices 0 h/6 h | 885 / 939 | ML +FCS 1 d/10 d | 1218 / 1026 | SW +FCS 1 d/10 d | 590 / 448 |
| Slices 0 h/1 d | 887 / 661 | FC/ML -FCS 1 d | 1612 / 1413 | FC/SW -FCS 1 d | 1920 / 1701 |
| Slices 0 h/2 d | 988 / 794 | ML -FCS 1 d/2 d | 157 / 212 | SW -FCS 1 d/2 d | 242 / 175 |
| FC/Susp. 2 h | 613 / 778 | ML -FCS 1 d/4 d | 362 / 371 | SW -FCS 1 d/4 d | 389 / 275 |
| FC/Susp. 4h | 738 / 819 | ML -FCS 1 d/6 d | 546 / 485 | SW -FCS 1 d/6 d | 532 / 356 |
| FC/Susp. 6 h | 898 / 1063 | ML -FCS 1 d/10 d | 590 / 457 | SW -FCS 1 d/10 d | 684 / 373 |
| FC/Susp. 1 d | 1064 / 1385 | | | | |

APPENDIX

Appendix 5: List of rat genes measured with TaqMan PCR for the verification of the microarray experiments

| Gene Symbol | Gene name | Accession Nr. | Gene Symbol | Gene name | Accession Nr. |
|---|---|---|---|---|---|
| Acox1 | acyl-Coenzyme A oxidase 1, palmitoyl | NM_017340 | Hnf4a | hepatocyte nuclear factor 4, alpha | NM_022180 |
| Actn1 | actinin, alpha 1 | NM_031005 | Hspa1b | heat shock 70kDa protein 1A | NM_212504 |
| Adk | adenosine kinase | NM_012895 | Jund | jun D proto-oncogene | XM_579658 |
| Afp | alpha-fetoprotein | NM_012493 | Abcb1 | ATP-binding cassette, sub-family B (MDR/TAP), member 1 | NM_012623 |
| Nr1i3 | nuclear receptor subfamily 1, group I, member 3 | NM_022941 | Abcb4 | ATP-binding cassette, sub-family B (MDR/TAP), member 4 | NM_012690 |
| Cdh1 | cadherin 1, type 1, E-cadherin (epithelial) | NM_031334 | Abcc2 | ATP-binding cassette, sub-family C (CFTR/MRP), member 2 | XM_577883 |
| Cebpa | CCAAT/enhancer binding protein (C/EBP), alpha | NM_012524 | Abcc3 | ATP-binding cassette, sub-family C (CFTR/MRP), member 3 | NM_080581 |
| Cebpb | CCAAT/enhancer binding protein (C/EBP), beta | NM_024125 | Myc | v-myc myelocytomatosis viral oncogene homolog (avian) | NM_012603 |
| Cpt1a | carnitine palmitoyltransferase 1A (liver) | NM_031559 | Oatp1 | Slco1a1 solute carrier organic anion transporter family, member 1a1 | XM_579394 |
| Ccnd1 | cyclin D1 | NM_171992 | Cdkn1a | cyclin-dependent kinase inhibitor 1A (p21, Cip1) | NM_080782 |
| Ccng1 | cyclin G1 | NM_012923 | Pck1 | Phosphoenolpyruvate carboxykinase | NM_198780 |
| Cyp1a2 | cytochrome P450, family 1, subfamily A, polypeptide 2 | NM_012541 | Alpi | alkaline phosphatase, liver/bone/kidney | NM_022665 |
| Cyp2c | cytochrome P450, family 2, subfamily C, polypeptide 8 | NM_019184 | Nr1i2 | nuclear receptor subfamily 1, group I, member 2 | NM_052980 |
| Cyp3a3 | cytochrome P450, family 3, subfamily A, polypeptide 4 | NM_013105 | Rgn | regucalcin (senescence marker protein-30) | NM_031546 |

# APPENDIX

| Fabp2 | fatty acid binding protein 1, liver | NM_013068 | Sod2 | superoxide dismutase 2, mitochondrial | NM_017051 |
|---|---|---|---|---|---|
| Fbp1 | fructose-1,6-bisphosphatase 1 | NM_012558 | Tgfa | transforming growth factor, alpha | NM_012671 |
| Gadd45a | growth arrest and DNA-damage-inducible, alpha | NM_024127 | Tgfb1 | transforming growth factor, beta 1 (Camurati-Engelmann disease) | NM_021578 |
| Gsn | gelsolin (amyloidosis, Finnish type) | NM_001004080 | Timp1 | TIMP metallopeptidase inhibitor 1 | NM_053819 |
| Gsta3 | glutathione S-transferase A1 | NM_031509 | Tnf | tumor necrosis factor (TNF superfamily, member 2) | NM_012675 |
| Gstp2 | glutathione S-transferase pi | NM_138974 | Txn2 | thioredoxin | NM_053331 |
| Hmox1 | heme oxygenase (decycling) 1 | NM_012580 | Ugt1a1 | UDP glucuronosyltransferase 1 family, polypeptide A6 | NM_012683 |
| Tcf1 | transcription factor 1, hepatic; LF-B1, hepatic nuclear factor (HNF1), albumin proximal factor | NM_012669 | | | |

# APPENDIX

Appendix 6: List of rat genes measured with TaqMan PCR for the verification of the microarray experiments

| Gene Symbol | Gene name | Accession Nr. | Gene Symbol | Gene name | Accession Nr. |
|---|---|---|---|---|---|
| ACTN1 | actinin, alpha 1 | NM_001102 | TCF1 | transcription factor 1, hepatic; LF-B1, hepatic nuclear factor (HNF1) | NM_000545 |
| ADK | adenosine kinase | NM_001123 | HNF4A | hepatocyte nuclear factor 4, alpha | NM_000457 |
| AFP | alpha-fetoprotein | NM_001134 | JUND | jun D proto-oncogene | NM_005354 |
| ALPI | alkaline phosphatase, liver/bone/kidney | NM_000478 | ABCB1 | ATP-binding cassette, sub-family B (MDR/TAP), member 1 | NM_000927 |
| CEBPA | CCAAT/enhancer binding protein (C/EBP), alpha | NM_004364 | ABCB4 | ATP-binding cassette, sub-family B (MDR/TAP), member 4 | NM_000443 |
| CEBPB | CCAAT/enhancer binding protein (C/EBP), beta | NM_005194 | ABCC2 | ATP-binding cassette, sub-family C (CFTR/MRP), member 2 | NM_000392 |
| CPT1A | carnitine palmitoyltransferase 1A (liver) | NM_001031847 | ABCC3 | ATP-binding cassette, sub-family C (CFTR/MRP), member 3 | NM_003786 |
| CCND1 | cyclin D1 | NM_053056 | MYC | v-myc myelocytomatosis viral oncogene homolog | NM_002467 |
| CCNG1 | cyclin G1 | NM_004060 | CDKN1A | cyclin-dependent kinase inhibitor 1A (p21, Cip1) | NM_000389 |
| CYP1A2 | cytochrome P450, family 1, subfamily A, polypeptide 2 | NM_000761 | RGN | regucalcin (senescence marker protein-30) | NM_004683 |
| CDH1 | cadherin 1, type 1, E-cadherin (epithelial) | NM_004360 | SOD2 | superoxide dismutase 2, mitochondrial | NM_000636 |
| FABP2 | fatty acid binding protein 1, liver | NM_001443 | TGFA | transforming growth factor, alpha | NM_003236 |
| GADD45A | growth arrest and DNA-damage-inducible, alpha | NM_001924 | TGFB1 | transforming growth factor, beta 1 (Camurati-Engelmann disease) | NM_000660 |
| FBP1 | fructose-1,6-bisphosphatase 1 | NM_000507 | TXN2 | thioredoxin | NM_003329, BC054866 |
| GSN | gelsolin (amyloidosis, Finnish type) | NM_000177 | TIMP1 | TIMP metallopeptidase inhibitor 1 | NM_003254 |
| GSTA3 | glutathione S-transferase A1 | NM_145740 | TNF | tumor necrosis factor (TNF superfamily, member 2) | NM_000594 |
| HMOX1 | heme oxygenase (decycling) 1 | NM_002133 | UGT1A1 | UDP glucuronosyltransferase 1 family, polypeptide A6 | NM_001072 |

# APPENDIX

Appendix 7: Genes induced in expression after the perfusion of rat liver. Listed are only genes more than 2-fold deregulated and with a pV<0.01.

| Symbol | Accession | Fold change | Symbol | Accession | Fold change | Symbol | Accession | Fold change |
|---|---|---|---|---|---|---|---|---|
| Acy1 | XM_579142.1 | 2.0 | Jun | NM_021835.2 | 5.2 | Okl38 | NM_138504.2 | 2.6 |
| Adamts7_pred | XM_236471.3 | 2.5 | Junb | NM_021836.2 | 10.2 | Per2 | NM_031678.1 | 2.1 |
| Ankrd9_pred. | XM_576103.1 | 2.1 | LOC246266 | NM_144750.1 | 2.0 | Pex14 | NM_172063.1 | 2.2 |
| Anpep | NM_031012.1 | 2.4 | LOC287419 | XM_213367.3 | 2.0 | Phgdh | NM_031620.1 | 2.0 |
| Apba3 | NM_031781.1 | 2.1 | LOC287452 | XM_213357.3 | 2.1 | Pmvk | NM_001008352 | 2.0 |
| Atf3 | NM_012912.1 | 5.5 | LOC288659 | XM_213769.3 | 2.2 | Ppp1r10 | XM_579471.1 | 2.1 |
| Bat3 | NM_053609.1 | 2.3 | LOC290500 | XM_214256.3 | 2.6 | Ppp4c | XM_341929.2 | 2.1 |
| Besh3 | XM_346854.2 | 2.2 | LOC291905 | XM_214652.3 | 2.0 | Prodh2_pred. | XM_341825.2 | 2.5 |
| Bhlhb2 | NM_053328.1 | 6.1 | LOC293689 | XM_215181.3 | 2.1 | Ptges2_pred. | XM_231144.3 | 2.1 |
| Btd_pred. | XM_577477.1 | 2.1 | LOC296733 | XM_216063.3 | 2.1 | Ptov1 | NM_001008304 | 2.2 |
| Btg2 | NM_017259.1 | 12.0 | LOC297388 | XM_216181.2 | 2.2 | Rab11b | NM_032617.2 | 2.2 |
| Cbara1 | NM_199412.1 | 2.1 | LOC300043 | XM_216963.3 | 2.0 | RGD1305860_pred | XM_343183.2 | 2.3 |
| Ccs | NM_053425.1 | 2.0 | LOC303677 | XM_221119.3 | 2.0 | RGD1311324_pred | XM_343028.2 | 2.3 |
| Cd14 | NM_021744.1 | 2.1 | LOC310395 | XM_227134.3 | 2.7 | Rgs3 | NM_019340.1 | 2.2 |
| Cdc20 | NM_171993.1 | 2.0 | LOC310585 | XM_227366.3 | 2.0 | Rhob | NM_022542.1 | 2.3 |
| c-fos | XM_234422.3 | 5.0 | LOC360919 | XM_341193.2 | 2.2 | Ring1 | NM_212549.1 | 2.0 |
| Creb3l3_pred. | XM_576179.1 | 2.2 | LOC361184 | XM_341467.2 | 2.1 | Rps6ka1 | NM_031107.1 | 2.0 |
| Creld1_pred. | XM_232270.3 | 2.1 | LOC361523 | XM_341808.2 | 2.7 | Scarb1 | NM_031541.1 | 2.2 |
| Cry1 | NM_198750.1 | 2.4 | LOC362196 | XM_342497.2 | 4.6 | Scrn2_pred. | XM_573186.1 | 2.2 |
| Cxxc5 | NM_001007628 | 2.1 | LOC362287 | XM_342601.2 | 2.0 | Sds | NM_053962.2 | 2.4 |
| Cyp2t1 | NM_134369.1 | 2.2 | LOC362840 | XM_343168.2 | 2.4 | Sfrs9 | NM_001009255.1 | 2.0 |
| Cyr61 | NM_031327.2 | 3.1 | LOC362899 | XM_343227.2 | 2.5 | Slc13a3 | NM_022866.1 | 2.1 |
| Ddx56 | NM_001004211 | 2.3 | LOC362983 | XM_343313.2 | 2.0 | Slc16a11_pred. | XM_213334.3 | 2.7 |
| Dgkz | NM_031143.1 | 2.1 | LOC497733 | XM_579432.1 | 2.5 | Slc16a13 | NM_001005530.1 | 2.1 |
| Dhcr24_pred. | XM_216452.3 | 2.5 | LOC497875 | XM_573059.1 | 2.4 | Slc25a25 | NM_145677.1 | 2.8 |
| Dom3z | NM_212497.1 | 2.1 | LOC498703 | XM_573985.1 | 2.3 | Slc27a1 | NM_053580.2 | 2.2 |
| Dp1l1_pred. | XM_343163.2 | 2.4 | LOC499072 | XM_574354.1 | 2.2 | Slc29a1 | NM_031684.2 | 2.1 |
| Dusp1 | NM_053769.2 | 3.3 | LOC499823 | XM_575162.1 | 40.7 | Slc39a3 | NM_001008356.1 | 2.1 |
| Dusp5 | NM_133578.1 | 2.1 | LOC499837 | XM_580023.1 | 2.1 | Slc6a12 | NM_017335.1 | 2.3 |
| Egr1 | NM_012551.1 | 11.1 | LOC500019 | XM_575373.1 | 3.3 | Snf1lk | NM_021693.1 | 3.6 |
| Egr2 | NM_053633.1 | 2.1 | LOC502714 | XM_578213.1 | 2.7 | Soat2 | NM_153728.2 | 2.0 |
| Fam20a_pred. | XM_573215.1 | 2.1 | LOC503325 | XM_578859.1 | 4.1 | Socs2 | NM_058208.1 | 2.7 |
| Fgf21 | NM_130752.1 | 3.7 | Mafb | NM_019316.1 | 2.4 | Srebf1 | XM_213329.3 | 2.2 |
| Gadd45a | NM_024127.1 | 2.3 | Man2c1 | NM_139256.1 | 2.1 | Srm | NM_053464.1 | 2.3 |
| Gadd45g_pred | XM_237999.3 | 9.0 | Mbd6_pred. | XM_343219.2 | 2.0 | Srms_pred. | XM_575301.1 | 2.0 |
| Gdf15 | NM_019216.1 | 14.4 | Mclc | NM_133414.1 | 2.4 | Stard4_pred. | XM_214592.3 | 2.2 |
| Gfra3 | XM_341593.2 | 2.0 | Minpp1 | XM_342044.2 | 2.0 | Stub1_pred. | XM_213270.3 | 2.1 |
| Gpaa1 | NM_001004240 | 2.4 | Mtch1_pred. | XM_215358.3 | 2.3 | Tieg | NM_031135.1 | 2.1 |
| Grina | NM_153308.1 | 2.0 | Myc | NM_012603.2 | 3.2 | Tmem7_pred. | XM_236656.3 | 3.1 |
| Hes1 | NM_024360.2 | 2.7 | Myd116 | NM_133546.1 | 4.6 | Tomm40 | NM_212520.1 | 2.0 |
| Hspbp1 | NM_139261.1 | 2.0 | Napa | NM_080585.1 | 2.1 | Tst | NM_012808.1 | 2.4 |
| Ier2 | NM_001009541 | 4.8 | Nat8 | NM_022635.1 | 2.9 | Ube2m_pred. | XM_341790.2 | 2.4 |
| Igfals | NM_053329.1 | 3.2 | Ndufv3l | NM_022607.1 | 2.0 | Wbscr16_pred. | XM_341066.2 | 2.0 |
| Igfbp1 | NM_013144.1 | 5.3 | Nfil3 | NM_053727.2 | 2.2 | Zfp36 | NM_133290.2 | 4.0 |

# APPENDIX

Appendix 8: Genes reduced in expression after the perfusion of rat liver. Listed are only genes more than 2-fold deregulated and with a pV<0.01.

| Symbol | Accession | Fold change | Symbol | Accession | Fold change | Symbol | Accession | Fold change |
|---|---|---|---|---|---|---|---|---|
| Sept7 | NM_022616 | -2.4 | Cmkor1 | NM_053352 | -2.1 | Fcna | NM_031348 | -3.9 |
| 1200013a08rik | NM_001007002 | -2.1 | Col14a1_pred | XM_235308 | -8.1 | Fli1_pred | XM_235979 | -2.1 |
| Acadsb | NM_013084 | -2.7 | Col1a2 | NM_053356 | -13.8 | Folr2_pred | XM_215013 | -2.1 |
| Acsl4 | NM_053623 | -2.3 | Col3a1 | NM_032085 | -8.4 | Frg1_pred | XM_341442 | -2.0 |
| Adamts1 | NM_024400 | -3.4 | Col4a1_pred | XM_214400 | -2.4 | Fstl1 | NM_024369 | -5.3 |
| Adamts9_pred | XM_232202 | -2.1 | Col5a1 | NM_134452 | -2.6 | Gbp2 | NM_133624 | -3.6 |
| Adcy4 | NM_019285 | -2.1 | Col5a2 | XM_343564 | -4.2 | Ghr | NM_017094 | -3.7 |
| Adn | XM_343169 | -4.9 | Col6a3_pred | XM_346073 | -2.0 | Gja1 | NM_012567 | -6.8 |
| Adora2a | NM_053294 | -2.5 | Col8a1_pred | XM_221536 | -2.7 | Gja4 | NM_021654 | -3.1 |
| Adora3 | NM_012896 | -2.2 | Coro1a | NM_130511 | -3.3 | Glipr1_pred | XM_576223 | -2.2 |
| Ahr | XM_579375 | -2.6 | Ctbp2 | NM_053335 | -2.1 | Gmfg | NM_181091 | -2.4 |
| Aif1 | NM_017196 | -6.0 | Ctgf | NM_022266 | -5.2 | Gna12 | NM_031034 | -2.1 |
| Akr1b4 | NM_012498 | -3.7 | Ctse | NM_012938 | -2.2 | Gnai2 | NM_031035 | -2.0 |
| Alp1 | NM_199097 | -2.5 | Ctss | NM_017320 | -8.5 | Gng11 | NM_022396 | -4.0 |
| Anxa1 | NM_012904 | -5.3 | Cxcl9 | NM_145672 | -2.0 | Gpr105 | NM_133577 | -4.2 |
| Anxa2 | NM_019905 | -2.2 | Cyba | NM_024160 | -4.5 | Gpx3 | NM_022525 | -2.4 |
| Anxa3 | NM_012823 | -8.8 | Cybb | NM_023965 | -2.6 | Gstp1 | XM_579338 | -2.8 |
| Anxa5 | NM_013132 | -2.0 | Cyp2a1 | NM_012692 | -2.2 | Gstp2 | NM_138974 | -4.3 |
| Aox2 | XM_579191 | -2.3 | Cyp3a3 | NM_013105 | -4.7 | Gucy1b3 | NM_012769 | -3.5 |
| App | NM_019288 | -2.7 | Cyp4b1 | NM_016999 | -3.4 | Gzma | NM_153468 | -3.1 |
| Arhgdib | NM_001009600 | -5.2 | Dab2 | NM_024159 | -4.4 | Hba-a1 | NM_013096 | -120.3 |
| Asah3l_pred | XM_233138 | -2.2 | Dcir3 | XM_579150 | -3.3 | Hbb | NM_033234 | -106.2 |
| Atp6v1a1_pred | XM_340987 | -2.4 | Dcn | NM_024129 | -7.8 | Hla-dmb | NM_198740 | -2.4 |
| B4galt6 | XM_579528 | -2.0 | Ddah2 | XM_579741 | -2.0 | Hod | NM_133621 | -2.3 |
| Bak1 | NM_053812 | -2.7 | Ddx3x | XM_228701 | -2.1 | Ibtk_pred | XM_236481 | -2.6 |
| Bcl2a1 | NM_133416 | -2.6 | Dnase1l3 | NM_053907 | -3.8 | Icam2 | NM_001007725 | -2.7 |
| Bcl6_pred | XM_221333 | -3.4 | Ecm1 | NM_053882 | -5.9 | Ifi44_pred | XM_227821 | -2.2 |
| Bgn | NM_017087 | -2.0 | Ednrb | NM_017333 | -4.5 | Ifitm1_pred | XM_215117 | -3.5 |
| Bucs1_pred | XM_341917 | -3.2 | Ehd3 | NM_138890 | -2.1 | Igfbp3 | NM_012588 | -8.6 |
| C1qa | NM_001008515 | -4.7 | Eif1a_pred | NM_001008773 | -2.9 | Igfbp7_pred | XM_214014 | -8.8 |
| C1qb | NM_019262 | -3.5 | Eif3s6_pred | XM_576262 | -2.0 | Igj_pred | XM_341195 | -3.6 |
| C1qg | NM_001008524 | -3.0 | Eif4g2_pred | XM_341907 | -3.7 | Ik | NM_001005537 | -2.0 |
| C1qr1 | NM_053383 | -5.2 | Eltd1 | NM_022294 | -2.5 | Il1a | NM_017019 | -2.6 |
| Casp1 | NM_012762 | -4.4 | Emcn | NM_001004228 | -3.9 | Il1b | NM_031512 | -2.0 |
| Ccl19_pred | XM_342824 | -2.4 | Emilin1_pred | NM_238447 | -2.3 | Itgb2_pred | XM_228072 | -2.2 |
| Ccl5 | NM_031116 | -5.5 | Emp1 | NM_012843 | -2.3 | Krt1-19 | NM_199498 | -2.4 |
| Ccl6 | NM_001004202 | -4.4 | Emp3 | NM_030847 | -2.4 | Lamb1-1_pred | XM_216679 | -3.4 |
| Ccr5 | NM_053960 | -2.7 | Emr1 | XM_579174 | -4.4 | Laptm5 | NM_053538 | -2.5 |
| Cd163_pred | XM_232342 | -3.3 | Esam | NM_001004245 | -2.2 | Lcp1_pred | XM_573816 | -4.0 |
| Cd36 | NM_031561 | -2.7 | Ets1 | NM_012555 | -2.7 | Ldb2_pred | XM_214054 | -2.4 |
| Cd48 | NM_139103 | -4.6 | Evl | XM_579484 | -2.3 | Lgals1 | NM_019904 | -2.0 |
| Cd53 | NM_012523 | -4.3 | F2r | NM_012950 | -3.2 | Lgals3 | NM_031832 | -4.0 |
| Cd68_pred | XM_213372 | -3.1 | F9 | XM_346365 | -6.4 | Lgmn | NM_022226 | -2.3 |
| Cd74 | NM_013069 | -2.6 | Fbln5 | NM_019153 | -3.1 | LOC259245 | NM_147213 | -2.7 |

# APPENDIX

| | | | | | | | | |
|---|---|---|---|---|---|---|---|---|
| Cd83_pred | XM_341509 | -3.4 | Fcgr1_pred | XM_215643 | -3.0 | LOC287029 | XM_212651 | -2.0 |
| Ceacam10 | NM_173339 | -2.2 | Fcgr2b | NM_175756 | -4.6 | LOC287167 | XM_213262 | -4.0 |
| Cklfsf6_pred | XM_579183 | -2.2 | Fcgr3a | NM_207603 | -2.3 | LOC287899 | XM_213548 | -3.9 |
| LOC289384 | XM_223076 | -2.0 | LOC362803 | XM_343130 | -2.0 | LOC499615 | XM_574941 | -3.2 |
| LOC289930 | XM_223826 | -2.0 | LOC362934 | XM_576293 | -2.5 | LOC499625 | XM_574949 | -2.2 |
| LOC291936 | XM_238042 | -2.8 | LOC363434 | XM_343756 | -2.1 | LOC499638 | XM_574960 | -4.2 |
| LOC293860 | XM_238167 | -4.1 | LOC363767 | XM_344015 | -2.3 | LOC499775 | XM_580014 | -2.0 |
| LOC294337 | XM_215375 | -3.7 | LOC365699 | XM_345167 | -2.5 | LOC499984 | XM_575338 | -3.1 |
| LOC294410 | XM_228157 | -2.1 | LOC365814 | XM_578024 | -2.1 | LOC499985 | XM_575339 | -2.9 |
| LOC294744 | XM_215486 | -3.4 | LOC366411 | XM_575861 | -2.2 | LOC500015 | XM_575369 | -2.5 |
| LOC294762 | XM_215491 | -2.1 | LOC366588 | XM_345652 | -3.3 | LOC500285 | XM_575635 | -2.9 |
| LOC294942 | XM_215541 | -2.2 | LOC367391 | XM_346122 | -2.2 | LOC500336 | XM_575687 | -2.1 |
| LOC295382 | XM_227605 | -2.0 | LOC367846 | XM_575151 | -2.0 | LOC500344 | XM_575696 | -2.4 |
| LOC295660 | XM_212955 | -2.7 | LOC497720 | XM_579423 | -2.1 | LOC500373 | XM_231625 | -2.1 |
| LOC295975 | XM_215794 | -2.2 | LOC497757 | XM_579393 | -5.1 | LOC500389 | XM_575748 | -2.2 |
| LOC297504 | XM_238366 | -2.7 | LOC497758 | XM_579454 | -4.8 | LOC500398 | XM_575757 | -3.3 |
| LOC300783 | XM_217180 | -2.3 | LOC497767 | XM_579388 | -3.4 | LOC500469 | XM_575833 | -2.4 |
| LOC301276 | XM_236965 | -2.6 | LOC497846 | XM_579586 | -3.3 | LOC500488 | XM_580072 | -2.7 |
| LOC302363 | XM_217566 | -3.4 | LOC497936 | XM_573123 | -2.3 | LOC500490 | XM_575855 | -2.0 |
| LOC302671 | XM_217618 | -2.6 | LOC497942 | XM_573130 | -2.1 | LOC500495 | XM_575859 | -2.7 |
| LOC303666 | XM_221094 | -2.4 | LOC497987 | XM_573183 | -2.2 | LOC500507 | XM_575869 | -2.5 |
| LOC304138 | XM_221702 | -2.4 | LOC498032 | XM_573233 | -2.5 | LOC500586 | XM_575955 | -3.5 |
| LOC306805 | XM_225198 | -2.0 | LOC498076 | XM_573278 | -2.5 | LOC500643 | XM_576018 | -2.4 |
| LOC307907 | XM_226529 | -2.4 | LOC498105 | XM_573309 | -4.2 | LOC500695 | XM_576077 | -2.2 |
| LOC308350 | XM_218261 | -4.4 | LOC498162 | XM_573377 | -2.3 | LOC500788 | XM_576174 | -2.3 |
| LOC308654 | XM_218706 | -2.1 | LOC498241 | XM_573464 | -2.6 | LOC500829 | XM_576219 | -3.2 |
| LOC310760 | XM_227556 | -2.8 | LOC498245 | XM_573468 | -3.6 | LOC500916 | XM_576325 | -2.4 |
| LOC310926 | XM_227769 | -20.6 | LOC498276 | XM_573502 | -3.7 | LOC500941 | XM_576351 | -2.2 |
| LOC312102 | XM_231461 | -5.9 | LOC498277 | XM_573503 | -2.7 | LOC500949 | XM_576360 | -2.2 |
| LOC312924 | XM_232634 | -2.9 | LOC498279 | XM_573505 | -4.6 | LOC500988 | XM_576400 | -2.3 |
| LOC313304 | XM_233108 | -2.3 | LOC498371 | XM_573606 | -3.2 | LOC501091 | XM_576506 | -2.1 |
| LOC313308 | XM_233081 | -3.1 | LOC498375 | XM_573610 | -3.2 | LOC501187 | XM_576615 | -2.2 |
| LOC313391 | XM_233220 | -2.0 | LOC498378 | XM_573613 | -2.8 | LOC501224 | XM_576647 | -2.2 |
| LOC313445 | XM_233297 | -3.2 | LOC498452 | XM_573711 | -2.1 | LOC501245 | XM_576664 | -2.4 |
| LOC313974 | XM_233982 | -2.1 | LOC498557 | XM_573833 | -3.1 | LOC501393 | XM_576805 | -2.4 |
| LOC314075 | XM_234092 | -2.2 | LOC498644 | XM_573926 | -3.1 | LOC501396 | XM_576808 | -2.8 |
| LOC315352 | XM_235755 | -2.2 | LOC498669 | XM_573952 | -2.8 | LOC501553 | XM_576955 | -2.7 |
| LOC316186 | XM_236876 | -2.7 | LOC498690 | XM_573975 | -4.3 | LOC501562 | XM_576967 | -2.3 |
| LOC316406 | XM_237162 | -2.5 | LOC498799 | XM_574084 | -2.8 | LOC501610 | XM_577009 | -2.5 |
| LOC316481 | XM_237252 | -2.9 | LOC498829 | XM_574110 | -2.4 | LOC501619 | XM_577018 | -2.0 |
| LOC317218 | XM_228493 | -2.8 | LOC498973 | XM_574260 | -2.4 | LOC502490 | XM_577971 | -3.9 |
| LOC317312 | XM_228667 | -2.0 | LOC498989 | XM_574280 | -2.8 | LOC502953 | XM_578458 | -2.7 |
| LOC317599 | XM_229173 | -2.3 | LOC499300 | XM_574598 | -2.8 | LOC502954 | XM_578459 | -2.0 |
| LOC360602 | XM_340880 | -2.1 | LOC499321 | XM_574626 | -2.9 | LOC503409 | XM_578948 | -38.8 |
| LOC360627 | XM_340901 | -2.1 | LOC499481 | XM_574804 | -2.6 | Loxl2_pred | XM_214225 | -2.3 |
| LOC360690 | XM_340961 | -2.6 | LOC499526 | XM_579974 | -2.5 | Lpl | NM_012598 | -8.6 |
| LOC361117 | XM_341405 | -4.0 | LOC499531 | XM_574855 | -2.6 | Lrrn3 | NM_030856 | -2.0 |
| LOC361260 | XM_341544 | -2.5 | LOC499554 | XM_574879 | -2.3 | Ltbp1 | NM_021587 | -4.5 |
| LOC361283 | XM_341568 | -2.3 | LOC499560 | XM_574884 | -2.8 | Lum | NM_031050 | -2.0 |

# APPENDIX

| | | | | | | | | |
|---|---|---|---|---|---|---|---|---|
| LOC361885 | XM_342182 | -2.6 | LOC499564 | XM_574888 | -2.6 | Ly86_pred | XM_225636 | -2.5 |
| Mapre1 | NM_138509 | -2.5 | Prss23 | NM_001007691 | -5.7 | Tagln | XM_579512 | -2.3 |
| MGC105601 | NM_001009620 | -2.7 | Psma1 | NM_017278 | -2.1 | Tagln2_pred | XM_222906 | -3.8 |
| MGC72614 | NM_199105 | -2.6 | Ptgds2 | NM_031644 | -2.8 | Tax1bp1 | NM_001004199 | -2.1 |
| MGC72973 | NM_198776 | -28.1 | Pthr1 | NM_020073 | -3.9 | Tcf21 | XM_341737 | -4.9 |
| MGC94010 | NM_001007732 | -4.5 | Ptprb_pred | XM_235156 | -5.7 | Tcf4 | NM_053369 | -2.2 |
| MGC94782 | NM_001004282 | -2.2 | Ptprc | NM_138507 | -2.1 | Tde2 | NM_182951 | -2.5 |
| MGC95001 | NM_001007619 | -3.2 | Ptpro | NM_017336 | -2.8 | Tek | XM_342863 | -2.2 |
| Mgp | NM_012862 | -12.6 | Ramp2 | NM_031646 | -2.4 | Timp1 | NM_053819 | -3.0 |
| Mpeg1 | NM_022617 | -2.6 | Rasa1 | NM_013135 | -2.1 | Tnfrsf11b | NM_012870 | -4.7 |
| Mrc1_pred | XM_225585 | -4.4 | Rasip1_pred | XM_214916 | -2.4 | Tpbg | NM_031807 | -2.2 |
| Ms4a11_pred | XM_342028 | -4.4 | Rbbp7 | NM_031816 | -2.3 | Tpm4 | NM_012678 | -3.9 |
| Ms4a6b | NM_001006975 | -3.3 | Rcn_pred | XM_342481 | -4.1 | Tspan3 | NM_001005547 | -2.3 |
| Mthfs | NM_001009349 | -2.4 | Rcn2 | NM_017132 | -2.4 | Ttpa | NM_013048 | -2.1 |
| Mx1 | NM_173096 | -2.5 | Rcn3_pred | NM_001008694 | -2.5 | Tuba1 | NM_022298 | -5.6 |
| Napsa | NM_031670 | -2.7 | Reck_pred | XM_233371 | -3.7 | Txndc1_pred | XM_343076 | -2.0 |
| Nfib | XM_342854 | -2.6 | Reln | NM_080394 | -9.2 | Txnip | NM_001008767 | -2.5 |
| Nid2_pred | XM_573694 | -2.2 | RGD1308143_pred | XM_237468 | -2.1 | Tyrobp | NM_212525 | -2.8 |
| Nkg7 | NM_133540 | -3.0 | RGD1308373_pred | XM_344268 | -2.6 | Ube1c | NM_057205 | -2.1 |
| Nol5 | NM_021754 | -2.0 | RGD1310191_pred | XM_341102 | -2.4 | Ucp2 | NM_019354 | -4.2 |
| Npy | NM_012614 | -2.6 | Rgs10 | XM_341936 | -2.5 | Ugcg | XM_579533 | -2.3 |
| Nritp | XM_341519 | -2.2 | Rgs18_pred | XM_222692 | -2.4 | Vcam1 | NM_012889 | -3.4 |
| Nrp1 | NM_145098 | -3.9 | Rgs2 | NM_053453 | -2.7 | Vim | NM_031140 | -13.6 |
| Oasl2_pred | XM_579310 | -2.0 | Rock1 | NM_031098 | -2.4 | Vwf | XM_342759 | -2.3 |
| Ogn_pred | XM_214441 | -6.1 | RT1-Ba | XM_579226 | -2.9 | Waspip | NM_057192 | -3.9 |
| Oit3 | NM_001001507 | -4.6 | RT1-Da | XM_579241 | -8.3 | Wfdc1 | NM_133581 | -3.1 |
| Pam | NM_013000 | -4.6 | RT1-Db1 | XM_579272 | -2.7 | Xlkd1_pred | XM_219001 | -4.5 |
| Pde2a | NM_031079 | -2.1 | S100a11 | XM_215598 | -5.8 | Zfp354a | NM_052798 | -3.3 |
| Pdia3 | NM_017319 | -2.9 | S100a6 | NM_053485 | -4.4 | | | |
| Pf4 | NM_001007729 | -3.2 | Sart2_pred | XM_345110 | -3.1 | | | |
| Pfc | XM_216784 | -2.7 | Scd2 | NM_031841 | -3.1 | | | |
| Pigr | NM_012723 | -3.4 | Sdcbp | NM_031986 | -2.1 | | | |
| Pla2g2a | NM_031598 | -2.3 | Sdccag1_pred | XM_216724 | -2.3 | | | |
| Pla2g4a | NM_133551 | -2.6 | Sema6a_pred | XM_341612 | -2.3 | | | |
| Plac8_pred | XM_341188 | -4.9 | Serpinb6 | NM_199085 | -4.0 | | | |
| Plat | NM_013151 | -2.5 | Serpine2 | XM_343604 | -2.1 | | | |
| Plek_pred | XM_344267 | -3.3 | Slc25a4 | NM_053515 | -3.7 | | | |
| Plscr1 | NM_057194 | -2.2 | Slc28a2 | NM_031664 | -3.4 | | | |
| Pltp_pred | XM_215939 | -2.3 | Slfn3 | NM_053687 | -5.1 | | | |
| Plvap | NM_020086 | -3.6 | Slpi | NM_053372 | -6.3 | | | |
| Plxdc2_pred | XM_341567 | -2.2 | Smoc2_pred | XM_214777 | -4.9 | | | |
| Plxnd1_pred | XM_232283 | -2.5 | Snx5_pred | XM_215872 | -2.1 | | | |
| Pmp22 | NM_017037 | -2.4 | Sod3 | NM_012880 | -7.3 | | | |
| Pnutl2_pred | XM_573172 | -3.0 | Sparc | NM_012656 | -6.6 | | | |
| Ppt | NM_022502 | -2.1 | Sparcl1 | NM_012946 | -4.8 | | | |
| Prkcb1 | NM_012713 | -3.3 | Ssg1 | XM_573284 | -5.9 | | | |
| Prkch | NM_031085 | -2.2 | Sv2b | NM_057207 | -3.6 | | | |
| Prnp | XM_579340 | -3.8 | Tacc1a | NM_001004107 | -2.9 | | | |

## APPENDIX

Appendix 9: Summary of gene expression changes in primary rat hepatocytes culture measured with TaqMan PCR. Only genes 2-fold deregulated are shown.

| Gene Symbol | Accession Nr. | Susp 1d | Slices 1d | M+ 1d | M+ 6d | M+ 10d | M- 1d | M- 6d | M- 10d | S+ 1d | S+ 6d | S+ 10d | S- 1d | S- 6d | S- 10d | FaO |
|---|---|---|---|---|---|---|---|---|---|---|---|---|---|---|---|---|
| Acox1 | NM_017340 | -15.8 | 2.8 | -2.2 | -2.1 | -2.6 | 3.8 | 89.9 | 79.4 | 2.1 | 37.4 | 35.6 | 2.3 | 2.6 | 2.2 | 6.4 |
| Actn1 | NM_031005 | -3.7 | 8.7 | 6.8 | 195.4 | 140.3 | 2.3 | | | -2.1 | | | 2.3 | 21.1 | 15.7 | -2.2 |
| Adk | NM_012895 | -3.2 | | -2.2 | | -2.0 | 3.6 | | | -2.8 | -2.3 | | 5.2 | | | 23.7 |
| Afp | NM_012493 | | 3.0 | | | | | | | -5.5 | -11.4 | -5.1 | -4.0 | | | -18.7 |
| Nr1i3 | NM_022941 | -5.9 | 2.0 | -4.1 | 5.8 | 5.1 | | -2.6 | 6.9 | 4.0 | 3.4 | 3.9 | | 2.5 | 5.5 | |
| Cdh1 | NM_031334 | -6.4 | | 5.5 | | -3.3 | | 7.0 | | | | | | 4.6 | 3.6 | -2.0 |
| Cebpa | NM_012524 | -3.3 | 6.2 | -2.5 | | | 2.5 | -2.1 | 2.0 | | | | -2.3 | | 6.0 | 2.4 |
| Cebpb | NM_024125 | 2.7 | 2.9 | | | | | | | | | 2.4 | -2.2 | 2.4 | | 2.1 |
| Cdt1a | NM_031559 | -19.7 | | -5.1 | 12.6 | 2.9 | | | 2.3 | -6.1 | 5.6 | 8.2 | -5.6 | | 2.5 | 6.4 |
| Ccnd1 | NM_171992 | | | | 25.5 | 20.7 | -7.8 | 30.1 | 2.2 | | 7.4 | 9.1 | -13.4 | -2.3 | 2.0 | 3.7 |
| Ccng1 | NM_012923 | | 6.4 | 14.0 | -72.5 | 23.1 | 16.0 | | 2.2 | 9.3 | | | 13.1 | 7.4 | -3.4 | |
| Cyp1a2 | NM_012541 | -4.7 | 3.5 | -2.7 | -869.8 | -515.5 | | -153.7 | -57.0 | -4.9 | -107.2 | -95.7 | -2.2 | -154.6 | 4.8 | -194.5 |
| Cyp2c | NM_019184 | -27.7 | -4.7 | -5.5 | -883.7 | -347.5 | -5.1 | -6.7 | -13.6 | -7.1 | -126.0 | -352.6 | -5.3 | -5.1 | -101.0 | 68.3 |
| Cyp3a3 | NM_013105 | -8.4 | | | | -2208.5 | | | | -2.3 | -96.2 | -498.6 | | 8.5 | -4.4 | -3539.8 |
| Fabp2 | NM_013068 | | 4.9 | 2.6 | | -2.3 | 4.1 | 2.7 | 3.3 | | 4.3 | 7.2 | -4.7 | 3.3 | 7.1 | 4.9 |
| Ftp1 | NM_012558 | -43.8 | | | -18.1 | -28.7 | -3.4 | -3.5 | -3.6 | | -2.3 | -2.5 | -4.1 | | 2.1 | -16.2 |
| Gadd45a | NM_024127 | 4.5 | 14.8 | 45.5 | 67.8 | 38.8 | 28.7 | 35.8 | 23.2 | 33.2 | 25.1 | 19.7 | 32.3 | 15.5 | 9.6 | 2.8 |
| Gsn | NM_001004080 | | 2.0 | -6.7 | 8.1 | 18.5 | -13.2 | | 2.5 | -6.7 | | 5.1 | -19.5 | | -2.7 | -67.2 |
| Gsta3 | NM_031509 | -11.3 | | | | | | | | | | | | | | | 58.7 |
| Gstp2 | NM_138974 | 13.9 | 13.6 | 16.1 | 53.4 | 37.8 | 2.9 | 15.5 | 28.8 | 10.7 | 54.6 | 54.1 | 47.3 | 10.4 | 10.0 | 38.8 |
| Hmox1 | NM_012580 | 12.2 | 84.6 | 49.5 | 38.0 | 37.3 | 30.3 | 10.4 | 8.1 | 58.0 | 16.3 | 31.2 | | 3.8 | | 5.2 |
| Tcf1 | NM_012669 | | 3.9 | | 2.2 | | 2.6 | 2.2 | | | | | | | | |
| Hnf4a | NM_022180 | -43.2 | 4.6 | | | | 2.2 | | | | | | | | | | 72.4 |
| Hspa1b mapped | NM_212504 | 472.9 | 43.8 | 10.6 | 16.9 | 13.5 | 8.2 | 7.7 | 9.5 | 17.2 | 3.6 | 3.6 | 7.6 | 5.5 | 4.4 | 17.3 |
| Jund | XM_579658 | 4.4 | 6.5 | 7.9 | 13.0 | 11.3 | 6.6 | 10.6 | 9.7 | 4.7 | 6.2 | 5.2 | 6.8 | 6.5 | 6.2 | |
| Abcb1 | NM_012623 | 51.1 | 1187.0 | 343.0 | 1295.3 | 490.8 | 143.2 | 1523.4 | 951.8 | 184.4 | 788.8 | 822.4 | 101.2 | 570.6 | 246.1 | 58.9 |
| Abcb4 | NM_012690 | | | | -2.0 | -2.2 | -2.2 | | | | -3.1 | | -2.2 | 2.4 | 2.2 | -2.2 |
| Abcc2 | XM_577883 | -5.3 | | | | | | 3.1 | 3.0 | | | | | | | | |
| Abcc3 | NM_080581 | 13.5 | 25.1 | 12.6 | 24.2 | 16.6 | 4.1 | 31.1 | 34.3 | 11.0 | 20.0 | 21.5 | 2.3 | 31.5 | 37.9 | 21.6 |
| Myc | NM_012603 | | 78.3 | 76.6 | 117.7 | 36.0 | 47.9 | 50.9 | 37.5 | 42.8 | 39.5 | 27.4 | 52.8 | 33.1 | 28.2 | 49.9 |
| OATP1 | XM_579394 | -32.1 | -2.7 | -8.1 | -70.9 | -68.4 | -5.0 | -4.0 | -7.0 | -11.4 | -4.2 | 4.9 | -5.0 | -2.4 | -3.4 | -9041.6 |
| Cdkn1a | NM_080782 | 2.1 | 6.0 | 8.2 | 26.0 | 18.5 | 14.5 | 17.1 | 14.9 | 4.4 | 5.7 | 5.3 | 11.3 | 9.2 | 7.1 | 4.4 |
| Pck1 | NM_198780 | -120.2 | -8.8 | -244.8 | -119.7 | -300.0 | -165.7 | -77.5 | -31.4 | -101.1 | -177.3 | -104.9 | -79.7 | -120.4 | -95.4 | -4.7 |
| Alpi | NM_022665 | | 27.6 | 26.2 | 8.1 | 5.1 | 25.2 | 15.9 | 16.6 | 37.4 | 15.3 | 17.3 | 28.6 | 20.0 | 23.0 | 4.1 |
| Nr1i2 | NM_052980 | -11.4 | | -2.3 | | -2.3 | 2.6 | | | -2.1 | | | | 2.7 | | -4.3 |
| Ran | NM_031546 | -185.6 | -16.6 | -14.7 | 37.6 | -52.8 | -18.2 | -42.5 | -57.4 | -19.5 | -59.5 | -60.8 | -14.1 | -90.4 | -129.4 | -11.1 |
| Sod2 | NM_017051 | -10.9 | 11.3 | 14.1 | 5.3 | 2.2 | 14.0 | 3.9 | | 14.5 | 4.6 | 3.3 | 8.9 | 4.0 | | -3.5 |
| Tdra | NM_012671 | | 4.1 | 5.6 | 9.6 | 6.5 | 4.1 | 5.9 | 4.8 | 2.6 | 3.0 | 3.2 | 2.8 | 7.2 | 4.8 | 7.1 |
| Tgfb1 | NM_021578 | -14.4 | 3.5 | -5.0 | 7.7 | 10.6 | -6.0 | | | -5.2 | | 3.8 | -9.1 | -6.1 | -3.3 | -3.7 |
| Timp1 | NM_053819 | 3.3 | 16.3 | 8.9 | 68.0 | 60.5 | 4.0 | 9.7 | 12.0 | | 17.1 | 28.8 | | 3.2 | 3.1 | 30.8 |
| Tnf | NM_012675 | | 387.4 | 114.7 | 338.0 | 507.1 | 16.3 | | 23.3 | 368.1 | 170.4 | 312.1 | | | | 2.0 |
| Txn2 | NM_053331 | -18.1 | 2.1 | | | | | | | | | | 6.3 | 2.3 | | |
| Ugt1a1 | NM_012683 | -3.6 | 5.7 | 3.5 | | | 6.5 | 6.7 | 5.1 | | | | 5.1 | 14.9 | 12.2 | 2.1 |

# APPENDIX

Appendix 10: Summary of gene expression changes in primary rat hepatocytes culture measured with Illumina BeadChips. Only genes 2-fold deregulated and with a pValue lower than 0.05 are shown.

| Gene Symbol | Accession Nr. | Susp 1d | Slices 1d | M+ 1d | M+ 6d | M+ 10d | M- 1d | M- 6d | M- 10d | S+ 1d | S+ 6d | S+ 10d | S- 1d | S- 6d | S- 10d | FaO |
|---|---|---|---|---|---|---|---|---|---|---|---|---|---|---|---|---|
| Acox1 | NM 017340 | | | -2.7 | -4.6 | -4.1 | | | | -2.5 | | | -3.3 | | | -3.2 |
| Actn1 | NM 031005 | | | 2.2 | 4.9 | 5.1 | | 4.0 | 4.3 | | 2.8 | 2.1 | | | | |
| Adk | NM 012895 | | | -3.2 | -3.0 | -4.0 | | | | -3.4 | -2.0 | -2.3 | | | | |
| Afp | NM 012493 | | -2.6 | -2.7 | -4.7 | -5.9 | -2.0 | | -2.1 | -2.4 | -2.4 | -2.7 | -2.4 | | | -9.0 |
| Nr1i3 | NM 022941 | | -5.2 | -5.7 | -13.1 | -13.1 | -2.5 | -6.6 | -4.8 | -4.7 | -8.2 | -8.0 | -4.6 | | | -7.3 |
| Cdh1 | NM 031334 | -5.6 | | | | | | | | | | | | | | -5.2 |
| Cebpa | NM 012524 | | | | -6.1 | -6.0 | | | | | | | | | | |
| Cebpb | NM 024125 | | | | | | 2.1 | | | | | | 2.2 | | | -2.2 |
| Cpt1a | NM 031659 | -2.0 | -4.0 | -8.2 | -2.2 | 5.4 | -3.0 | -2.2 | | -5.5 | | | -5.8 | | | 2.1 |
| Ccnd1 | NM 171992 | -3.0 | | 7.1 | 2.6 | 10.9 | -8.8 | -2.3 | 9.9 | 5.5 | 5.1 | 2.6 | -10.3 | -4.8 | -4.1 | 2.3 |
| Ccng1 | NM 012923 | 2.5 | 4.4 | -5.4 | 8.5 | -100.4 | 7.8 | 9.8 | -70.8 | -8.4 | -92.6 | 5.6 | 11.0 | 6.1 | 4.9 | -53.9 |
| Cyp1a2 | NM 012541 | | | -2.6 | -138.7 | -188.6 | -3.5 | -103.5 | -7.0 | -2.8 | -36.8 | -83.9 | -4.3 | -64.7 | -69.2 | -448.8 |
| Cyp2c | NM 019184 | -4.7 | -3.7 | -2.4 | -276.3 | -233.4 | -2.5 | -4.7 | | -2.4 | -47.1 | -119.5 | -2.4 | -3.0 | -2.4 | -254.1 |
| Cyp3a3 | NM 013105 | -3.7 | -5.4 | | -278.7 | -4.1 | | | | | 2.2 | -78.9 | -4.0 | -3.2 | -2.5 | -4.1 |
| Fabp2 | NM 013068 | | | -3.5 | -4.0 | -61.8 | -3.7 | -8.1 | -7.4 | -2.4 | -3.5 | 2.5 | -6.2 | 5.3 | 3.8 | -17.2 |
| Fbp1 | NM 012558 | -2.7 | -5.1 | 13.8 | -54.1 | 10.4 | -6.0 | 8.3 | 6.9 | 14.5 | 9.7 | -4.0 | 12.1 | | | 2.5 |
| Gadd45a | NM 024127 | 6.2 | 6.5 | | 11.4 | 3.0 | 9.8 | | | | | 6.6 | | | | |
| Gsn | NM 001004080 | | | | | | | | | | | | | | | |
| Gsta3 | NM 031509 | | | | | | | | | | | | | | | |
| Gstp2 | NM 138974 | 4.2 | 4.8 | 17.6 | 29.7 | 34.8 | 4.1 | 15.3 | 21.4 | 18.3 | 38.0 | 40.5 | 2.4 | 10.9 | 10.8 | 22.0 |
| Hmox1 | NM 012580 | 8.4 | | 11.3 | 4.3 | 7.0 | 7.3 | | | 22.9 | 4.1 | 7.9 | 17.0 | | | 3.7 |
| Tcf1 | NM 012669 | | | | -2.1 | -3.1 | | | | | | -2.0 | | | | |
| Hnf4a | NM 022180 | | | | -4.3 | -3.8 | | -2.4 | | | -2.4 | -2.2 | | | | |
| Hspa1b mapped | NM 212504 | | | | | | | | | | | | | | | |
| Jund | XM 579658 | 73.7 | 25.9 | 2.5 | 2.4 | 2.2 | 2.5 | 2.3 | 2.4 | 2.2 | 2.2 | 2.1 | 2.3 | 2.3 | 2.4 | 2.1 |
| Abcb1 | NM 012623 | | -2.5 | 49.9 | 98.0 | 61.7 | 17.6 | 97.4 | 95.1 | 29.2 | 91.4 | 81.5 | 8.4 | 54.0 | 38.5 | 12.2 |
| Abcb4 | NM 012590 | | | | -4.8 | -4.2 | | | | | -4.5 | -3.9 | -2.2 | | | -2.5 |
| Abcc2 | XM 577883 | | 7.7 | 3.2 | 3.6 | -2.4 | | 5.5 | 6.2 | | 4.7 | -2.1 | -2.1 | | | |
| Abcc3 | NM 080581 | 3.6 | | 12.9 | 11.8 | 2.7 | 9.8 | 7.0 | 6.8 | 4.0 | 8.6 | 4.4 | 12.2 | 6.4 | -2.2 | 6.6 |
| Myc | NM 012603 | 6.3 | | | | 6.0 | | | | 10.6 | | 5.7 | | 6.1 | 7.8 | 4.9 |
| OATP1 | XM 579394 | | | | 2.1 | 2.5 | 3.9 | 2.8 | 2.7 | | 4.9 | | 5.1 | 2.4 | 7.4 | |
| Cdkn1a | NM 080782 | -9.2 | -31.9 | -82.1 | -126.8 | -180.5 | -65.4 | -60.0 | -25.0 | -52.6 | -120.7 | -91.8 | -41.5 | -51.3 | -59.8 | -3.8 |
| Pck1 | NM 198780 | | | | -5.7 | -5.7 | | | | -2.9 | -2.7 | -2.7 | -11.1 | | | -10.5 |
| Alb | NM 022665 | -2.3 | -3.8 | -4.0 | -69.3 | -71.7 | -19.2 | -62.6 | -69.6 | -21.1 | -48.3 | -53.8 | 4.0 | -71.8 | -69.9 | -12.8 |
| Nr1i2 | NM 052980 | -41.4 | -53.9 | -16.8 | | | 3.3 | | | 7.2 | | | | | | |
| Rgn | NM 031646 | 3.4 | | 4.0 | | | | | | | | | | | | 2.1 |
| Sod2 | NM 017051 | | | | | | | | | | | | | | | |
| Tat | NM 012671 | 2.4 | | 2.3 | 3.4 | 4.6 | | | 2.6 | | 4.9 | 7.3 | | | 2.1 | |
| Tgfb1 | NM 021578 | 7.5 | | | 11.2 | 13.4 | | | | | | | -2.4 | | | |
| Timp1 | NM 053819 | | | | | | | | | | | | | | | |
| Tnf | NM 012675 | | | | | -2.6 | | -2.0 | -2.2 | | | | | -2.4 | | |
| Txn2 | NM 053331 | | | -2.2 | -2.7 | | | | | | | | | | | |
| Ugt1a1 | NM 012683 | | | | | | | | | | | | | 8.5 | | |

# APPENDIX

Appendix 11: Summary of gene expression changes in primary human hepatocytes culture measured with TaqMan PCR. Only genes 2-fold deregulated are shown.

| Gene Symbol | Accession Nr. | HepaRG_DMSO 1d | HepaRG_DMSO 2d | HepaRG_DMSO 9d | HepaRG_basal 1d | HepaRG_basal 2d | HepaRG_basal 9d | Susp_24h | M_2d | M_7d | M_11d | S_2d | S_7d | S_11d |
|---|---|---|---|---|---|---|---|---|---|---|---|---|---|---|
| ACTN1 | NM_001102 | | | | 3.3 | 3.2 | | | 2.4 | 3.0 | 3.3 | | 2.1 | 2.8 |
| ADK | NM_001123 | | | | | | | -4.6 | -2.7 | -2.4 | -3.0 | -6.5 | -3.8 | -4.6 |
| AFP | NM_001134 | -2.0 | | -3.6 | | | | -10.2 | | -21.1 | -15.5 | -67.2 | | |
| ALPI | NM_000478 | -5.4 | -7.2 | | | | | -6.1 | -3.8 | -10.2 | -6.7 | -2.8 | -5.3 | -5.1 |
| CEBPA | NM_004364 | | | | | | | | -4.1 | | 2.3 | | | 3.6 |
| CEBPB | NM_005194 | | | | | | | | | | 2.1 | | | |
| CPT1A | NM_0010318 | | | | | | -2.0 | -7.5 | -7.7 | -3.1 | | -13.8 | -5.2 | -3.2 |
| CCND1 | NM_053056 | -2.9 | -2.4 | -3.6 | | 2.1 | | -5.0 | -5.2 | -2.4 | -2.5 | -8.8 | -5.3 | -4.5 |
| CCNG1 | NM_004060 | | | | | | 2.1 | | | | | -3.7 | -2.9 | -3.3 |
| CYP1A2 | NM_000761 | -280.5 | -357.8 | -151.0 | -588.5 | -1009.6 | | -11.4 | -17.7 | -2.0 | -4.7 | -14.0 | | -3.4 |
| CDH1 | NM_004360 | -4.2 | -3.3 | -4.5 | | | | -9.9 | -3.6 | -3.4 | | -5.6 | -3.8 | |
| FABP2 | NM_001443 | -7.5 | -5.1 | -22.2 | -3.6 | -3.9 | -4.5 | -10.8 | -134.2 | -15.9 | -15.4 | -83.7 | -9.1 | -7.9 |
| GADD45A | NM_001924 | 11.2 | 14.7 | 10.2 | 12.0 | 11.5 | 8.5 | -2.7 | | 4.3 | 3.5 | | 6.3 | 6.4 |
| FBP1 | NM_000507 | | -2722.9 | -3427.4 | | -1613.6 | | -11.4 | -16.3 | -9.0 | -8.5 | -11.6 | -3.8 | -4.4 |
| GSN | NM_000177 | 5.7 | 3.9 | 5.8 | 13.6 | 11.7 | 6.9 | | 2.9 | 5.0 | 4.3 | 2.8 | 5.1 | 8.1 |
| GSTA3 | NM_145740 | | | | | | | -9.4 | -11.3 | -12.1 | -9.1 | -15.0 | -11.6 | -9.0 |
| HMOX1 | NM_002133 | | | | | -2.1 | | 3.9 | | 3.5 | 2.9 | 2.2 | 2.3 | 2.1 |
| TCF1 | NM_000545 | | | | | | | | | | | | | |
| HNF4A | NM_000457 | | | | | | | -2.0 | | | | | | |
| JUND | NM_005354 | | | | | | | | | | | | | |
| ABCB1 | NM_000927 | | | | | | | | | | | | 2.1 | 2.1 |
| ABCB4 | NM_000443 | -3.0 | -3.1 | -3.8 | -3.6 | | -3.0 | -13.4 | -20.4 | -35.5 | -42.1 | -5.5 | -2.2 | -55.2 |
| ABCC2 | NM_000392 | | | | | | -2.1 | -2.3 | | | | -37.7 | -63.7 | |
| ABCC3 | NM_003786 | 2.8 | 3.0 | 2.9 | 5.3 | 4.9 | 2.8 | -3.8 | 3.7 | 3.1 | 4.4 | -4.2 | -2.1 | |
| MYC | NM_002467 | | | | 2.1 | | | | 3.0 | 7.2 | 11.8 | -2.2 | | 2.2 |
| CDKN1A | NM_000389 | 2.6 | 2.3 | 2.4 | 3.7 | 1.9 | | | | | | 3.0 | 5.9 | 12.7 |
| RGN | NM_004683 | -6.7 | -5.2 | -8.1 | -4.7 | -6.7 | -7.4 | -13.0 | -21.0 | -14.4 | -16.5 | -21.1 | -10.7 | -12.5 |
| SOD2 | NM_000636 | 2.3 | | 2.1 | 4.4 | 5.4 | 2.2 | 9.7 | 14.1 | 4.8 | 3.5 | 8.9 | 2.6 | 2.4 |
| TGFA | NM_003236 | 3.6 | 3.8 | 3.7 | 5.4 | 6.4 | 5.6 | | -2.6 | -2.3 | 2.5 | -2.2 | -2.2 | 2.6 |
| TGFB1 | NM_000660 | 3.7 | 3.3 | 3.9 | 6.5 | 7.0 | 4.7 | | 3.4 | 3.2 | | 2.8 | | |
| TXN2 | NM_003329, | 2.7 | 2.2 | 2.7 | 8.1 | 4.5 | 5.0 | | -2.1 | | 3.2 | -2.2 | -2.2 | 3.6 |
| TIMP1 | NM_003254 | 6.3 | 5.5 | 5.5 | 8.8 | 7.5 | | | -3.2 | | -3.9 | -2.2 | 3.1 | |
| TNF | NM_000594 | | | | | | | | -3.8 | | | -6.4 | | |
| UGT1A1 | NM_001072 | | 2.2 | | | | | -4.2 | | | | | | |

APPENDIX

Appendix 12: Summary of gene expression changes in primary human hepatocytes culture measured with Illumina BeadChips. Only genes 2-fold deregulated and with a pValue lower than 0.05 are shown.

| Gene Symbol | Accession Nr. | HepaRG DMSO 1d | HepaRG DMSO 2d | HepaRG DMSO 9d | HepaRG basal 1d | HepaRG basal 2d | HepaRG basal 9d | Susp 24h | M_2d | M_7d | M_11d | S_2d | S_7d | S_11d |
|---|---|---|---|---|---|---|---|---|---|---|---|---|---|---|
| ACTN1 | NM_001102 | | | | | | | | | | | | | |
| ADK | NM_001123 | | | | | | | | | | | | | |
| AFP | NM_001134 | -4.8 | -4.9 | -4.6 | -3.4 | -4.8 | -2.6 | -4.5 | -6.5 | | | -5.7 | -6.4 | -5.6 |
| ALPI | NM_000478 | -3.0 | -2.1 | -2.9 | -3.6 | | -2.3 | | -3.4 | | | | -2.3 | -3.2 |
| CEBPA | NM_004364 | | | | | | | | | | | | | |
| CEBPB | NM_005194 | | | | | | | | | | | | | |
| CPT1A | NM_0010318 | | | | | | | | | | | | | |
| CCND1 | NM_053056 | -3.6 | -2.6 | -3.3 | | | | -3.4 | -4.5 | -3.4 | -4.6 | -5.3 | | |
| CCNG1 | NM_004060 | | | | | | | | | | | -2.8 | | |
| CYP1A2 | NM_000761 | -47.5 | -37.0 | -39.5 | -49.3 | -62.8 | -54.5 | -8.0 | -13.1 | -2.4 | -3.0 | -7.0 | | |
| CDH1 | NM_004360 | | | | | | | | | | | | | |
| FABP2 | NM_001443 | | | | | | | | | | | | | |
| GADD45A | NM_001924 | | | | | | | | 2.3 | | | | | |
| FBP1 | NM_000507 | -273.0 | -220.1 | -234.5 | -250.3 | -275.3 | -268.2 | -5.5 | -14.3 | -11.1 | -13.3 | -7.1 | -6.1 | -7.6 |
| GSN | NM_000177 | 7.6 | 6.4 | 8.4 | 11.0 | 10.3 | 7.2 | 2.2 | 4.4 | 5.4 | 4.5 | 4.9 | 6.5 | 3.4 |
| GSTA3 | NM_145740 | | | | | | | | | | | | | |
| HMOX1 | NM_002133 | -3.3 | -3.3 | -2.4 | -4.0 | -4.9 | -5.5 | 2.6 | | | | | | |
| TCF1 | NM_000545 | | | | | | | | | | | | | |
| HNF4A | NM_000457 | | | | | | | | | | | | | |
| JUND | NM_005354 | -2.0 | | | -2.6 | | -2.4 | | | | | | | |
| ABCB1 | NM_000927 | | | | | | | | | | | | | |
| ABCB4 | NM_000443 | -2.8 | -2.8 | -3.1 | -4.4 | -2.2 | -3.5 | -5.9 | -7.1 | -7.0 | -10.5 | -8.3 | -8.6 | -8.1 |
| ABCC2 | NM_000392 | | | | | -2.2 | | | | | | | | |
| ABCC3 | NM_003786 | | | | | | | | | | | | | |
| MYC | NM_002467 | | | | | | | 2.2 | 2.2 | | | 2.5 | | |
| CDKN1A | NM_000389 | 2.6 | 2.6 | 3.1 | 2.6 | 2.5 | 2.6 | 2.6 | 3.9 | 4.4 | 5.2 | 3.2 | 3.7 | 4.3 |
| RGN | NM_004683 | -4.3 | -2.9 | -6.0 | -4.6 | -6.3 | -9.0 | -3.6 | -14.1 | -12.3 | -15.0 | -7.3 | -8.4 | -10.5 |
| SOD2 | NM_000636 | 5.4 | 4.5 | 5.8 | 7.4 | 7.5 | 5.9 | 15.3 | 12.1 | 9.0 | 7.7 | 13.4 | 8.0 | 9.0 |
| TGFA | NM_003236 | | | | | | | | | | | | | |
| TGFB1 | NM_000660 | | | | | | | | | | | | | |
| TXN2 | NM_003329 | | | | | | | | | | | | | |
| TIMP1 | NM_003254 | 3.3 | 3.8 | 4.1 | 3.6 | 2.9 | 3.3 | | | | | | | |
| TNF | NM_000594 | | | | | | | | | | | | | |
| UGT1A1 | NM_001072 | 2.6 | 3.5 | 2.8 | | | -2.1 | | | | | | 3.2 | |

Appendix 13: Gene set with the 724 top ranked genes of the predictive model giving the best classification results of the experiments 9 d after treatment

| Gene Symbol | Accession-Nr | Gene Symbol | Accession-Nr | Gene Symbol | Accession-Nr |
|---|---|---|---|---|---|
| Abca3_predicted | XM_220219 | Clic5 | NM_053603 | Frg1_predicted | XM_341442 |
| Abca8a_predicted | XM_221100 | Cnot6l_predicted | XM_341191 | Fusip1_predicted | XM_342948 |
| Abcg4_predicted | XM_236186 | Cobll1_predicted | XM_229988 | Fxc1 | NM_053371 |
| Abl1 | XM_231137 | Col18a1 | XM_241632 | G2an_predicted | XM_215144 |
| Acbd3 | NM_182843 | Colec10_predicted | XM_235330 | Gata4 | NM_144730 |
| Adar | NM_031006 | Commd5 | NM_139108 | Gbp2 | NM_133624 |
| Aer61 | XM_579302 | Cops5_predicted | XM_232615 | Gcipip | NM_133417 |
| Aes | NM_019220 | Coq3 | NM_019187 | Ghitm | NM_001005908 |
| Akna_predicted | XM_342848 | Cox7b | NM_182819 | Gla | XM_343817 |
| Akt1s1_predicted | XM_238103 | Cryl1 | NM_175757 | Gluld1 | NM_181383 |
| Alg5_predicted | XM_215561 | Csprs_predicted | XM_237360 | Gm83_predicted | XM_343231 |
| Amid_predicted | XM_342137 | Ctla4 | NM_031674 | Gnb1 | NM_030987 |
| Ankrd24_predicted | XM_216841 | Cubn | NM_053332 | Gpr61_predicted | XM_227581 |
| Ankrd5_predicted | XM_215854 | Cxxc1_predicted | XM_238016 | Gps2_predicted | XM_220615 |
| Anpep | NM_031012 | Cycs | NM_012839 | Grtp1_predicted | XM_341463 |
| Ap1g1 | XM_341686 | Cyp11a1 | NM_017286 | Gsta4_predicted | XM_217195 |
| App | NM_019288 | Cyp17a1 | NM_012753 | Gtf2b | NM_031041 |
| Aprin_predicted | XM_221833 | Cyp1a1 | NM_012540 | Gucy1b2 | NM_012770 |
| Areg | NM_017123 | Cyp2e1 | NM_031543 | Hadh2 | NM_031682 |
| Arhgap21_predicted | XM_225628 | Cyp2r1_predicted | XM_341909 | Hagh | NM_033349 |
| Arhgap8_predicted | XM_576323 | Dclre1b_predicted | XM_227537 | Hdh | XM_573634 |
| Arsb | XM_345140 | Ddt | NM_024131 | Herc2_predicted | XM_218720 |
| Arvcf_predicted | XM_221276 | Ddx24 | NM_199119 | Hexa | NM_001004443 |
| Ascc1 | NM_001007632 | Ddx3x | XM_228701 | Hgd_predicted | XM_573291 |
| Atad2_predicted | XM_235326 | Dgka | NM_080787 | Hibch_predicted | XM_217395 |
| Atp13a_predicted | XM_214310 | Diablo | NM_001008292 | Hmgb1 | NM_012963 |
| Atp5g1 | NM_017311 | Dnm2 | NM_013199 | Hoxc4 | XM_235703 |
| Atp5h | NM_019383 | Dnmt1 | NM_053354 | Hpd | NM_017233 |
| Atp6ap1 | NM_031785 | Drap1_predicted | XM_215177 | Hsd17b9 | NM_173305 |
| Bap1_predicted | XM_224614 | Dscr1 | NM_153724 | Idh1 | NM_031510 |
| Bat2 | NM_212462 | Dzip1_predicted | XM_344460 | Igbp1 | NM_031624 |
| Bcl2l2 | NM_021850 | Echs1 | NM_078623 | Igf2r | NM_012756 |
| Bmp4 | NM_012827 | Egf | NM_012842 | Ikbkap | NM_080899 |
| Bmp7 | XM_342591 | Ehmt1_predicted | XM_342379 | Ikbkb | NM_053355 |
| Brd2 | NM_212495 | Eif4b | NM_001008324 | Inppl1 | NM_022944 |
| Btc | NM_022256 | Elmo2_predicted | XM_342579 | Ipo13 | NM_053778 |
| Bwk1 | NM_198743 | Eml1_predicted | XM_343109 | Itm2b | NM_001006963 |
| Cacnb4 | XM_215742 | Eno3 | NM_012949 | Itpa | XM_230604 |
| Cadps | NM_013219 | Ensa | NM_021842 | Jam3 | NM_001004269 |
| Calmbp1_predicted | XM_213891 | Entpd4_predicted | XM_341346 | JSAP1 | XM_220232 |

# APPENDIX

| Gene Symbol | Accession-Nr | Gene Symbol | Accession-Nr | Gene Symbol | Accession-Nr |
|---|---|---|---|---|---|
| Camta2_predicted | XM_213362 | Epb4 | XM_345535 | Kcng1 | XM_215951 |
| Ccr7 | NM_199489 | Eps8l3_predicted | XM_215677 | Kctd5_predicted | XM_220224 |
| Cd59 | XM_579359 | Exosc5_predicted | XM_218343 | Khdrbs1 | NM_130405 |
| Cdc14a_predicted | XM_227618 | Fadd | NM_152937 | Kidins220 | NM_053795 |
| Cdc26_predicted | XM_345540 | Fah | NM_017181 | Kif3b_predicted | XM_215883 |
| Cdk7 | XM_215467 | Falz_predicted | XM_221050 | L3mbtl2_predicted | XM_235769 |
| Cdk9 | NM_001007743 | Fbxo33_predicted | XM_234205 | Lactb2_predicted | XM_216316 |
| Cetn2 | XM_215222 | Fdx1 | NM_017126 | Lama5 | XM_215963 |
| Chd4 | XM_232354 | Fkbp4 | XM_342763 | Laptm4b_predicted | XM_235393 |
| Chd7_predicted | XM_232671 | Fkbp9 | NM_001007646 | Ldhb | NM_012595 |
| Cipar1 | NM_173114 | Fkbpl | NM_001002818 | Leng1_predicted | XM_214797 |
| Ckap4_predicted | XM_343189 | Flrt2_predicted | XM_234361 | Lnk | XM_579519 |
| Clasp2 | NM_053722 | Frap1 | NM_019906 | LOC245925 | NM_139093 |
| Cldn10_predicted | XM_214250 | Freq | NM_024366 | LOC287101 | XM_213222 |
| LOC287115 | XM_213235 | LOC298842 | XM_216656 | LOC317604 | XM_229179 |
| LOC287250 | XM_220370 | LOC299179 | XM_216763 | LOC360531 | XM_340803 |
| LOC287388 | XM_213328 | LOC299199 | XM_234416 | LOC360596 | XM_340876 |
| LOC287477 | XM_213394 | LOC299264 | XM_216764 | LOC360664 | XM_340940 |
| LOC287541 | XM_213403 | LOC299315 | XM_238474 | LOC360668 | XM_340943 |
| LOC287962 | XM_213588 | LOC299713 | XM_235021 | LOC360681 | XM_340953 |
| LOC288089 | XM_221431 | LOC299949 | XM_216928 | LOC360760 | XM_346914 |
| LOC288309 | XM_213675 | LOC300126 | XM_217016 | LOC360826 | XM_341099 |
| LOC288396 | XM_221799 | LOC300160 | XM_235581 | LOC361140 | XM_341426 |
| LOC288455 | XM_213700 | LOC300361 | XM_217080 | LOC361174 | XM_341459 |
| LOC288646 | XM_222167 | LOC300441 | XM_217094 | LOC361340 | XM_341623 |
| LOC288772 | XM_222316 | LOC300444 | XM_235926 | LOC361460 | XM_341739 |
| LOC288978 | XM_213864 | LOC300644 | XM_217113 | LOC361475 | XM_341753 |
| LOC289182 | XM_213922 | LOC300783 | XM_217180 | LOC361543 | XM_341829 |
| LOC289264 | XM_222923 | LOC300839 | XM_217189 | LOC361578 | XM_341861 |
| LOC290500 | XM_214256 | LOC301137 | XM_236799 | LOC361606 | XM_341884 |
| LOC290706 | XM_214341 | LOC301711 | XM_237538 | LOC361646 | XM_341925 |
| LOC290825 | XM_212786 | LOC302092 | XM_229666 | LOC361649 | XM_341928 |
| LOC290916 | XM_225053 | LOC302559 | XM_217599 | LOC361774 | XM_342068 |
| LOC290999 | XM_214433 | LOC302898 | XM_579268 | LOC361797 | XM_347003 |
| LOC291000 | XM_214432 | LOC303100 | XM_220372 | LOC361871 | XM_342165 |
| LOC291034 | XM_214448 | LOC303730 | XM_221185 | LOC361990 | XM_342290 |
| LOC291290 | XM_225531 | LOC304349 | XM_221990 | LOC362127 | XM_342428 |
| LOC291952 | XM_226397 | LOC304860 | XM_222736 | LOC362294 | XM_347039 |
| LOC291974 | XM_214666 | LOC304863 | XM_222746 | LOC362295 | XM_342608 |
| LOC292195 | XM_217716 | LOC305122 | XM_223143 | LOC362370 | XM_342695 |
| LOC292811 | XM_214901 | LOC305332 | XM_223397 | LOC362526 | XM_342844 |
| LOC293156 | XM_215012 | LOC305452 | XM_223536 | LOC362559 | XM_342878 |
| LOC293509 | XM_219352 | LOC306007 | XM_224329 | LOC362662 | XM_575960 |

| Gene Symbol | Accession-Nr | Gene Symbol | Accession-Nr | Gene Symbol | Accession-Nr |
|---|---|---|---|---|---|
| LOC293699 | XM_212887 | LOC306586 | XM_224997 | LOC362725 | XM_343047 |
| LOC293711 | XM_219546 | LOC307235 | XM_225730 | LOC362776 | XM_343103 |
| LOC294560 | XM_215428 | LOC308758 | XM_218817 | LOC362801 | XM_343127 |
| LOC294722 | XM_226796 | LOC308765 | XM_218824 | LOC362938 | XM_343266 |
| LOC294925 | XM_226988 | LOC309081 | XM_219424 | LOC363000 | XM_343330 |
| LOC295015 | XM_227132 | LOC310137 | XM_226853 | LOC363069 | XM_343397 |
| LOC295090 | XM_215580 | LOC311114 | XM_230006 | LOC363129 | XM_343464 |
| LOC295161 | XM_215594 | LOC311218 | XM_230305 | LOC363162 | XM_343501 |
| LOC295234 | XM_215630 | LOC311355 | XM_230503 | LOC363289 | XM_343631 |
| LOC295952 | XM_215788 | LOC311382 | XM_230560 | LOC363309 | XM_343649 |
| LOC296050 | XM_215787 | LOC311591 | XM_230798 | LOC363332 | XM_343670 |
| LOC296300 | XM_215885 | LOC312728 | XM_232372 | LOC363476 | XM_343795 |
| LOC296318 | XM_215910 | LOC312946 | XM_232647 | LOC363555 | XM_343870 |
| LOC296320 | XM_215906 | LOC313346 | XM_233144 | LOC363611 | XM_343905 |
| LOC296761 | XM_216066 | LOC313373 | XM_233199 | LOC363817 | XM_344036 |
| LOC297388 | XM_216181 | LOC313842 | XM_233805 | LOC363937 | XM_344119 |
| LOC297402 | XM_216190 | LOC313982 | XM_233989 | LOC363962 | XM_573437 |
| LOC297514 | XM_238368 | LOC314196 | XM_234264 | LOC363974 | XM_344134 |
| LOC297890 | XM_216348 | LOC314660 | XM_234947 | LOC364006 | XM_577273 |
| LOC297971 | XM_216368 | LOC314927 | XM_235252 | LOC364060 | XM_344178 |
| LOC298282 | XM_216446 | LOC315434 | XM_235833 | LOC364136 | XM_344230 |
| LOC298384 | XM_216480 | LOC315463 | XM_235924 | LOC364139 | XM_573586 |
| LOC298490 | XM_216527 | LOC316228 | XM_236927 | LOC364253 | XM_344296 |
| LOC298496 | XM_233477 | LOC317346 | XM_228716 | LOC364258 | XM_344301 |
| LOC298787 | XM_216638 | LOC317405 | XM_228821 | LOC364343 | XM_344366 |
| LOC364381 | XM_344404 | LOC499316 | XM_574620 | Lpin2_predicted | XM_237521 |
| LOC364535 | XM_344495 | LOC499401 | XM_574716 | Lrp10_predicted | XM_224170 |
| LOC364577 | XM_573906 | LOC499411 | XM_579965 | Lsm8_predicted | XM_216102 |
| LOC364613 | XM_573924 | LOC499525 | XM_574850 | Man2b1 | NM_199404 |
| LOC364823 | XM_344652 | LOC499561 | XM_574885 | Map3k3_predicted | XM_221034 |
| LOC365300 | XM_574483 | LOC499581 | XM_574906 | Mapkapk2 | XM_579712 |
| LOC365314 | XM_344924 | LOC499617 | XM_574942 | Mark2 | NM_021699 |
| LOC365580 | XM_577905 | LOC499660 | XM_574984 | Mbd1_predicted | XM_574171 |
| LOC365664 | XM_574847 | LOC499700 | XM_575029 | Mcmdc1_predicted | XM_342146 |
| LOC365924 | XM_345284 | LOC499755 | XM_575090 | Mcpt1l4 | XM_573784 |
| LOC365949 | XM_345296 | LOC499809 | XM_575149 | Mesdc1_predicted | XM_218853 |
| LOC366248 | XM_575286 | LOC499856 | XM_575197 | Metap1_predicted | XM_215717 |
| LOC366315 | XM_345503 | LOC499905 | XM_575251 | MGC94056 | NM_001004258 |
| LOC366461 | XM_345576 | LOC499931 | XM_575276 | MGC94221 | NM_001004224 |
| LOC366468 | XM_345581 | LOC499950 | XM_575298 | MGC94326 | NM_001007709 |
| LOC366565 | XM_578532 | LOC499956 | XM_575304 | MGC94413 | NM_001007745 |
| LOC367030 | XM_576362 | LOC500005 | XM_575359 | MGC95208 | NM_001005552 |
| LOC367109 | XM_345951 | LOC500148 | XM_575500 | MGC95210 | NM_001005532 |
| LOC367171 | XM_576473 | LOC500196 | XM_575548 | Mgst2_predicted | XM_215562 |

# APPENDIX

| Gene Symbol | Accession-Nr | Gene Symbol | Accession-Nr | Gene Symbol | Accession-Nr |
|---|---|---|---|---|---|
| LOC367205 | XM_578768 | LOC500382 | XM_575740 | Mki67_predicted | XM_225460 |
| LOC367761 | XM_346284 | LOC500506 | XM_575868 | Mlc3 | NM_020104 |
| LOC367806 | XM_346310 | LOC500553 | XM_575916 | Mnt_predicted | XM_220698 |
| LOC367944 | XM_346362 | LOC500606 | XM_575979 | Mocs1_predicted | XM_236911 |
| LOC497703 | XM_579683 | LOC500650 | XM_576028 | Mocs2 | NM_001007633 |
| LOC497706 | XM_579538 | LOC500662 | XM_576040 | Mrpl22_predicted | XM_213307 |
| LOC497717 | XM_579724 | LOC500814 | XM_576201 | Mrpl27_predicted | XM_213439 |
| LOC497754 | XM_579458 | LOC500819 | XM_576208 | Mrpl42_predicted | XM_216882 |
| LOC497832 | XM_579562 | LOC500869 | XM_576267 | Mrpl49_predicted | XM_219525 |
| LOC497886 | XM_573071 | LOC500981 | XM_576391 | Mrps17_predicted | XM_213762 |
| LOC497904 | XM_573090 | LOC501002 | XM_576412 | Ms4a8b_predicted | XM_342026 |
| LOC497974 | XM_573168 | LOC501058 | XM_576474 | Mss4 | NM_001007678 |
| LOC498002 | XM_573198 | LOC501064 | XM_576479 | Mybph | NM_031813 |
| LOC498058 | XM_573255 | LOC501172 | XM_576599 | Myc | NM_012603 |
| LOC498229 | XM_573449 | LOC501204 | XM_576630 | Myo1 d | NM_012983 |
| LOC498230 | XM_573451 | LOC501326 | XM_576737 | Myr8 | NM_138893 |
| LOC498268 | XM_579805 | LOC501351 | XM_576762 | Nap1l3 | NM_133402 |
| LOC498374 | XM_573609 | LOC501363 | XM_576776 | Ncdn | NM_053543 |
| LOC498411 | XM_573658 | LOC501370 | XM_576783 | Ncor2_predicted | XM_341072 |
| LOC498435 | XM_573687 | LOC501397 | XM_576809 | Ndufa8_predicted | XM_216044 |
| LOC498729 | XM_574003 | LOC501514 | XM_576915 | Ndufb9_predicted | XM_216929 |
| LOC498747 | XM_574026 | LOC501534 | XM_576934 | Ndufs3_predicted | XM_215776 |
| LOC498759 | XM_574044 | LOC501621 | XM_577021 | Ndufv2 | NM_031064 |
| LOC498805 | XM_574089 | LOC501655 | XM_577050 | Nedd4a | XM_343427 |
| LOC498819 | XM_574101 | LOC501952 | XM_577379 | Negr1 | NM_021682 |
| LOC498837 | XM_574121 | LOC502201 | XM_577662 | Neo1 | XM_343402 |
| LOC498899 | XM_574186 | LOC502393 | XM_577872 | Neu1 | NM_031522 |
| LOC499009 | XM_574302 | LOC502686 | XM_578183 | Nfatc4_predicted | XM_240184 |
| LOC499018 | XM_574311 | LOC502743 | XM_578243 | Nfe2l2 | NM_031789 |
| LOC499031 | XM_574321 | LOC502858 | XM_578358 | nidd | NM_213627 |
| LOC499071 | XM_574352 | LOC502935 | XM_578437 | Nisch_predicted | XM_240330 |
| LOC499087 | XM_574374 | LOC503000 | XM_578512 | Nosip_predicted | XM_214926 |
| LOC499255 | XM_574549 | LOC503197 | XM_578721 | Notch1 | XM_342392 |
| LOC499262 | XM_574557 | LOC503351 | XM_578889 | Npl4 | NM_080577 |
| LOC499288 | XM_574587 | Loc65027 | XM_573762 | Npy | NM_012614 |
| Nr3c1 | NM_012576 | Prlph | NM_021580 | RGD1359460 | NM_001006959 |
| Nucb1 | NM_053463 | Psma2 | NM_017279 | RGD1359600 | NM_001007688 |
| Nudt6 | NM_181363 | Psma4 | NM_017281 | Rgs14 | NM_053764 |
| Nyw1 | XM_230288 | Psma5 | NM_017282 | Rhcg | NM_183053 |
| Ogfrl1_predicted | XM_237000 | Psma6 | NM_017283 | Ripk5 | NM_199463 |
| Olr1024_predicted | NM_001000068 | Psma7 | XM_579184 | Rnf111_predicted | XM_236380 |
| Olr1242_predicted | NM_001000450 | Psmb1 | NM_053590 | Rnf153_predicted | XM_215286 |
| Olr1340_predicted | XM_236174 | Psmb3 | NM_017285 | Rpl3l_predicted | XM_213231 |

| Gene Symbol | Accession-Nr | Gene Symbol | Accession-Nr | Gene Symbol | Accession-Nr |
|---|---|---|---|---|---|
| Olr1592_predicted | NM_001000084 | Psmb4 | NM_031629 | Rpo2tc1 | NM_001009618 |
| Olr1690_predicted | NM_001000274 | Psmb6 | NM_057099 | Rps12 | NM_031709 |
| Olr1751_predicted | NM_001000492 | Psmb7 | NM_053532 | Rragc_predicted | XM_216515 |
| Olr29_predicted | NM_001000691 | Psmc1 | NM_057123 | RSB-11-77 | NM_182669 |
| Olr495_predicted | NM_001000310 | Psmc2 | NM_033236 | S100a1 | XM_579178 |
| Olr535_predicted | NM_001000672 | Psmc3 | NM_031595 | Sdhc | NM_001005534 |
| Olr552_predicted | NM_001001055 | Psmc5 | NM_031149 | Sec14l2 | NM_053801 |
| Olr818_predicted | NM_001000844 | Psmd1 | NM_031978 | Sec24b_pred. | XM_215706 |
| Pabpc4_predicted | XM_216517 | Psmd11_predicted | XM_220754 | Sema3b_pred. | XM_343479 |
| Pacs1 | NM_134406 | Psmd7_predicted | XM_226439 | Sema3f_predicted | XM_236623 |
| Pafah1b3 | NM_053654 | Pspn | NM_013014 | Serpinh1 | NM_017173 |
| Pafah2 | NM_177932 | Ptbp1 | NM_022516 | Setdb1_predicted | XM_227444 |
| Pam | NM_013000 | Ptgfrn | NM_019243 | Siahbp1 | XM_343268 |
| Pax2_predicted | XM_239083 | Ptk2 | NM_013081 | Skp1a | NM_001007608 |
| Pcdhga8_predicted | XM_344668 | Ptms | NM_031975 | Slc12a4 | NM_019229 |
| Perq1_predicted | XM_222024 | Ptpn21 | NM_133545 | Slc1a3 | NM_019225 |
| Pgpep1 | NM_201988 | Pus1_predicted | XM_222267 | Slc24a4_predicted | XM_234470 |
| Phb | XM_579541 | Pycs_predicted | XM_342048 | Slc25a11 | NM_022398 |
| Phr1_predicted | XM_214245 | Pygb | XM_342542 | Slc28a2 | NM_031664 |
| Pias3 | NM_031784 | Rab6b_predicted | XM_343459 | Slc30a8_predicted | XM_235269 |
| Pigh_predicted | XM_343083 | Rac2 | NM_001008384 | Slc35b4_predicted | XM_216122 |
| Pigq | NM_001007607 | Rarsl_predicted | XM_216367 | Slc35e1_predicted | XM_224707 |
| Pip5k2c | NM_080480 | Rasip1_predicted | XM_214916 | Slc37a1_predicted | XM_574727 |
| Plcb1 | XM_342524 | Rassf5 | NM_019365 | Slc39a6_predicted | XM_214607 |
| Plec1 | NM_022401 | Rce1_predicted | XM_219685 | Slc39a8_predicted | XM_575042 |
| Plekhb2_predicted | XM_217372 | Rfx1_predicted | XM_222456 | Slc6a8 | XM_579415 |
| Plekhf2_predicted | XM_342803 | RGD1305327_predicted | XM_343285 | Slc7a1 | NM_013111 |
| Plekhm2_predicted | XM_233611 | RGD1305649_predicted | XM_575926 | Slit2 | XM_346464 |
| Plk3 | XM_342888 | RGD1305679_predicted | XM_341511 | Smad1 | NM_013130 |
| Plod3 | NM_178101 | RGD1305793_predicted | XM_219958 | Smndc1_predicted | XM_213506 |
| Plp2_mapped | NM_207601 | RGD1306284 | NM_001008283 | Snapc1_predicted | XM_234299 |
| Podxl | NM_138848 | RGD1307423 | NM_001008334 | Snx11_predicted | XM_573185 |
| Poldip2_predicted | XM_237790 | RGD1307481 | NM_001008327 | Spr | XM_342714 |
| Pole4_predicted | XM_342710 | RGD1307512_predicted | XM_343357 | Spred2_predicted | XM_223647 |
| Polr2j_predicted | XM_213753 | RGD1307599_predicted | XM_233692 | Srd5a1 | NM_017070 |
| Pom210 | NM_053322 | RGD1307648_predicted | XM_215262 | Ssr1_predicted | NM_001008891 |
| Pomc | NM_139326 | RGD1308009_pred | XM_226233 | Ssrp1 | NM_031121 |

# APPENDIX

| Gene Symbol | Accession-Nr | Gene Symbol | Accession-Nr | Gene Symbol | Accession-Nr |
|---|---|---|---|---|---|
| Pp | XM_215416 | RGD1308054_predicted | XM_214834 | Stard3nl | NM_001008298 |
| Ppie_predicted | XM_216524 | RGD1308350_predicted | XM_343116 | Sulf2_predicted | XM_230861 |
| Ppm1 d_predicted | XM_213418 | RGD1308600_predicted | XM_342393 | Supt4h2_predicted | XM_213415 |
| Ppp5c | NM_031729 | RGD1309207_predicted | XM_343064 | Syngr1 | NM_019166 |
| Pprc1_predicted | XM_215259 | RGD1309256_predicted | XM_214087 | Tacc2 | NM_001004415 |
| Prcc_predicted | XM_227476 | RGD1309721 | NM_001009670 | Tacc2 | NM_001004418 |
| Prdm13_predicted | XM_345509 | RGD1309906 | NM_001009246 | Taok2 | NM_022702 |
| Prkaca | XM_341661 | RGD1310022_predicted | XM_214983 | Tcam1 | NM_021673 |
| Prkcdbp | NM_134449 | RGD1311745 | NM_001008329 | Tceb3bp1_predicted | XM_576183 |
| Tcerg1_predicted | XM_225983 | Trim21_predicted | XM_219011 | Vps13 d_predicted | XM_233792 |
| Tcf2 | NM_013103 | Trim28 | XM_344861 | Vps39_predicted | XM_575216 |
| Tcf8 | XM_341539 | Trpv6 | NM_053686 | Vwf | XM_342759 |
| Tcof1_predicted | XM_214552 | Tsga10ip | XM_579136 | Wdr22_predicted | XM_234345 |
| Tep1 | NM_022591 | Tspyl_predicted | XM_228225 | Wfdc3_predicted | XM_215938 |
| Terf1_predicted | XM_238387 | Tst | NM_012808 | Xpo6_predicted | XM_574559 |
| Tex27_predicted | XM_574725 | Ttyh3_predicted | XM_221962 | Xylt1 | XM_341912 |
| Tfdp2_predicted | XM_217232 | Tubb5 | NM_173102 | Zbtb7a | NM_054002 |
| Tfpi | NM_017200 | Tubgcp3_predicted | XM_225013 | Zc3hdc5_predicted | XM_340939 |
| Tfrc | XM_340999 | Txk_predicted | XM_223365 | Zc3hdc6_predicted | XM_230592 |
| Tgfb1 | NM_021578 | Txn2 | NM_053331 | Zdhhc2 | NM_145096 |
| Tgfb2 | NM_031131 | Txndc9 | NM_172032 | Zfp262_predicted | XM_233529 |
| Timm17a | NM_019351 | Txnl5_predicted | XM_213382 | Zfp282_predicted | XM_216140 |
| Timm22 | XM_340856 | Ua20 | NM_144742 | Zfp367_predicted | XM_573970 |
| Tinf2 | NM_001006962 | Ube2r2_predicted | XM_216864 | Zmynd12_predicted | XM_233458 |
| Tjp4_predicted | XM_236932 | Ufc1 | NM_001003709 | Zmynd15_predicted | XM_213338 |
| Tlr6 | NM_207604 | Ufd1l | NM_053418 | Znf500_predicted | XM_343376 |
| Tmc4_predicted | XM_218186 | Uhrf1_mapped | NM_001008882 | | BC093384 |
| Tmprss7_predicted | XM_221464 | Uqcrh | NM_001009480 | | AY724519 |
| Tnfrsf6 | NM_139194 | Urod | XM_342887 | | AY724532 |
| Tnn_predicted | XM_222794 | Uros_predicted | XM_574579 | | BC079376 |
| Tor1b_predicted | XM_231146 | Usp12_predicted | XM_341033 | | BC100083 |
| Tpi1 | XM_579468 | Usp7_predicted | XM_340747 | | CO382628 |
| Trim14_predicted | XM_232992 | V1rj6 | NM_001009507 | | DN935439 |
| Trim2_predicted | XM_342268 | Vmac | XM_579064 | | DV728079 |

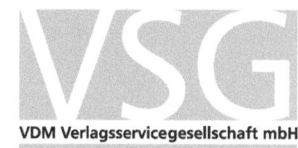

Die VDM Verlagsservicegesellschaft sucht für wissenschaftliche Verlage abgeschlossene und herausragende

## Dissertationen, Habilitationen, Diplomarbeiten, Master Theses, Magisterarbeiten usw.

für die kostenlose Publikation als Fachbuch.

Sie verfügen über eine Arbeit, die hohen inhaltlichen und formalen Ansprüchen genügt, und haben Interesse an einer honorarvergüteten Publikation?

Dann senden Sie bitte erste Informationen über sich und Ihre Arbeit per Email an *info@vdm-vsg.de*.

### Sie erhalten kurzfristig unser Feedback!

VDM Verlagsservicegesellschaft mbH
Dudweiler Landstr. 99
D - 66123 Saarbrücken

Telefon +49 681 3720 174
Fax +49 681 3720 1749

**www.vdm-vsg.de**

Die VDM Verlagsservicegesellschaft mbH vertritt

 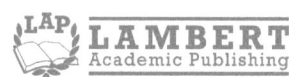 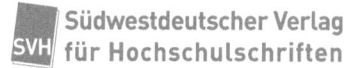

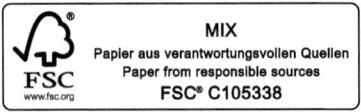

Printed by Books on Demand GmbH, Norderstedt / Germany